Manual of Orthopaedics

Fifth Edition

Manual of Orthopaedics
Fifth Edition

Editor

Marc F. Swiontkowski, MD
Professor and Chair
Department of Orthopaedic Surgery
University of Minnesota

LIPPINCOTT WILLIAMS & WILKINS
A **Wolters Kluwer** Company
Philadelphia · Baltimore · New York · London
Buenos Aires · Hong Kong · Sydney · Tokyo

Acquisitions Editor: James Merritt
Developmental Editor: Keith Donnellan
Production Editor: Jeff Somers
Manufacturing Manager: Colin Warnock
Cover Designer: Patricia Gast
Compositor: Circle Graphics
Printer: R.R. Donnelley–Crawfordsville

Library of Congress Cataloging-in-Publication Data

Manual of orthopaedics / editor, Marc F. Swiontkowski.—5th ed.
    p. ; cm.
    Rev. ed. of: Manual of acute orthopaedic therapeutics / Larry D. Iversen, Marc F. Swiontkowski. 4th ed. c1995.
    Includes bibliographical references and index.
    ISBN 0-7817-2441-4 (alk. paper)
    1. Orthopedics—Handbooks, manuals, etc. 2. Musculoskeletal system—Wounds and injuries—Handbooks, manuals, etc. 3. Fractures—Handbooks, manuals, etc. I. Swiontkowski, Marc F. II. Iversen, Larry D. Manual of acute orthopaedic therapeutics.
    [DNLM: 1. Musculoskeletal System—injuries—Handbooks. 2. Fractures—rehabilitation—Handbooks. 3. Orthopedics—Handbooks. WE 39 M2938 2001]
    RD732.5 .I96 2001
    676.7—dc21
                                                                                    2001029279

Care has been taken to confirm the accuracy of the information presented and to describe generally accepted practices. However, the authors, editor, and publisher are not responsible for errors or omissions or for any consequences from application of the information in this book and make no warranty, expressed or implied, with respect to the currency, completeness, or accuracy of the contents of the publication. Application of this information in a particular situation remains the professional responsibility of the practitioner.

The authors, editor, and publisher have exerted every effort to ensure that drug selection and dosage set forth in this text are in accordance with current recommendations and practice at the time of publication. However, in view of ongoing research, changes in government regulations, and the constant flow of information relating to drug therapy and drug reactions, the reader is urged to check the package insert for each drug for any change in indications and dosage and for added warnings and precautions. This is particularly important when the recommended agent is a new or infrequently employed drug.

Some drugs and medical devices presented in this publication have Food and Drug Administration (FDA) clearance for limited use in restricted research settings. It is the responsibility of the health care provider to ascertain the FDA status of each drug or device planned for use in their clinical practice.

10 9 8 7 6 5 4 3 2 1

Editors to Previous Editions

D. Kay Clawson, MD
Larry D. Iverson, MD
First, Second, and Third Editions

Larry D. Iverson, MD
Marc F. Swiontkowski, MD
Fourth Edition

CONTENTS

Contributing Authors ix

Preface xi

1. The Diagnosis and Management of Musculoskeletal Trauma 1

2. Complications of Musculoskeletal Trauma 19

3. Prevention and Management of Acute Musculoskeletal Infections 29

4. Acute Nontraumatic Joint Conditions 40

5. NonAcute Pediatric Orthopaedic Conditions 57

6. Common Types of Emergency Splints 78

7. Cast and Bandaging Techniques 85

8. Orthopaedic Unit Care 104

9. Traction 115

10. Operating Room Equipment and Techniques 131

11. Acute Spinal Injury 161

12. Disorders and Diseases of the Spine 178

13. Fractures of the Clavicle 185

14. Sternoclavicular and Acromioclavicular Joint Injuries 187

15. Acute Shoulder Injuries 192

16. NonAcute Shoulder Disorders 197

17. Fractures of the Humerus 203

18. Elbow and Forearm Injuries 214

19. Wrist and Hand Injuries 227

20. NonAcute Elbow, Wrist, and Hand Conditions 242

21. Fractures of the Pelvis 259

22. Hip Dislocations, Femoral Head Fractures, and Acetabular Fractures 266

23. Fractures of the Femur 275

24. Knee Injuries: Acute and Overuse 295

25. Fractures of the Tibia 314

26. Ankle Injuries 325

27. Fractures and Dislocations of the Foot 334

28. Overuse and Miscellaneous Conditions of the Foot and Ankle 345

Appendix A. Joint Motion Measurement 354

Appendix B. Muscle Strength Grading 375

Appendix C. Dermatomes and Cutaneous Distribution of Peripheral Nerves 376

Appendix D. Desirable Weights of Adults 379

Appendix E. Surgical Draping Techniques 382

Appendix F. Electromyography and Nerve Conduction Studies 387

Appendix G. Approaches for Injection and Aspiration of Joints 390

Subject Index 397

CONTRIBUTING AUTHORS

Elizabeth A. Arendt, M.D.
Department of Orthopaedic Surgery, University of Minnesota, Box 492,
420 Delaware Street, S.E., Minneapolis, Minnesota 55455
Knee Injuries: Acute and Overuse

Daniel D. Buss, M.D.
Department of Orthopaedic Surgery, University of Minnesota, Box 492,
420 Delaware Street, S.E., Minneapolis, Minnesota 55455
Fractures of the Clavicle, Sternoclavicular and Acromioclavicular Joint Injuries,
Acute Shoulder Injuries, NonAcute Shoulder Conditions, Fractures of the Humerus

J. Chris Coetzee, M.D., F.R.C.S.C.
Department of Orthopaedic Surgery, University of Minnesota, Box 492,
420 Delaware Street, S.E., Minneapolis, MN 55455
Overuse and Miscellaneous Conditions of the Foot and Ankle

Matthew Putnam, M.D.
Department of Orthopaedic Surgery, University of Minnesota, Box 492,
420 Delaware Street, S.E., Minneapolis, Minnesota 55455
NonAcute Elbow, Wrist, and Hand Conditions

Andrew H. Schmidt, M.D.
Department of Orthopaedic Surgery, Hennepin County Medical Center,
701 Park Avenue, Minneapolis, Minnesota 55455
HCMC Treatment Protocols

Marc F. Swiontkowski, M.D.
Professor and Chair, Department of Orthopaedic Surgery, University of Minnesota
Medical School, Minneapolis, Minnesota

Ensor E. Transfeldt, M.D.
Department of Orthopaedic Surgery, University of Minnesota, Box 492,
420 Delaware Street, S.E., Minneapolis, Minnesota 55455
Disorders and Diseases of the Spine

Dean T. Tsukayama, M.D.
Department of Medicine, Division on Infectious Diseases, Hennepin County Medical
Center, 701 Park Avenue S., Minneapolis, Minnesota 55415
Prevention and Management of Acute Musculoskeletal Infections

Thomas F. Varecka, M.D.
Department of Orthopaedic Surgery, Hennepin County Medical Center,
701 Park Avenue, Minneapolis, Minnesota 55455
HCMC Treatment Protocols

Kevin R. Walker, M.D.
Department of Orthopaedic Surgery, University of Minnesota, Box 492, 420 Delaware
Street, S.E., Minneapolis, Minnesota 55455; Gillett Children's Specialty Healthcare,
200 East University Ave., St. Paul, Minnesota 55101
NonAcute Pediatric Othopaedic Conditions

PREFACE

The fifth edition of the manual formerly known as The *Manual of Acute Orthopaedic Therapeutics* brings several substantive changes over the prior four editions, including the change in title to The *Manual of Orthopaedics*. A detailed list of the changes and rationale will follow but it is worthwhile to review the history of this useful "spiral notebook" to place these changes in context.

The *Manual of Acute Orthopaedic Therapeutics* was the creation of Dr. Larry Iversen who worked out its basic framework and conceptualization with his orthopaedic mentor, Dr. D. Kay Clawson. Dr. Iversen was at the time a senior resident working closely with Dr. Clawson who was the first professor and Chairman of the Department of Orthopaedic Surgery at the University of Washington. The orthopaedic services at the University Hospital and King County Hospital (later renamed Harborview Medical Center) were active and focused mainly around the management of injured patients. Drs. Clawson and Iversen saw the need for a manual that would improve teaching and patient care in these institutions. These were days when the management of long bone fractures was in transition from traction and casting to operative techniques and the University of Washington Orthopaedic department was at the forefront with wonderful, dedicated, and creative clinicians like Drs. Robert Smith and Sigvard Hansen. Care was primarily delivered by junior housestaff, interns, and students and they needed information readily at hand. So the manual provided the "how-to's" for traction, casting, and pre- and postoperative care while explaining the rationale for treatment decisions and providing an excellent reference list for later review and in-depth study. This manual was a labor of love for Dr. Iversen and Clawson; the two would often work on the manuscripts for three straight weeks seated around the dining room table in Dr. Clawson's home. Little Brown publishers liked the concept of the book and added it to its growing list of subspecialty spiral manuals; the book enjoyed broad acceptance.

Each of the first three editions brought a review of the contents and reference list for each chapter as the field continued to evolve. In 1987, I returned to the University of Washington where I had done my training (and used the second edition) to assume a position at Harborview Medical center. In 1991, I was a new Professor in the department and chief of the orthopaedic service, and Dr. Clawson asked me to assume his place with the Manual. It then became Dr. Iversen and I who labored for two weeks in the medical school library revising the chapters, updating the reference lists, adding sections of historical references, changing several illustrations, and adding fresh chapters on infection and rheumatologic conditions. As such we began to broaden the scope of the manual to include conditions that were nonacute and nontrauma-related in order to make the manual more useful for students and interns as well as to provide a more comprehensive tool for primary care physicians. The changes in care delivery moved strongly in favor of attending delivered/supervised care in academic centers where the manual was in widespread use. As such the chapters evolved drastically as the push towards management of fractures had dramatically changed the way trauma patients were managed—for the better, we believe.

For this fifth edition, Dr. Iversen, with a mature, busy private practice in Bremerton, Washington, has chosen to step aside. I moved from the University of Washington to assume the Chair of the Orthopaedic Department at the University of Minnesota in 1997 and brought the project along. We made a major philosophical shift in the manual, moving it to a more comprehensive position in covering nearly all of orthopaedic surgery in new chapters. Members of the Department of Orthopaedic Surgery at the University of Minnesota agreed to support the project by authoring new chapters on pediatric orthopaedics, nontraumatic hand and shoulder surgery, spine, and nonacute lower extremity conditions. Also new to this edition are treatment protocols preferred by the attending staff at Hennepin County Mecial Center, where the University of Minnesota staff and residents provide care. These protocols, "HCMC Treatment Recommendations," are found at the ends of appropriate chapters and provide a set of principles for decision-making which may serve as a starting point for developing a treatment plan for an injured patient. The manual has moved from a two-author project to a multiple-author, single-department project in the evolution toward greater usefulness for students, housestaff, and primary care MD's.

The purpose of the manual is to provide a well-thought out approach to problems related to the musculoskeletal system, both acute and chronic. The discussions and reference lists are not meant to be comprehensive, rather to provide an initial starting point in approaching an individual patient problem. Every student and resident is encouraged to delve more deeply into the study of the condition: both the reference list and historical references will be useful in gaining more information for personal gratification or for preparing for teaching conference discussions. Commonly there is no single way to manage an orthopaedic injury or condition: we have attempted to provide scholarly discussions which cover the gamut of approaches while informing the reader of what we think is the best current method. We have tried to be clear about which conditions can be appropriately managed by primary care practitioners and which need orthopaedic subspecialist care.

No individual in the department will receive personal remuneration for this project. Rather we will use the funds derived from the sale of the book to further student and resident education and research—a move that rings true to the initial motivation of Drs. Clawson and Iversen in creating the manual. It is to these two fine surgeons and educators that this fifth edition is dedicated as well as to the many students at all levels who will benefit from the *Manual of Orthopaedics.*

Manual of Orthopaedics

Fifth Edition

1. THE DIAGNOSIS AND MANAGEMENT OF MUSCULOSKELETAL TRAUMA

I. A team approach to trauma. In trauma centers, the care of the patient with potential injuries to more than one organ system is handled by a **team of specialists** (1). The general surgeon with special expertise in the management of the trauma patient is the captain of the team. The captain is responsible for managing the patient's injuries efficiently and effectively. Care is organized in three stages: primary survey, secondary survey, and definitive management.

    A. The **primary survey** is concerned with the preservation of life.

        1. Initial resuscitation. The first steps in managing the trauma patient follow the ABCs (airway, breathing, and circulation). It is important to correct each of these problems in sequence (be sure the airway is clear before assessing the patient's breathing, then check the circulation). These initial steps generally have been performed by the paramedic team, but the surgeon in charge should follow the established sequence.

            a. Airway. The most common cause of preventable death in accidents is airway obstruction, so the trauma leader must immediately check that the patient's airway is adequate. Any obstruction (e.g., vomitus, tongue, blood, dentures) must be removed. If necessary, airway obstruction can be prevented by lifting the mandible forward, by using an oral airway, or by intubation. Caution should be taken to avoid overextending the neck during intubation. An **endotracheal tube** can be inserted orally or nasally by the team captain or consulting anesthesiologist to support the airway and prevent aspiration of vomitus. Ideally, two people should perform this procedure, with one person inserting the tube and the other stabilizing the neck. They must make certain the endotracheal tube is not in a mainstem bronchus by auscultating both sides of the chest and by obtaining a chest roentgenogram. Orotracheal intubation is preferred unless there is significant oral or mandibular trauma. Contraindications to nasal intubation include significant midface trauma where fractures may be present. An endotracheal tube may be left in place for 7–14 days, during which time the decision to perform a tracheotomy can be made. Emergency tracheotomy or cricothyroidotomy should be performed if passage of an endotracheal tube is impossible. Tracheotomy is accompanied by a long list of complications and should not be used merely as a convenient method of gaining control of the airway. Cricothyroidotomy is contraindicated in children younger than 12 years old.

            b. Breathing. After airway obstruction has been ruled out or controlled, the patient's ventilation should be assessed. The major life-threatening problems are tension pneumothorax, massive hemothorax, and flail chest. A tension pneumothorax is diagnosed by signs of massive pneumothorax plus positive pressure in the intrapleural space, causing mediastinal shift and decreasing venous blood return. This condition produces a rapidly worsening respiratory and cardiovascular status and requires immediate aspiration of the air to relieve symptoms. Frequently, this must be done before a roentgenographic diagnosis is available. If the patient can ventilate but has persistent cyanosis and dyspnea, a **flail chest** may be the cause. This condition, which is diagnosed by discordant motion of the chest wall, can be controlled by ventilator assistance. Trauma patients are generally placed on supplemental oxygen therapy, either by mask, if adequate ventilatory effort is present, or via the ventilator.

            c. Circulation. The cardiovascular status must be immediately evaluated and supported. Prompt determination of vital signs is essential. Control of **external bleeding** is accomplished by direct pressure and

Table 1-1. Glasgow Coma Scale

Criteria	Score
Eye opening (E)	
Spontaneous	4
To speech	3
To pain	2
Nil	1
Verbal response (V)	
Oriented	5
Confused conversation	4
Inappropriate words	3
Incomprehensible sounds	2
Nil	1
Best motor response (M)	
Obeys	6
Localizes	5
Withdraws	4
Abnormal flexion	3
Extensor response	2
Nil	1
Coma Score (E + M + V) = 3 to 15	

bandage. Elevation of the lower extremities helps prevent venous bleeding from the limbs and increase cardiac venous return and preload. The classic Trendelenburg (head down) position is not used for more than a few minutes because it can interfere with respiratory exchange.

d. **Disability.** A rapid, organized neurologic examination should be performed. This is critical in the awake patient. In the unconscious patient, the Glasgow Coma Scale score is rapidly computed based on pupil response to light, motor activity, and withdrawal to painful stimuli (Table 1-1).

2. **Members** of the trauma team can begin to treat **shock** by inserting one or two large-bore (14 gauge) venous catheters if not already initiated by the paramedic team. The infusion rate depends on the length and internal diameter of the catheters (Table 1-2).

Table 1-2. Infusion time for 1 L of Ringer's lactate or whole blood through various size catheters

	Ringer's lactate (3.5-ft elevation)	Whole blood (300 mm Hg pressure)
24-in large (14-gauge needle) catheter (as for CVP line)	38 min	25 min
8-in large (14-gauge needle) catheter (as for subclavian)	19 min	14 min
2.5-in 14-gauge plastic catheter (catheter of choice)	7.5 min	7 min

CVP, central venous pressure.

a. The **first choice** for the type and location of IV catheters is for one or two 14-gauge catheters to be inserted percutaneously in the arm veins, the external jugular veins, or in extraordinary circumstances, the saphenous veins of the ankle.

b. If percutaneous catheters cannot be inserted because the veins have collapsed or are too small, then the **second choice** depends on the physician's expertise with subclavian or femoral vein percutaneous puncture versus a cutdown approach to a vein.

   (1) If no veins are available in the extremities for percutaneous puncture or a cutdown catheterization, then **bilateral subclavian or internal jugular or femoral percutaneous puncture** can be performed using the Seldinger technique of a catheter over a guidewire. Subclavian puncture carries the risk of pneumothorax.

   (2) An alternative approach is to use **two cutdown catheterizations** of the cephalic or saphenous veins. Long-term placement of catheters into veins in the lower extremities should be avoided because of the potential of thrombophlebitis.

c. Place two large-bore IV catheters **even if the patient has no signs of impending or actual significant shock.** Do not use veins that drain through the site of injury.

d. A **central venous catheter** for monitoring central venous pressure is of value when significant fluid or blood component therapy is required or in elderly patients who may have preexisting cardiac disease.

e. Venous blood is often taken for **typing and cross-matching.** The emergency use of O-negative blood even with a low anti-A titer is discouraged. It generally takes only a few minutes to obtain the specific typed, cross-matched blood. O-negative blood must be used in female patients of child-bearing age when type-specific blood is unavailable.

   (1) Until cross-matched blood is available, rapidly infuse 1–2 L of isotonic Ringer's lactate or normal saline solution. If **blood loss is minimal,** then blood pressure should return to normal and remain that way with only a maintenance amount of balanced saline solution.

   (2) If **blood loss is severe** or the hemorrhage is continuing, then the evaluation of blood pressure and the decrease in pulse rate that occurs with the rapid infusion of Ringer's lactate will be transient. By the time this assessment is made, typed and cross-matched whole blood should be available.

   (3) In general, hypotension in a trauma patient should not be attributed to a femur or other long bone fracture; another source must be sought. The following gross **estimates of localized blood loss** (in units) from adult closed fractures can be useful in establishing baseline blood replacement requirements:

Humerus	1.0–2.0
Pelvis	1.5–4.5
Knee	1.0–1.5
Elbow	0.5–1.5
Hip	1.5–2.5
Tibia	0.5–1.5
Forearm	0.5–1.0
Femur	1.0–2.0
Ankle	0.5–1.5

   (4) Extracellular fluid may also be lost to the intracellular space. This occurs with shock when the cell membrane fails. Blood alone does not replace the **lost extracellular fluid.** This fluid loss should be replaced by Ringer's lactate. Overhydration can occur. Central venous monitoring alone is of little value in detecting crystalloid overload. When fluid management is a problem, insertion of a Swan-Ganz catheter allows measurement of the more useful pulmonary artery pressure, pulmonary capillary wedge pressure, and cardiac output as a guide to hemodynamic status and fluid therapy. The use of diuretics simply to produce urine, however, has no sound physiologic basis and is detrimental because these agents further deplete the intravascular and extravascular extracellular fluids.

f. If large quantities (>8 units) of blood are required, then dilution of platelet and coagulation factors occurs. The platelet count, prothrombin time, partial thromboplastin time, and fibrinogen level should be determined. As blood is stored, the amount of 2,3-diphosphoglycerate (2,3-DPG) markedly decreases. This substance is the prime regulator of oxygen binding and oxygen release from hemoglobin. When 2,3-DPG is decreased, as it is in aged red blood cells, the cells lack the full capacity to deliver oxygen to the tissues.

g. Urine output is an essential guide to adequate organ perfusion. Therefore, the insertion of an indwelling catheter and the monitoring of urinary output are necessary for treating shock. Adequate renal perfusion is indicated by a urine output greater than 40 mL per hour.

3. A **flow sheet** should be established to monitor patient resuscitation.

B. Secondary survey

1. The **history** should include a careful account of the accident, a description of the mechanism of injury, and a statement of the degree of violence involved. Concomitant medical disease, drug abuse, and alcoholism should be considered as contributing factors. The transporting paramedic team or member of the accompanying family should be interviewed for these details when the patient is unconscious or has been intubated. A useful mnemonic to guide the initial history is based on the word **AMPLE:**

   A. Allergies (e.g., penicillin)

   M. Medications (e.g., steroids, anticoagulants)

   P. Past illness (e.g., asthma, heart disease, diabetes)

   L. Last meal (e.g., vomiting, aspiration)

   E. Events of accident (e.g., recall, position)

2. The **initial physical examination** of the multiply injured patient must be a meticulous, fully documented, head-to-toe examination. The patient must be completely undressed for the second survey.

   a. The **level of consciousness** and the response to stimuli, coherence, orientation, and so on should be carefully noted. This is best done by using the Glasgow Coma Scale (Table 1-1). This information is frequently obtained by the medics who perform the field rescue, initiate treatment, and transport the patient. They also note the position of the patient at the scene of the accident, especially the head, and whether all limbs were moving actively.

   b. Injury to the bone rarely occurs without significant **soft-tissue injury.** Because soft-tissue trauma is not readily demonstrable with roentgenograms, the orthopaedist must pay special attention to the physical examination for the proper diagnosis and treatment of soft-tissue injuries.

   c. The primary survey should be performed before **roentgenography.** After the primary survey is done, any patient who is involved in high-energy trauma, has head injuries, or is intoxicated should have chest roentgenograms, a lateral C-spine roentgenogram (showing the inferior endplate of C7), and an anteroposterior roentgenogram of the pelvis. During the secondary survey, additional radiographs may be required. Special views, in addition to two different plane views, may be necessary.

      (1) When **gross deformity and crepitation** are present, further examination of the fracture site is not necessary. Otherwise,

all four limbs should be palpated thoroughly and each joint placed through a passive range of motion. Any obvious **fractures or deformities are splinted**, and any **open wounds are covered** with sterile dressings. A more detailed description of fracture wound management is given later in this chapter (see **III**).

(2) **In the absence of these classic findings**, carefully examine for **point bony tenderness** in the alert patient.

d. Carefully palpate **skull and facial bones** and look for **small lacerations** hidden in the hair. Roentgenograms of facial bones are difficult to interpret unless previous clinical examination suggests the presence of trauma.

e. Beware of the **association between cervical spine and head injuries**. In a conscious patient, any neck spasm is a cervical spine fracture or dislocation until it is roentgenographically disproved. In the unconscious patient, protect the neck until bony injury is ruled out by cervical films and ligamentous injury is ruled out by physical examination.

f. **Hemothorax** and **pneumothorax** often cause preventable deaths. The improved blood pressure and pulmonary air flow subsequent to resuscitation can also precipitate the development of a hemothorax or pneumothorax. Therefore, the chest should be examined carefully and the examination repeated frequently. The chest roentgenogram from the trauma series must be carefully scrutinized.

g. **Abdominal injury** is also a common cause of preventable death. The imprint of clothes or a contusion of the abdominal wall from the seat belt suggests intraabdominal injury. Airbags have altered patterns of injury in frontal collision (7). If intraperitoneal bleeding is suspected, peritoneal lavage (Fig. 1-1), the most sensitive and rapid test for determination of peritoneal bleeding, is indicated (10). In the hemodynamically stable patient in whom injury is suspected, computed tomography (CT) scanning of the abdomen is more specific. Low back pain, pubic tenderness, or pain with compression of the iliac crest can indicate a pelvic ring injury. Pelvic fractures may cause severe internal bleeding, and transfusion can be necessary for significant pelvic fractures. A severe backache can be an indication of retroperitoneal bleeding. A rectal examination must be done in all patients with spine or pelvic injury to check for blood reflecting injury or loss of tone indicative of neurologic injury. A bimanual pelvic examination is appropriate in female patients to rule out open fractures in the vagina.

h. Carefully log roll the patient and **palpate the back** to detect tenderness or defects of the interspinous ligaments. An increase in the interspinous distance accompanied by local swelling may signify injury.

i. Major injury to the limbs usually is obvious. However, the likelihood of **multiple fractures and joint injuries occurring in the same limb** increases with the velocity of the injury. Carefully evaluate the circulation of the limb distal to any fracture and record the presence of all wounds after applying a sterile dressing.

j. A detailed **neurologic examination** is related to the type of injury suspected. In the alert patient, perform a careful peripheral nerve examination with any limb fracture. In the case of a spinal injury, the examination must be complete, emphasizing the level of the neurologic lesion and including a description of all sensory findings. Frequently evaluate and record muscle power, tone, tendon reflexes, and cutaneous reflexes. Chart the neurologic examination with illustrations for sensory deficits and mark sensory levels on the skin so that all changes are easily recognized during the subsequent hours.

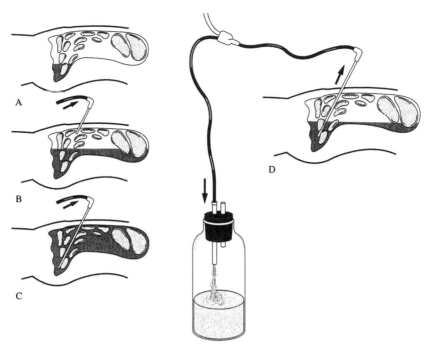

FIG. 1-1. Diagnostic peritoneal lavage. **A.** Small amount of free intraperitoneal fluid gravitates toward the cul-de-sac, the most dependent portion of the peritoneal cavity in the supine position. **B** and **C.** Intraperitoneal administration of Ringer's lactate. The fluid has a tendency to collect posteriorly as the air-containing viscera move anteriorly. The intraperitoneal fluid gives the intestines more mobility. **D.** Catheter directed toward cul-de-sac. Nearly quantitative return is possible because of a siphoning effect. In theory, the amount of blood in the last 50 mL of dialysate removed is most apt to represent the "true" amount of blood in the peritoneal cavity. Initial recovery of a blood-tinged dialysate followed by clear dialysate is highly suggestive of catheter-related abdominal wall bleeding in a patient who would otherwise have had a negative lavage.

> **k. Maintain accurate records** with repeated monitoring. Notations of pupil size, level of consciousness, and vital signs may be critically important in documenting changes in the patient's status that might require immediate operation. As a rule, severely injured patients are minimally medicated and maximally oxygenated. Accompany the patient to the radiology department or obtain portable films in the emergency department so that continued monitoring is maintained.
>
> l. The following is a list of **commonly overlooked injuries** that must be ruled out with any multiply injured patient.
>> (1) **Basilar skull fracture**
>> (2) **Zygomatic arch and orbital fractures**
>> (3) **Fracture of the odontoid process**
>> (4) **Injury to the C7 vertebra** (generally overlooked as the result of an inadequate radiologic evaluation)
>> (5) **Posterior dislocation of the shoulder** (physical examination shows that the patient has no external rotation)

    (6) Scaphoid, lunate, or perilunate dislocation
    (7) Fracture of the radial head
    (8) Seatbelt fracture (T12 or L1)
    (9) Pelvis fracture
    (10) Femoral neck fracture
    (11) Posterior dislocation of the hip
    (12) Tibial plateau fracture. (A knee hemarthrosis often is present with fat globules, which rise to the surface of the aspirate. Oblique roentgenograms of the tibial plateau usually show the fracture.)
    (13) Fracture of the talus that is minimally displaced.

3. Roentgenograms of **any suspected limb fracture** should be made, including the joints above and below the injury on the film. The following special points should be emphasized:

    a. A radiograph of the **chest, lateral cervical spine, and pelvis** should be obtained in all multiply injured patients after the primary survey.

    b. If a **spine fracture is detected,** then a complete spinal series including anteroposterior, lateral, and odontoid cervical views and thoracic plus lumbar spine view is mandatory. CT or tomography may be required to rule out upper cervical fractures. The documented incidence of multiple level spine fractures is 7%–12%. A full spine series should be obtained in the unconscious trauma victim.

    c. Head CT scans are mandatory for patients with loss of consciousness or external evidence of **head trauma.** Patients with femur fractures and head injury should generally have the femur fracture stabilized (8).

    d. An Intravenous pyelogram (IVP), cystogram, and abdominal-pelvic CT scan are indicated in the presence of fractures of the pelvis. Bloody urine or the **inability to void** raises the suspicion of a urethral injury, so a retrograde urethrogram should be considered before a catheter is inserted (1). In male patients, blood at the penile meatus or a "high-riding" prostate seen on rectal examination is a clear indication for a obtaining a retrograde urethrogram before Foley catheterization. If the catheter does not pass easily, then it should not be forced, and the urologist should be consulted. If a bladder injury is suspected, then it is essential to insert an indwelling catheter, unless the patient is voiding clear urine.

    e. Computed axial tomography might be necessary in complex fractures to delineate the fracture pattern fully. Tomography is most useful for spine, pelvis, calcaneus, and proximal and distal tibia fractures.

    f. Aggressive stabilization for femur and pelvic fractures has a favorable effect on pulmonary function following blunt trauma (9). In general, fixation of femur fractures with an interlocking nail is indicated in the multiply injured patient (2,3,8).

4. Use **maximal monitoring** and **minimal medication.**

  C. Definitive management. In the management of the multiply injured patient, the repair phase includes various operations and procedures carried out by **appropriate specialty groups.** The specialist involved should be cognizant of all injuries and should discuss the timing, type, and extent of operative procedures with the trauma team leader.

II. Principles of fracture healing (4)

  A. Normal bone is highly vascular and has a great ability to resist infection and to repair itself. On the other hand, avascular bone cannot participate in the reparative process. Therefore, treatment must be directed toward the prevention of further devascularization to create an environment that improves the vascularity of the region and promotes osseous healing. The following **principles** are applicable in the treatment of most fractures.

1. **Intraarticular fractures** require anatomic reduction, if possible, and early initiation of range of motion of the involved point.
2. **Metaphyseal fractures** have an abundant blood supply to ensure bone healing. A special type of pediatric metaphyseal injury is called a **torus fracture,** or buckle fracture. For most metaphyseal fractures in adults, treatment should be directed toward the following:
   a. **Adequate joint alignment**
   b. **Early** passive and active **movement** of the joint
3. **Diaphyseal fractures** have relatively poor blood supply and require more strict attention to proper stabilization (4). Reduction must be adequate to ensure full function after the fracture heals. Adequate stability of the fracture must be achieved to allow motion of the adjacent joints.
4. When performing an open reduction of a closed fracture, **disturb as little of the periosteal or the endosteal blood supply as possible.** When the treatment of choice is an open reduction and internal fixation, some diaphyseal fractures may also be considered for an **autogenous cancellous bone graft.**

B. **Factors generally reported with delayed union and non-union** (12)
1. **Too much motion** destroys the vascular budding into the fracture hematoma and interferes with revascularization. Adequate stabilization of the fracture, therefore, is mandatory (12).
2. **Distraction** decreases the surrounding vascularity as well as increases the length of the bony bridge necessary to heal the fracture.
3. **Open fracture** (or the surgical opening of fresh fractures) often results in the loss of the fracture hematoma and viable osteoblasts or preosteoblastic cells. The wide displacement that occurs to produce these injuries also strips the soft tissues at the long bone, which prolongs healing time.
4. **Infection** interferes with the blood supply and fracture healing.
5. **Patient factors** include smoking, diabetes, steroid medications, and poor nutrition.

III. **Management of open fractures and large soft-tissue wounds**
A. Early and careful treatment of wounds is necessary to restore function and prevent infection. Wounds, large or small, should immediately be covered with a sterile dressing. Open fractures should be splinted following reduction. Many authorities believe that it is worthwhile to **cover the wound with a moist dressing** of a balanced electrolyte solution or aqueous benzalkonium chloride in a 1:5,000 dilution. **Do not probe or blindly use surgical hemostats in the wound. Do not push or stuff extruded soft tissue or bone back into the wound. Do not soak the wound.** Externalized material is contaminated and will contaminate deeper recesses if replacement into the wound is attempted outside the operating environment.
B. The diagnosis of any neurovascular injury is made by careful **physical examination** of the distal motor, sensory, and circulatory function. The surgeon should assume that a laceration communicates with any fracture in the nearby area. A helpful diagnostic sign is elicited by a gentle squeeze over the fracture: If the blood coming from the wound shows fat droplets or marrow elements, this is a confirmatory sign. A bloody joint aspirate with fat droplets accumulating on the surface is a diagnostic sign of joint involvement by a fracture. The surgeon should assume that lacerations over a joint extend into the joint until the contrary is proved in the operating room. Air in the joint noted on roentgenography is a sign that a laceration extends into the joint.
C. With all wounds, including surgical wounds, consider **tetanus prophylaxis,** which is discussed later (see **V. I.**).
D. With any open fracture or major wound, start parenteral **bactericidal antibiotics** immediately in the emergency department (6). The bead pouch technique elevates normal levels of antibiotic (6).
1. **Cephalosporins** are the drug of choice for prophylaxis. If a cephalosporin is used, the preparations and dosages commonly recom-

mended by the authors are cefazolin (Kefzol or Ancef), 1 g IV (or IM) q6–8h. For all practical purposes, patients who are allergic to penicillin (excluding history of anaphylaxis) usually may receive cephalosporins; a small test dose is recommended before giving the entire dose. To obtain an adequate concentration of antibiotics in the fracture hematoma, begin the antibiotic therapy as soon as possible. To avoid many of the side effects of antibiotics, such as superinfections, limit the duration of prophylactic antibiotic therapy to 1–2 days.

2. An acceptable alternative is **vancomycin** 1 g IV initially and then 500 mg IV q6h for 2 days. Use this drug only if there is both penicillin and cephalosporin allergy or history of anaphylaxis as the isolates of resistant strains of bacteria have increased in number recently and this drug is the mainstay of treatment for methicillin-resistant *Staphylococcus aureus* (MRSA).

3. For type III open wounds with marked contamination, an aminoglycoside should also be given, and for barnyard injuries, penicillin is added as a third agent against clostridia. A more detailed discussion of the use of antibiotics in orthopaedics is presented in Chap. 3, **II.G.**

E. **Open fractures** are generally **classified** using Gustilo's system (Table 1-3). With increasing severity, the complications of deep infection, non-union, and amputation increase. A type IIIB open fracture requires a muscle flap for wound closure.

F. **All large wounds, open fractures, and nerve disruptions, and most tendon lacerations should be debrided and repaired in the operating room.**
   1. The dressing should be left on the wound while the **surrounding area is shaved** for the purpose of extending the wound with surgical incisions.
   2. A chlorhexidine (Hibiclens), hexachlorophene (pHisoHex), or povidone-iodine (Betadine) **scrub of the surrounding skin** is carried out before removing the dressing.
   3. The dressing is removed, and the entire area is **re-prepared** with aseptic techniques. A 1% tincture of iodine may be used to prepare the skin after the initial scrub, but great care must be taken to keep the iodine out of the wound because it causes further tissue damage.
   4. **Debridement** means removal of all foreign matter and devitalized tissue in or about a lesion. Irrigation with large quantities of Ringer's lactate

Table 1-3. Classification of open fractures

Grade I	Small wounds (1 cm or less) caused by low-energy trauma (e.g., the protrusion of a bony fragment through the skin or the entrance wound of a low-velocity bullet lodged in the soft tissues), resulting in minimal soft-tissue damage
Grade II	Extensive wounds with little or no avascular or devitalized soft tissue and relatively little contamination by foreign material
Grade III	Moderate or massive wounds with considerable area of devitalized soft tissue and/or contamination by foreign material, or a traumatic amputation
Grade IIIA	Wounds with extensive soft-tissue lacerations or flaps, or high-energy wounds with adequate remaining soft tissues to cover the fractured bone
Grade IIIB	Wounds with extensive soft-tissue injury or loss, periosteal stripping, and bone exposure
Grade IIIC	Open fractures associated with arterial injuries requiring repair

Adapted from Gustilo RB, Mendoza RM, Williams DM. Problems in management of type III open fractures. A new classification of type III open fractures. *J Trauma* 1984;24·742.

solution does not replace the need for proper surgical debridement technique. Pulsating saline lavage is a useful adjunct to good debridement.
5. The wound should be **debrided from the outside in.** The skin edges are sharply trimmed in a circular manner. The debridement is then continued into the depth of the wound until the entire damaged area has been identified and resected.
6. With an open fracture, all **devitalized bone** (bone without enough soft-tissue attachments to maintain adequate blood supply) is generally removed. Large cortical fragments that seem essential for stability are debrided if they do not have good soft-tissue attachments. Great care must be taken not to devitalize the bone further. Initial internal fixation of open fractures is preferable if rigid stabilization is provided without significantly jeopardizing the blood supply (6).

G. Open fractures should generally be treated by a **delayed primary closure** (3–5 days). An exception may be made for uncomplicated hand fractures, wounds that enter joints, or small wounds with no extensive hemorrhage. **The burden of proof rests with the surgeon electing to close the wound.** Cover all exposed tendons, nerves, and bone but not at the expense of compromising blood supply to injured skin and subcutaneous tissues. Acute consultation with an orthopaedic or plastic surgeon skilled in myoplasty is indicated.

IV. **Stress fractures**
   A. Normal bone might undergo fatigue or stress fractures when subjected to unaccustomed use. This condition can range from a stress fracture of a fibula in a runner who has recently increased his or her training distance or in an older person who is being mobilized after having been confined to a chair or bed. A **history** of having done something out of one's normal routine, followed by pain, should raise the question of stress fracture in the mind of the physician. Common sites of stress fracture include the metatarsals after unusually long walks or running, the distal fibula in runners, the tibia in football players (frequently misdiagnosed as shin splints), and the femoral neck in both young and older patients.
   B. The **physical examination** reveals tenderness to pressure on the bone at the site of the fracture. Occasionally, swelling and erythema are present. Radiographic examination usually is negative in the first 10–14 days, after which a small, radiolucent line can usually be seen in association with increasing adjacent bone sclerosis. A bone scan shows radioactive uptake earlier and may be indicated in the competing athlete, particularly if the suspected fracture is in the tibia or femoral neck, both of which have a high incidence of complete fracture if the athlete continues competition. Magnetic resonance imaging (MRI) can definitively identify a stress fracture. Healing stress fractures have been mistaken for bone tumors (5).
   C. **Treatment** should be based on the relief of symptoms unless there is danger of complete fracture under normal use. Under such circumstances, the injury should be treated like any undisplaced fracture.

V. **Repair of soft-tissue injuries**
   A. **Skin.** Leaving only viable skin is most important in treating musculoskeletal trauma. Damaged or devitalized skin provides a source of nutrition as well as a hiding place for bacteria. The following **principles of skin closure** are emphasized for musculoskeletal lacerations:
      1. **Major nerves and vessels should be covered by skin,** even if this requires transposition of the structures or construction of skin flaps, except when the skin coverage causes so much tension that it compromises blood supply to the skin edges.
      2. Although exposed bone can survive if it is not allowed to dry, every reasonable effort to ensure **soft-tissue coverage over exposed bone** should be made. Again, the soft-tissue coverage should not create enough tension to cause any devitalization from a lack of blood supply.

3. Whenever skin closure necessitates **tension** on the suture, follow one of two courses:
    a. Dress the wound with a saline moistened dressing and perform a **delayed primary closure.** This closure should be carried out within 5 days for hand wounds.
    b. Close the wound by **turning a flap or making a relaxing incision** only after consultation with a surgeon trained in these reconstruction techniques.
4. Use **monofilament sutures** for skin closure, not braided wire or multifilament synthetic, cotton, or silk sutures. Adequate control of bone bleeding may be difficult, so the surgeon should use either a loose skin closure that allows exodus of some of the hematoma or a skin closure combined with a suction drain.

B. **Musculotendinous junction injury**
    1. Diagnosis (11)
        a. **First-degree strain** (mild)
            (1) The **etiology** is trauma to a portion of the musculotendinous unit from excessive forcible use of stretch.
            (2) **Symptoms** include local pain that is aggravated by movement or by tension of the muscle.
            (3) **Signs** of injury include mild spasm, swelling, ecchymosis, local tenderness, and minor loss of function and strength.
            (4) **Complications** include recurrence of the strain, tendonitis, and periostitis at the tendinous insertion site.
            (5) **Pathologic changes** cause a low-grade inflammation and some disruption of muscle-tendon fibers by no appreciable hemorrhage.
        b. **Second-degree strain** (moderate) (11)
            (1) The **etiology** is trauma to a portion of the musculotendinous unit from violent contraction or excessive forcible stretch.
            (2) **Symptoms and signs** include local pain that is aggravated by movement or tension of the muscle, moderate spasm, swelling, ecchymosis, local tenderness, and impaired muscle function.
            (3) **Complications** include a recurrence of the strain.
            (4) The **pathologic findings** consist of hemorrhage and the tearing of muscle-tendon junction fibers without complete disruption.
        c. **Third-degree strain** (severe) (11)
            (1) **Symptoms and signs** include severe pain and disability, severe spasm, swelling, ecchymosis, hematoma, tenderness, and loss of muscle function, and usually a palpable defect. An avulsion fracture at a tendinous insertion may mimic a severe strain.
            (2) A **complication** is prolonged disability.
            (3) **Roentgenograms** can demonstrate an avulsion fracture at the tendinous attachment as well as soft-tissue swelling.
            (4) The **pathology** consists of a ruptured muscle or tendon with the resultant separation of muscle from muscle, muscle from tendon, or tendon from bone.
    2. **Treatment.** Direct treatment toward immobilization, with the disrupted tissue ends approximated. In some settings, this requires removal of devitalized tissue and repair by the sites and type of suture that will not cause further devitalization. When possible, sutures are placed in the surrounding fascia and not in the muscle itself.
C. **Tendon**
    1. Tendons are relatively avascular structures and do not handle infection well. At sites where they course along long synovial tunnels, **blood supply** is via the long axis of the tendon or vincula. Trauma or sheath infections can jeopardize nutrition of the tendon.

2. As a **general principle,** a lacerated or ruptured tendon should be repaired primarily with a nonreactive material and a suture technique to ensure continued approximation of the tendon ends. Even with prophylactic antibiotics, primary repair of tendons in wounds more than 12 hours old carries considerable risk. A nonreactive synthetic suture or braided wire is the suture of choice. If the tendon is expected to glide subsequently, then handling the tendon with sponges and forceps is avoided because this causes further trauma and may be associated with dense adhesions.
3. Any involved **tendon sheath** should be opened in a longitudinal fashion so that the tendon is unroofed for the entire excursion of a repaired laceration site to
   a. **Prevent "triggering"** of the enlarged sutured site
   b. **Allow for revascularization** of the tendon at the suture site
   c. **Prevent fixation** on the relatively immobile sheath
4. Only those with special training in hand surgery should repair **digital flexor tendons in the hand.**

D. **Ligaments**
1. **Types of injury**
   a. **First-degree sprain** (mild)
      (1) **Signs** include mild point tenderness, no abnormal motion, little or no swelling, minimal hemorrhage, and minimal functional loss.
      (2) **Complications** include a tendency toward recurrence.
      (3) The **pathology** consists of minor tearing of the ligamentous fibers.
   b. **Second-degree sprain** (moderate)
      (1) **Signs** include point tenderness, moderate loss of function, slight-to-moderate abnormal motion, swelling, and localized hemorrhage.
      (2) **Complications** can include a tendency toward recurrence, persistent instability, and traumatic arthritis.
      (3) This **pathology** is a partial tear of a ligament.
   c. **Third-degree sprain** (severe)
      (1) **Signs** include a loss of function, marked abnormal motion, possible deformity, tenderness, swelling, and hemorrhage.
      (2) **Complications** can involve persistent instability and traumatic arthritis.
      (3) **Stress roentgenograms** demonstrate abnormal motion when pain is adequately relieved.
      (4) The **pathology** is a complete tear of a ligament.
2. **Diagnosis** of the extent of the ligamentous injury presents one of the major problems in orthopaedics. Rupture may be suspected from the mechanism of injury or from physical examination, which reveals tenderness over the ligament. If the patient is seen shortly after injury, a gap may be felt where the ligament is normally located. The injury might be fairly painless, especially if the ligament is completely disrupted. Once hemorrhage and swelling occur, this diagnostic possibility is eliminated. Another diagnostic aid is a stress roentgenogram, but it must be compared with the opposite and normal side. Such films should be made when the pain is inhibited by regional or general anesthesia. Arthroscopy or arthrography can provide pertinent information and a diagnosis, but a skilled arthroscopist should first be consulted. An MRI scan can be used to make the diagnosis.
3. **Treatment** of a complete ligamentous rupture is in essence the treatment of a dislocated joint after the dislocation has been reduced. In general, preserving motion is most important and early mobilization is the treatment of choice. Ligaments are relatively avascular, so healing is slow. The larger ligaments must be protected until the scar matures (8–16 weeks).

4. There often is no clear answer when operative repair of ligaments is essential, but **open repair** is indicated in the following instances:
   a. Whenever the joint **cannot be anatomically reduced**
   b. When there is reasonable evidence of **infolding or turning of the ligament** on itself so that with any closed treatment the ends of the torn ligament would not be in close proximity
   c. When ligaments are injured **about a joint that has no internal stability** (relies primarily on ligamentous structure for its stability)

E. **Nerves**
   1. Nerve injuries are of **three types:** contusion or **neurapraxia,** crush or **axonotmesis,** and complete division or **neurotmesis.** Blunt injuries and those associated with fractures tend to be either neurapraxia or axonotmesis. For this reason, the fracture should be treated in its usual manner and the nerve injury observed. If it is neurapraxia, recovery will be complete within 6 to 12 weeks. If it is an axonotmesis, recovery from the trauma site to the next muscle to be innervated should be followed, keeping in mind that the expected recovery rate is 1 mm/day or 1 inch/month. If reinnervation does not occur on time, exploration is indicated. When the distance from the site of trauma to the next innervated muscle that can be assessed causes a 6-month delay, early exploration is indicated. An electromyogram shows reinnervation approximately 1 month before it can be detected clinically, but one is dependent on the skill of the electromyographer for interpretation (see **App. F**). A traction injury is usually a mixed lesion with a large element of neurotmesis of individual axons at various places along the nerve. A nerve injury associated with sharp trauma is usually neurotmesis, and surgical repair is indicated. The **brachial plexus** presents a special diagnostic and treatment problem. Injuries from lacerations, especially in children, should be repaired primarily. Most brachial plexus injuries, however, are caused by traction and are either an avulsion of the root from the cord or the typical tearing of the axons at multiple levels along the nerve. MRI is essential for differentiation. If the lesion is an avulsion injury, no recovery is possible, and the patient should be started early on rehabilitation. If the lesion is the typical traction injury, the patient should be followed up to document recovery. If no recovery appears at the appropriate time intervals, exploration and possible suture or nerve graft should be considered.
   2. As a general principle, **secondary repair** (3–6 weeks after injury) is preferable to primary repair for the following reasons:
      a. The repair is done as an **elective procedure** by the first team. The surgeon is rested and prepared for the procedure.
      b. There is **less hesitancy in extending the incision** for proper mobilization of the nerve.
      c. It is easier to delineate the **extent of damage** along the nerve.
      d. The **epineurium** has some degree of scarring and hence holds the suture better.
      e. The **distal axon tubules** are open because wallerian degeneration has occurred, and regeneration has a chance to proceed.
   3. There are many **exceptions** to the preference for **secondary repair,** such as suturing
      a. A **digital nerve**
      b. A **nerve in the brachial plexus**
      c. An isolated nerve injury **less than 8–12 hours old** inflicted by a razor or **sharp** knife
   4. **Nerve surgery should not be performed at any time by a surgeon inexperienced in microscopic techniques.**

F. **Hematomas**
   1. **Treatment** of large hematomas (large compared to the area of confinement) whether subcutaneous or in muscle, usually should consist of evacuation as an elective procedure in the operating room. A hematoma

is not absorbed but undergoes organization, fibrosis, and scarring. Aspiration of a clot is not possible, so a large hematoma is evacuated by open drainage. Before considering this, the surgeon must be sure the hematoma is not expanding or the cause of shock. If it is, vascular surgery consultation is mandatory to consider primary repair.

G. **Gunshot wounds and fractures**
   1. As with any other wounds, **check** the status of the **neurovascular structures.**
   2. If possible, **identify** the caliber and type of **weapon.** This information helps determine whether the wound was caused by a high- or low-velocity weapon.
   3. **High-velocity weapons** have a muzzle velocity greater than 610 m/sec or an impact velocity of 2,000–2,500 ft/sec. These weapons cause severe cavitation within the wound and always make debridement necessary.
   4. Wounds and fractures from **low-velocity weapons** can be treated without extensive debridement, but it is safer to debride and inspect when in doubt. Most civilian weapons are low-velocity; however, big-game rifles, such as a .30–.30 or a .30–.06, can approach this high-velocity impact energy, and wounds from them must be treated accordingly.
   5. Most gunshot wounds with fractures inflicted by civilian weapons may be **treated** as follows:
      a. With **tetanus prophylaxis**
      b. With 1–2 days of **antibiotics**
      c. With **cleansing** of the skin adjacent to the wound
      d. With **debridement** of the skin edges
      e. With superficial **irrigation** of the wound
      f. By application of a **sterile dressing**
      g. By **leaving the wound open**
      h. By **immobilizing** any fractures
   6. If there is any doubt about the **type of weapon** used, the examination often indicates the degree of debridement required. Gunshot wounds of high-impact energy cause marked comminution of the fracture and leave a gaping exit wound. These wounds require formal debridement as outlined previously for open fractures.
   7. If the bullet **enters a joint,** formal **debridement** is indicated. Similarly, **shotgun wounds** require debridement.
   8. If the bullet tract passes close to a major vessel, the **distal circulation** must be carefully checked. This should be done initially by palpation and noting blood pressure indices in the ankle or arm. If this value is less than 90% of the uninjured side, then duplex ultrasound or arteriography is indicated. If a significant injury is then identified, immediate surgical repair is necessary.

H. **Traumatic amputation** of a finger or an entire extremity calls for a planned team approach to assess the possibility of replantation. The proximal stump is first dressed with Ringer's lactate soaked dressing and a pressure dressing is applied. A tourniquet is to be avoided. The amputated part is wrapped in Ringer's lactate moistened sterile sponge and placed in a plastic bag. It should be cooled by placing it in a container with ice, which delays autolysis to allow time for transport to a center with a replantation team. The part must not be frozen or placed in direct contact with ice. If the travel distance by car is less than 2 hours, then this form of transport can be used. If not, arrangements should be made for air evacuation. Make no promises to the patient regarding whether replantation can be attempted or what the outcome will be. This assessment is left to a knowledgeable replantation team.

I. **Tetanus prophylaxis.** Although there are numerous recommended tetanus prophylaxis schedules, the authors generally follow the recommendations of the American College of Surgeons. Table 1-4 lists the current guidelines.

Table 1-4. Prophylactic treatment of tetanus[a]

Type of wound	Patient not immunized or partially immunized	Patient completely immunized—time since last booster dose	
		5[c]–10 yr	>10 yr
Clean minor	Begin or complete immunization per schedule; tetanus toxoid, 0.5 mL	None	Tetanus toxoid, 0.5 mL
Clean major or tetanus-prone	In one arm, human tetanus immunoglobulin, 250 units[b] In other arm, tetanus toxoid, 0.5 mL; complete immunization per schedule[b]	Tetanus toxoid, 0.5 mL	In one arm, tetanus toxoid, 0.5 mL[b] In other arm, human tetanus immunoglobulin, 250 units[b]
Tetanus-prone, delayed or incomplete debridement	In one arm, human tetanus immunoglobulin, 500 units[b] In other arm, tetanus toxoid, 0.5 mL; complete immunization per schedule thereafter[b]; antibiotic therapy	Tetanus toxoid, 0.5 mL; antibiotic therapy	In one arm, tetanus toxoid, 0.5 mL[b] In other arm, human tetanus immunoglobulin, 500 units[b]; antibiotic therapy

[a] With different preparations of toxoid, modify the volume of a single booster dose appropriately.
[b] Use different syringes, needles, and injection sites.
[c] No prophylactic immunization required if patient has had a booster within 5 years.
From Walt AJ, ed. *Early care of the injured patient.* Philadelphia: WB Sauders, 1982:70.

VI. Injuries in hemophiliacs
  A. Hemophilia includes a group of clinical states manifested by an abnormality of the coagulation mechanism and caused by absence or near absence deficiencies of specific clotting factors. Only two disorders are usually associated with sufficient bleeding to be clinically evident. The first is **classic hemophilia** (hemophilia A), in which there is a deficiency of factor VIII. The second is **Christmas disease** (hemophilia B), in which there is a deficiency of factor IX. Both deficiencies are sex-linked recessive disorders, manifested in the male and carried by the female. More rarely, **von Willebrand's disease,** in which both factor VIII deficiency and a functional platelet abnormality are present, causes significant musculoskeletal bleeding.
  B. Methods of replacing factors
    1. Concentrates from fresh-frozen plasma
      a. One contains **factor VIII and fibrinogen** and is used to treat classic hemophilia and von Willebrand's disease.
      b. The other contains **factors II, VII, IX, and X** and is used primarily for treatment of Christmas disease.
    2. Cryoprecipitate, the protein that precipitates in fresh-frozen plasma when it is thawed at 4°C, is rich in factor VIII and fibrinogen and is easily prepared and stored in ordinary blood banks.
    3. It is assumed that **1 unit of factor VIII** per kilogram of body weight raises the patient's plasma level of factor VIII activity by 2%, whereas **1 unit of factor IX** per kilogram of body weight raises the patient's plasma level by 1.5%.
    4. Maintenance levels are based on the plasma level desired, severity of the bleeding episode, length of time that replacement therapy is needed, the presence and amount of inhibitors, and the biologic half-life of the infused factor as determined by a survival study. In a patient who is not bleeding, the biologic half-life of factor VIII is 6–12 hours, whereas that of factor IX is 8–18 hours. Therefore, doses of factor VIII must be repeated q8h and doses of factor IX q12h.
  C. Treatment guidelines
    1. Secure initial hemostasis.
      a. A patient with severe hemophilia and a **fracture** should have plasma levels of 40%–60% of normal for the day of fracture and the next day, and up to 20%–30% of normal for approximately 1 week, depending on the degree of soft-tissue injury.
      b. Hemarthrosis generally requires a plasma level of 40%–50% of normal. This treatment is combined with resting the involved joint. Aspiration of a joint requires plasma levels of 30%–40%.
      c. Hematomas and muscle hemorrhages are usually controlled with 20%–30% of normal plasma levels when combined with compression and possibly ice. Treatment of bleeding into the gastrocsoleus muscle group often requires 40%–50% of normal plasma levels.
      d. A **team approach** with a knowledgeable hematologist is necessary to handle these cases in an ideal manner.
    2. Maintain proper hemostasis during healing.
    3. Provide rigid immobilization of fractures. Generally, treat the fracture itself in a normal manner, but avoid skeletal pins because there is likely to be oozing about the pins, requiring prolonged factor replacement therapy. Operative management requires 100% factor levels for 24–48 hours perioperatively.
VII. Pediatric musculoskeletal trauma
  A. Some brief **general principles** of fracture alignment in children follow:
    1. Up to **30 degrees of angulation** in the plane of joint motion is **acceptable** in metaphyseal fractures in young children. The **younger** the patient, the **greater the angulation acceptable.**
    2. If a **fracture deformity** is obvious on inspection, it should be **reduced.**
    3. Fractured femurs in the 3- to 8-year-old group can be allowed to have 1.0–1.5 cm of overlap.

4. As a general rule, **children do not experience stiffness of otherwise normal joints.**
B. **Epiphyseal plate injuries** are common in children. The epiphyseal plate is weakest at the site of cell degeneration and provisional calcification. This condition is seen particularly in children who have undergone a rapid growth spurt and in those who are excessively heavy for their skeletal maturity. **Salter** classified traumatic epiphyseal separations into the following functional groups:
   1. **Class 1.** This is a fracture through the zone of provisional calcification without fracture of bone. Such an injury does not involve a germinal layer unless associated with severe trauma either from the initial injury or from attempted reductions. Growth disturbances are rare but do occur.
   2. **Class 2.** A class 2 injury is an epiphyseal plate fracture with an associated fracture through the metaphysis. Such an injury falls into the same prognostic category as Class 1.
   3. **Class 3.** This is an epiphyseal plate fracture associated with fractures through the epiphysis. These fractures usually involve an articular surface; in addition, there is a fracture through the germinal layers. Accurate reduction is essential to prevent subsequent growth disturbance, but even so, alterations in growth are unpredictable. If the articular surface has more than 1 mm of "step off," then open reduction is indicated.
   4. **Class 4.** This is a fracture through the epiphysis, epiphyseal plate, and metaphysis. Such an injury almost invariably results in significant growth disturbance unless it is anatomically reduced. Open reduction and internal fixation are usually indicated.
   5. **Class 5.** This is an impact or "smash" injury that virtually destroys the epiphyseal plate and results in growth arrest. Close monitoring for remaining growth is essential. Surgical resection of the bone bridge and fat interposition are necessary if growth arrest results.
   6. With all types of injuries involving the epiphyseal plate, an accurate diagnosis as to the type of injury is important. The rule **"one doctor, one manipulation"** should be observed. Minor residual deformity in class 1 and 2 injuries correct themselves with subsequent growth, so open reduction is not usually indicated because the operation itself may cause more trauma.
C. **Diagnostic and therapeutic pitfalls** surrounding pediatric fractures
   1. **Treating accessory ossicles as fractures**
   2. **Missing an osteochondral fracture**
   3. **Forgetting that an upper tibial metaphyseal fracture in a child might progress into valgus**
   4. **Missing a stress fracture**
   5. **Confusing an epiphyseal fracture for a ligament injury, particularly at the knee**
   6. **Missing a tibial spine fracture**
   7. **Overdiagnosing instability of C2-3**
   8. **Overtreating an upper humeral fracture**
   9. **Failing to realize the instability of an apparently undisplaced lateral condylar fracture of the humerus**
   10. **Overlooking radial head dislocation**
   11. **Failing to appreciate the frequency of distal forearm fractures that lose initial reduction**
   12. **Overlooking abdominal injury in a child with a thoracolumbar flexion injury**

References
1. Bone LB, McNamara K, Shine B, et al. Mortality in multiple trauma patients with fractures. *J Trauma* 1994;37:262–264.
2. Bosse MJ, MacKenzie EJ, Reimer BL, et al. Adult respiratory distress syndrome, pneumonia, and mortality following thoracic injury and a femoral fracture treated

either with intramedullary nailing with reaming or with a plate: a comparative study. *J Bone Joint Surg (Am)* 1997;79:799–809.

3. DuWelius PJ, Huckfeldt R, Mullins RJ, et al. The effects of femoral intramedullary reaming on pulmonary function in a sheep lung model. *J Bone Joint Surg (Am)* 1997;79:194–202.

4. Einhorn TA. Enhancement of fracture healing. *J Bone Joint Surg (Am)* 1995; 77:940–956.

5. Eisele SA, Sammarco GJ. Fatigue fractures of the foot and ankle in the athlete. In: Heckman JD, ed. *Instructional course lectures,* 42, Rosemont, IL: American Academy of Orthopaedic Surgeons, 1993:175–183.

6. Henry SL, Osterman PA, Seligson D. The antibiotic bead pouch technique: the management of severe compound fractures. *Clin Orthop* 1993;295:54–62.

7. Loo GT, Siegel JH, Dischinger PC, et al. Airbag protection versus compartmental intrusion effect determines the pattern of injuries in multiple trauma motor vehicle crashes. *J Trauma* 1996;41:935–951.

8. McKee MD, Schemitsch EH, Vincent LO, et al. The effect of a femoral fracture on concomitant closed head injury in patients with multiple injuries. *J Trauma* 1997; 42:1041–1045.

9. Routt MI, Simonian PT, DeFalco AJ, et al. Internal fixation in pelvic fractures and primary repairs of associated genitourinary disruptions: a team approach. *J Trauma* 1996;40:784–790.

10. Shopnick RI, Brettler DB. Hemostasis: a practical review of conservative and operative care. *Clin Orthop* 1996;328:34–38.

11. Taylor DC, Dalton JD Jr, Seaber AV, et al. Experimental muscle strain injury: early functional and structural deficits and the increased risk for reinjury. *Am J Sport Med* 1993;21:190–194.

12. Weitzel PP, Esterhai JL Jr. Delayed union, nonunion and synovial pseudarthrosis. In: Brighton CT, Friedlaender GE, Lane JM, eds. *Bone formation and repair.* Rosemont, IL: American Academy of Orthopaedic Surgeons, 1994:505–527.

Selected Historical Readings

Godina M. Early microsurgical reconstruction of complex trauma of the extremities. *Plast Reconstr Surg,* 1986;78:285.

Gustilo RB, Mendoza RM, Williams DM. Problems in management of type III open fractures. A new classification of type III open fractures. *J Trauma* 1984;24:742.

Nash G, Blennerhassett JB, Pontoppidan H. Pulmonary lesions associated with oxygen therapy and artificial ventilation. *N Engl J Med* 1967;276:368.

Salter RB. Injuries involving the epiphyseal plate. *J Bone Joint Surg (Am)* 1963;45:587.

Shackford SR, et al. The effect of regionalization upon the quality of trauma care as assessed by concurrent audit before and after institution of a trauma system: a preliminary report. *J Trauma* 1986;26:812.

Subcommittee on Classification of Sports Injuries. *Standard nomenclature of athletic injuries.* Chicago: American Medical Association, 1976:99.

Tibbs PA, et al. Diagnosis of acute abdominal injuries in patients with spinal shock: value of diagnostic peritoneal lavage. *J Trauma,* 1980;20:55.

Traverso LW, et al. Fluid resuscitation after an otherwise fatal hemorrhage: I. Crystalloid solutions. *J Trauma* 1986;26:168.

Urbaniak JR, et al. The results of replantation after amputation of a single finger. *J Bone Joint Surg (Am)* 1985;67:611.

2. COMPLICATIONS OF MUSCULOSKELETAL TRAUMA

Every effort must be made to avoid the common complications of musculoskeletal trauma. Some complications are unavoidable, but prompt recognition and appropriate treatment decrease their severity and improve the outcome.

I. The fat embolism syndrome
- **A.** The fat embolism syndrome is generally a self-limited pulmonary disease that usually occurs within 3 days of a fracture. The **diagnosis** is suspected if the following symptoms and signs are present (4,10,16):
  1. **Skeletal injury**
  2. **Disturbances of consciousness** (i.e., confusion, delirium, coma)
  3. **Tachycardia and dyspnea**
  4. **History of hypovolemic shock**
  5. **Petechial hemorrhages**
- **B.** **Pertinent laboratory findings**
  1. Of all the laboratory values, a platelet count of less than 150,000 and a PaO_2 of less than 60 mm Hg are the **most useful diagnostic tests.** O_2 saturation of less than 96% by pulse oximetry is highly suggestive (18).
  2. **Electrocardiographic changes** may include tachycardia, a prominent S wave on lead I, a prominent Q wave on lead II, a shift in the transition zone to the left, arrhythmias, inverted T waves, depressed RST segments, and a right bundle branch block. Serial electrocardiograms are useful.
  3. **Increased serum lipase** is indicative.
  4. **Chest roentgenographic changes,** when present, are patchy pulmonary infiltrates. The clinical manifestations of fat embolism usually precede these changes.
  5. **Fat in the urine** is rarely observed. To investigate the presence of fat droplets in urine, a suggested method is to place the urine in a volumetric flask with enough water to bring the meniscus up to the neck of the flask without causing the urine to spill. Let the urine stand 6–12 hours in a refrigerator; then pass a freshly flamed loop (such as is used in microbiology) through the meniscus. Place the drop on a slide, add a drop of Sudan blue, and cover with a slide cover. The fat should be visible under the microscope.
- **C.** **Recommended treatment**
  1. **Respiratory support** is the cornerstone of prevention and treatment of fat embolism syndrome. Provide respiratory support with oxygen to keep the PaO_2 between 50 and 100 mm Hg. Intubate if necessary. Controlled volume ventilation with positive end-expiratory pressure helps inhibit the formation and presence of pulmonary edema. Early (within 24 hours) fixation of femur fractures helps limit the incidence of this complication (8,16).
  2. **Shock** is treated as outlined in Chap. 1 **(I.A.3).**
- **D.** **Other methods of treatment.** Historical recommendations include IV alcohol (1 L 5% dextrose and 5% ethanol q12h), corticosteroids (9), low-dose heparin therapy (3,000 units or 25 mg q6h, reducing the dosage by 3,000 units/day after the first 24 hours, and low-molecular-weight dextran (Rheomacrodex) (500–1000 mL/24 hours for no more than 5 days). The authors tend not to use any of these latter methods of treatment but rely on pulmonary support with oxygen and intubation with positive end-expiratory pressure when necessary.

II. Nerve compression syndromes
- **A.** **Carpal tunnel syndrome** (a median nerve entrapment at the wrist)
  1. The **diagnosis** is suspected with a history of pain, tingling, and subsequent numbness in the first three digits; the symptoms are usually worse

at night. When occurring as a complication of trauma, the condition is most commonly associated with distal radius fractures and can occur acutely. It must be recognized and treated emergently with carpal tunnel release. The syndrome is only rarely associated with acute trauma and is generally a chronic condition often associated with repetitive microtrauma (see Chap. 20).

B. **Ulnar nerve compression at the elbow** ("tardy" ulnar nerve palsy, acute ulnar palsy) is commonly associated with fractures around the elbow in children as well as adults.

1. One of the earliest **diagnostic signs** can be the inability to separate the fingers (interosseous weakness). There is usually decreased sensation in the fourth and fifth fingers. Light pressure on the cubital tunnel reproduces the pain. Nerve conduction studies show a slowing of the ulnar nerve conduction velocity as it crosses the elbow (see App. F); this test is not useful diagnostically until 3 weeks after injury.

2. If the neuropathy is minimal, the condition should be managed with observation and passive range of motion of the fingers. **Surgical therapy** consists of transposition of the ulnar nerve beneath the flexor muscle mass anterior to the medial epicondyle when the pattern of injury or fracture permits. This treatment usually stops any progressive neuropathy but does not guarantee complete regression of the neurologic symptoms or signs.

C. **Compression of the common peroneal nerve** occurs in the area of the fibular head or as the nerve enters the anterior compartment.

1. **Diagnosis** often is based on the motor loss, which includes weakness of dorsiflexion of the ankle and toes as well as eversion of the foot. History of a tibia, ankle, or foot injury is likely. Pain is usually on the lateral aspect of the leg and foot. Pressure over the nerve trunk may cause local pain as well as radiation into the sensory distribution of the nerve. Pressure over the nerve as it courses around the proximal fibula results from patient positioning in the operating room or intensive care unit or from poorly applied splints.

2. **Treatment.** If there is an operable cause, then neurolysis is rarely indicated. During the recovery stage, a lateral shoe wedge or plastic ankle-foot orthosis maintains eversion of the foot.

D. **Sciatic nerve** neuroproxia can accompany hip dislocation or fracture dislocation (acetabular fracture).

1. The main differentiating factor in the **diagnosis** of a sciatic neuropathy is an L5 or S1 traumatic injury resulting from pelvic or spine fracture. This factor often is difficult to assess, but a sciatic neuropathy must be suspected when multiple neurologic (L5-S3) segments are involved because multiple segments are rarely seen with disk herniation. A helpful differentiating test is straight-leg raising just short of discomfort; pain caused by a sciatic neuropathy is increased by internal rotation and relieved by external rotation of the hips. This reaction is not seen with lumbar radiculopathies.

2. **Treatment** is aimed at the cause of the sciatic neuropathy and the neuropathy itself is treated with observation. If the sciatic nerve is known to be damaged and is not improving, neurolysis may be indicated. In general, the tibial portion of the nerve recovers well, but the peroneal portion does not (2). This may relate to the fact that it is the peroneal portion that lies against the pelvis as it exits through the greater sciatic foramen.

III. **Compartmental syndromes.** A compartmental syndrome is defined as "a condition in which increased pressure within the space compromises the circulation to the contents of that space" (11). Other terms that have been used are Volkmann's ischemia, local ischemia, traumatic tension in muscles, impending ischemic contracture, exercise ischemia, exercise myopathy, anterotibial syndrome, medial tibial syndrome, rhabdomyolysis, and calf hypertension.

A. Locations
   1. In the **upper extremity**, typical locations include the volar and dorsal compartments of the forearm (Fig. 2-1). There are also several intrinsic compartments of the hand.
   2. In the **lower extremity,** typical locations include the anterior, lateral, superficial posterior (gastrocnemius, soleus), and deep posterior compartments of the leg (Figs. 2-2, 2-3). Compartmental syndromes are also seen in the thigh, buttocks (gluteal), hand and foot compartments (12).
B. Etiologies
   1. **Decreased compartment size,** such as closure of fascial defects, tight dressings, and localized external pressure, can precipitate a compartmental syndrome (20).
   2. **Increased compartment content** arises from
      a. **Bleeding** caused by a major vascular injury, massive crush, or a bleeding disorder
      b. **Increased capillary permeability** owing to shock, postischemic swelling, exercise, direct trauma, burns, intraarterial drugs, or orthopaedic surgery
      c. **Increased capillary pressure** from exercise or venous obstruction
      d. **Muscle hypertrophy**
      e. **Infiltrated infusion**
      f. **Application of excessive traction** (Fig. 2-4)
C. Increased **tissue pressure** is the key to compartmental syndromes. Once the pressure is elevated, it can compromise the local circulation by at least three mechanisms: decreased perfusion pressure, arteriolar closure, and reflex vasospasm (6). Muscle cell death begins at approximately 6 hours after the pressure begins to approach 20 mm Hg lower than the patients diastolic pressure.
D. The clinical approach
   1. **Identify** the patients at risk as early as possible and **examine them frequently.** If the risk is high, consider **prophylactic decompression.** Patients who have been hypotensive for any reason are at particular risk.
   2. Carefully **document** the time and findings of each examination.
   3. The appearance of excess **pain, sensory deficits,** or **muscle weakness** demands a thorough examination to rule out a compartmental syndrome (Table 2-1). Because the compartmental syndrome is usually progressive,

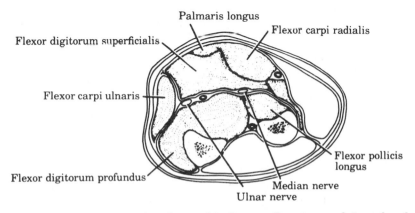

FIG. 2-1. Volar compartmental syndrome of the forearm. Symptoms and signs of weakness of finger and wrist flexion, pain on finger and wrist extension, hypesthesia of the volar aspect of the fingers, and tenseness of the volar forearm fascia.

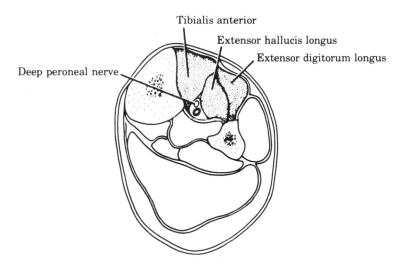

FIG. 2-2. Anterior compartmental syndrome of the leg. Symptoms and signs are weakness of toe extension and foot dorsiflexion, pain on passive toe flexion and foot plantar flexion, hypesthesia in the dorsal first web space, and tenseness of the anterior compartmental fascia.

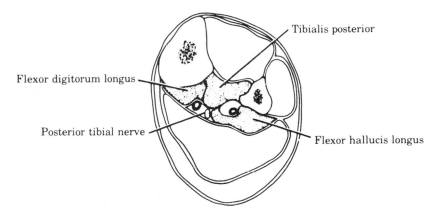

FIG. 2-3. Deep posterior compartmental syndrome of the leg. Symptoms and signs are weakness of toe flexion and foot inversion, pain on passive toe extension and foot eversion, hypesthesia of the plantar aspect of the foot and toes, and tenseness of the deep posterior compartmental fascia (between the tibia and Achilles tendon).

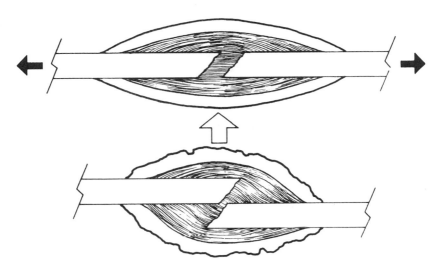

FIG. 2-4. Distraction of fracture fragments (excessive traction) can increase compartmental tissue pressure and be a cause of a compartmental syndrome.

frequent examination is indicated in questionable cases. Of the 5 "P's"
traditionally taught to be associated with compartmental syndrome
(pain, pulselessness, pallor, paresthesias, paralysis) pulselessness, pallor, and paralysis rarely occur.

   a. Check each potentially involved nerve using **two-point discrimination** and **light touch,** because both are more sensitive than the
commonly used pin.

   b. Grade the **strengths** of all potentially involved muscles (see App. B).

   c. The **passive muscle stretch** test causes severe pain if the muscle is
ischemic.

   d. **Palpation** of each compartment is important because tenseness is
a specific sign of a compartmental syndrome. This sign is obscured
unless the dressing and plaster are adequately opened. Warm and
red skin overlying the affected compartment suggests a cellulitis or
thrombophlebitis.

   e. The **peripheral pulse** frequently is normal in the presence of a
compartmental syndrome. If it is abnormal, the diagnosis of a major
arterial occlusion or compartmental syndrome must be entertained.

   f. **Laboratory findings** are nonspecific.

4. The **tissue pressure** can be accurately measured by the infusion or
wick techniques (Figs. 2-5, 2-6), which give similar pressure readings
(15). A simpler but less reliable measurement can be obtained by the
injection technique (Fig. 2-7). Tissue pressure readings in excess of
40 mm Hg are strongly suggestive of a compartmental syndrome. The
various techniques for pressure measurement are described by Whitesides
(20). Although these measuring techniques are useful, the clinician
should rely largely on the patient's history and ongoing (or repeat) examinations to establish the proper diagnosis and treatment program.
In the presence of head injury, intoxication, or an unreliable or uncon-
sciousness patient, these techniques are indispensable. The evaluation
should include measurement of the tissue pressure at multiple levels
in the compartment (5).

5. If the examination suggests a compartmental syndrome, **decompression** of the involved compartments should be performed within 12 hours
of the onset of symptoms; optionally within 6 to 8 hours of onset.

Table 2-1. Diagnostic factors in compartmental syndromes of the lower extremity

Compartment	Distribution of sensory changes	Muscles weakened	Painful passive movement	Location of tenseness
Anterior	Deep peroneal (first web space)	Toe extensors and tibialis anterior	Toe flexion	Anteriorly between tibia and fibula
Lateral	Superficial and deep peroneal (dorsum of foot)	Peronei	Inversion of foot	Laterally over fibula
Deep posterior	Posterior tibial (sole of foot)	Toe flexors and tibialis posterior	Toe extension	Posteromedially in distal half of leg between Achilles tendon and tibia
Superficial posterior	None	Gastrocnemius and soleus	Foot dorsiflexion	Over the bulk of the calf

Modified from Matsen III, FA. Compartmental syndrome. *Clin Orthop* 1976;113:8.

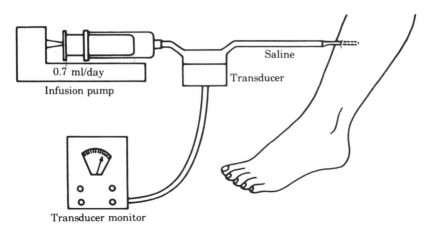

FIG. 2-5. Tissue pressure measured by the infusion technique.

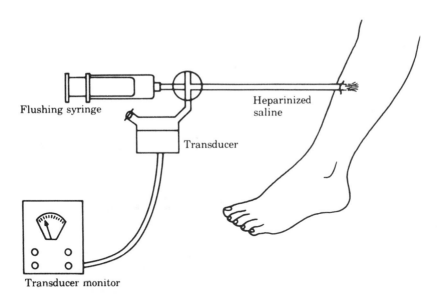

FIG. 2-6. Tissue pressure measured by the wick technique.

6. If decompression does not produce the expected improvement, one should consider the possibilities of inadequate decompression, another compartmental syndrome, incorrect diagnosis, or secondary arterial occlusion. Careful **reexploration** and possibly **arteriography** are indicated.

7. Because **myoglobinuria** and **renal failure** can complicate compartmental syndromes, adequate hydration and urinary output, with alkalinization of the urine using IV sodium bicarbonate, should be ensured. Dark urine may usually be attributed to myoglobinuria if the benzidine test is positive and in the absence of hematuria.

   If the compartment syndrome is recognized more than 24 hours after the onset, fasciotomy should not be performed. The risk of deep infection

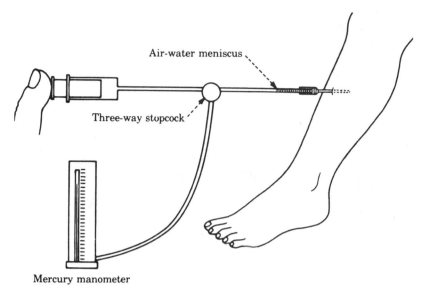

Air-water meniscus

Three-way stopcock

Mercury manometer

FIG. 2-7. Tissue pressure measured by the injection technique.

is high and often results in limb loss. When the time of onset is known to be 24 hours or longer, observation with urine alkalinization should be the recommendation (3).

IV. Sudeck's atrophy; reflex sympathetic dystrophy (RSD). Suspect early Sudeck's atrophy in any patient with persistent complaints of pain, hyperesthesia of the skin, or abnormal pseudomotor response. **For successful treatment, the diagnosis must be made before the classic signs** of thin shiny skin, excessive hair growth, attrition of nails, and diffuse osteoporosis are present. When the diagnosis is suspected, institute treatment immediately. Treatment consists of sympathetic blocks plus vigorous active physical therapy to mobilize any edema as well as to increase the muscle activity and the range of joint motion. The condition can occur in the upper extremity as well as in the lower extremity from the knee distally.

V. Myositis ossificans
  A. Heterotopic bone formation can occur in collagenous supportive tissue of skeletal muscles, tendons, ligaments, and fascia. There are **four clinical types:**
   1. **Myositis ossificans progressiva** is rare and can be genetic. It usually occurs between the ages of 5 and 10 years (younger than age 20) and proceeds relentlessly to progressive ossification of skeletal muscles. It is often present in the shoulders and neck as firm subcutaneous masses, which can be hot and tender and can undergo ossification. Often associated are microdactyly of the great toes and thumbs, ankylosis of the interphalangeal and metatarsophalangeal joints, and bilateral hallux valgus. Minor trauma often causes exacerbations. Treatment may include diphosphonate combined with surgery for severe joint malpositioning and functional impairment.
   2. **Myositis ossificans paralytica** occurs in proximal paralyzed muscles. The ossification occurs 1 to 10 months after a spinal cord injury. This process causes decreased passive range of motion. The three classic sites are in the vastus medialis, the quadratus femoris, and the hip

abductors. Surgical treatment is indicated only if the position and function of the extremity are unacceptable and when the ossification has matured. After excision, the dead space created must be drained by closed suction and the wound carefully observed for a hematoma.

3. **Myositis ossificans circumscripta** can be idiopathic but is more commonly caused by focal trauma and is common as a sports injury in the contact setting. It is more common in teenage or young adult males. It presents as an uncomfortable, indistinct mass that shows local induration and a local increase of temperature. The lesion occurs 80% of the time in the arm (biceps brachialis) but also occurs in the thigh (abductors and quadratus femoris). Roentgenograms show fluffy calcification 2 to 4 weeks after injury. In 14 weeks, the calcification has matured, and in 5 months, ossification has occurred. The differential diagnosis includes osteosarcoma and periosteal osteogenic sarcoma. Treatment is by excision, only if the lesion is unusually large or painful and after ossification is mature.

4. **Myositis ossificans traumatica** presents the same way as the circumscripta type except for a clear history of trauma, with ossification of a single muscle group in the traumatized area (7). Treatment is controversial but generally is aimed at the prevention of ossification by immediate application of cold and compression to the area of muscle injury. Later, heat is applied. An operation is indicated only when the ossification causes permanent impairment and only after the process has stabilized, often as soon as 6 to 8 months after injury.

B. The **sequence and roles of the different factors of myositis ossificans are not known. Preventive treatment** should be designed to stop the sequence of osteogenesis.

1. When the diagnosis of myositis ossificans is made, the extremity should be **splinted** for 2 to 3 weeks, after which, active range-of-motion exercises are slowly begun.

2. **Pharmacologic treatment** historically included bisphosphonates to inhibit hydroxyapatite crystallization, mithramycin to interfere with mobilization of calcium, and cortisone to decrease bone formation at the site of injury. None of these drugs, however, has proved to be an extremely beneficial therapeutic agent. Recently, indomethacin has been shown to help minimize posttraumatic heterotopic ossification associated with acetabular fractures and arthroplasty (13,14,17). Similarly, low-dose irradiation with 800 to 1,000 rad has been shown to be effective in these conditions (1).

3. When **surgical treatment** is indicated, traditional teaching has been to wait until the ossification is mature—that is, when the bone scan is negative and the alkaline phosphatase level is decreasing. Many authors have recently advocated earlier resection before these tests have returned to normal (19).

References

1. Bosse MJ, et al. Heterotopic ossification as a complication of acetabular fracture: prophylaxis with low-dose irradiation. *J Bone Joint Surg (Am)* 1988;70:1231.
2. Fassler PR, Swiontkowski MF, Kilroy AW, et al. Injury of the sciatic nerve associated with acetabular fracture. *J Bone Joint Surg (Am)* 1993;75:1157–116.
3. Finklestein JA, Hunter GA, Hu RW. Lower limb compartment syndrome: course after delayed fasciotomy. *J Trauma* 1996;40:342–344.
4. Ganong RB. Fat emboli syndrome in isolated fractures of the tibia and femur. *Clin Orthop* 1993;291:208–214.
5. Heckman MM, Whitesides TE, Greve SR, et al. Compartment pressure in association with closed tibia fractures—the relationship between tissue pressure, compartment and the distance from the site of fracture. *J Bone Joint Surg (Am)* 1994;76:1285–1292.
6. Heppenstall RB, Sapega AA, Scott R, et al. The compartment syndrome—an experimental and clinical study of muscular energy metabolism using phosphorous nuclear magnetic resonance spectroscopy. *Clin Orthop* 1988;226:138–155.

7. Hyder N, Shaw DL, Bouen SR. Myositis ossification: calcification of the entire tibialis anterior after ischaemic injury (compartment syndrome). *J Bone Joint Surg (Br)* 1995;78:318–319.

8. Johnson KD, Cadambi A, Seiber GB. Incidence of adult respiratory distress syndrome in patients with multiple musculoskeletal injuries: effect of early operative stabilization of fractures. *J Trauma* 1985;24:375.

9. Kallenbach J, et al. "Low-dose" corticosteroid prophylaxis against fat embolism. *J Trauma* 1987;27:1173.

10. Lindeque BGP, Schoeman HS, Dommisse OF, et al. Fat embolism and the fat embolism syndrome—a double blind therapeutic study. *J Bone Joint Surg (Br)* 1987; 69:128–131.

11. Matsen FA III. *Compartmental syndromes.* New York: Grune & Stratton, 1980.

12. Manoli A, Fakhouri AJ, Weber TG. Concurrent compartment syndromes of the foot and leg. *Foot Ankle* 1993;14:339–342.

13. Matta JM, Siebenrock KA. Does indomethacin reduce heterotopic bone formation after operations for acetabular fractures? A prospective randomized study. *J Bone Joint Surg (Br)* 1997;79:959–963.

14. Moed BR, Karzes DE. Prophylactic indomethacin for the prevention of heterotopic ossification after acetabular fracture in high risk patients. *J Orthop Trauma* 1993; 7:33–38.

15. Mubarak SJ, et al. Acute compartment syndromes: diagnosis and treatment with the aid of the Wick catheter. *J Bone Joint Surg (Am)* 1978;60:1091.

16. Miller C, Rahn BA, Pfister U, et al. The incidence, pathogenesis, diagnosis and treatment of fat embolism. *Orthopaedic Review* 1994;23:107–1171.

17. Schmidt SA, et al. The use of indomethacin to prevent the formation of heterotopic bone after total hip replacement: a randomized, double-blind clinical trial. *J Bone Joint Surg (Am)* 1988;70:834.

18. Schnaid E, et al. The early biochemical and hormonal profile of patients with long bone fractures at risk of fat embolism syndrome. *J Trauma* 1988;28:383.

19. Viola RW, Hanel DP. Early "simple" release of posttraumatic elbow contracture associated with heterotopic ossification. *J Hand Surg (Am)* 1999;24:370–380.

20. Whitesides TE, Heckman MM. Acute compartment syndrome: update on diagnosis and treatment. *J Am Acad Orthop Surg* 1996;4:209–218.

Selected Historical Readings

Bivins BA, et al. Fat embolism revisited. *South Med J* 1976;69:899.

Gelberman RH, et al. Compartment syndromes of the forearm: diagnosis and treatment. *Clin Orthop* 1981;161:252.

Gossling HR, Pellegrini VD. Fat embolism syndrome. *Clin Orthop* 1982;165:68.

Gurd AR, Wilson RI. The fat embolism syndrome. *J Bone Joint Surg (Br)* 1974;56:408.

Henk J, et al. Fat embolism in patients with an isolated fracture of the femoral shaft. *J Trauma* 1988;28:383.

Lilijedahl SO, Westemarks L. Etiology and treatment of fat embolism. *Acta Anaesthesiol Scand* 1967;11:177.

Matsen FA III, Winquist RA, Krugmire RB Jr. Diagnosis and management of compartmental syndromes. *J Bone Joint Surg (Am)* 1980;62:286,.

Murray DG, Raca GB. Fat-embolism syndrome (respiratory insufficiency syndrome). *J Bone Joint Surg (Am)* 1974;56:1338.

Patterson DC. Myositis ossificans circumscripta. *J Bone Joint Surg (Br)* 1970;52:296.

Peltier LF. Fat embolism. *Clin Orthop* 1969;66:241.

Peltier LF. Fat embolism. *Clin Orthop* 1984;187:3.

Riska EB, et al. Prevention of fat embolism by early internal fixation of fractures in patients with multiple injuries. *Injury* 1976;8:110.

Rorabeck CH, Bourne RB, Fowler PJ. The surgical treatment of exertional compartment syndrome in athletes. *J Bone Joint Surg (Am)* 1983;65:1245.

3. PREVENTION AND MANAGEMENT OF ACUTE MUSCULOSKELETAL INFECTIONS

Prevention of infection is the key to successful orthopaedic surgery. Meticulous attention to aseptic technique in the operating room, proper skin preparation and surgical scrub, the use of modern gown and mask techniques, planning the operation to shorten the time the tissues are exposed to air, laminar flow air, and prophylactic antibiotics (7–8,9,11) are all important in the prevention of infection. None, however, is as critical as meticulous debridement of wounds and the careful handling of tissues to prevent cell death (11). When infection does occur following an operation or from hematogenous origin, early diagnosis and prompt effective treatment can prevent disastrous complications.

I. **Prevention**
  A. **Elective surgery.** Refer to Chap. 1, **III**, and Chap. 10, **I,** for techniques described for the prevention of operative and posttraumatic infections.
  B. **Early diagnosis**
    1. Whenever a patient's postoperative or postinjury status does not follow the normal or expected course, the surgeon should be alert to the possibility of infection. A **respiratory problem** such as mild atelectasis may be a cause for persistent postoperative temperature elevation (this is especially common in patients who smoke), but such a potential diagnosis should not lull the surgeon into complacency. Wound infection may be the cause, or the two could be concurrent. Large hematomas can themselves be the cause of low-grade fever, but hematomas also represent the best culture media for bacteria and hence should be avoided or evacuated if present. Always obtain a culture of any evacuated hematoma.
    2. When there is concern regarding a wound infection, **inspect the wound and document the findings** at least daily, using sterile technique. Inspect the wound for swelling, erythema, and serous or bloody drainage. Culture any drainage. Tense skin, erythema, and abnormal tenderness or swelling frequently are signs of low-grade inflammation and infection.
    3. If the patient does not respond promptly to treatment or if the wound remains indurated, then **aspiration** should be carried out using aseptic technique with a large needle inserted into the wound area but away from the suture line.
    4. A low-grade fever in patients who have had antibiotics is not uncommon. In such instances, the temperature rarely exceeds 100°F (37.8°C) and may show a mild afternoon elevation. The erythrocyte sedimentation rate (ESR) is often abnormal. The patient frequently feels lethargic and has mild anorexia. If the **low-grade inflammatory process** involves a joint, the patient complains of pain to passive motion of the joint, which should alert the surgeon to the possibility of a septic joint.
    5. Be alert to the possibility of infection. **Establish the diagnosis through cultures** whenever possible, and treat the infection aggressively. If in doubt, the best course is generally to return the patient to the operating room and open the wound, irrigate and debride it to remove hematoma and necrotic wound tissue, and reclose the wound using the most "tissue friendly" suture technique (see Chap. 10). Consultation with another experienced surgeon can be helpful.
  C. **Treatment.** Once the diagnosis of a musculoskeletal infection has been established, treatment proceeds as for acute osteomyelitis or septic arthritis. The principles of treatment include removal of all dead tissue and any hematoma along with appropriate antibiotic therapy. The wound is nearly always left open for secondary closure, except when the infection involves a joint. If the wound is closed, a suction drain is mandatory.

29

II. Bone and joint infections

A. Bones and joints represent special problems for the host defense mechanisms. Normal bone has an excellent blood supply, although there is slowing of the circulation in the metaphyseal region in children. **Once pus forms under pressure, the vascular supply to bone is lost** because of its rigid structure, resulting in areas of infected, devitalized bone. Septic emboli in bone or vascular thrombosis can cause additional devascularization. Ligaments and tendons are relatively avascular structures and do not handle infection well. Joints, with their avascular cartilage and menisci, pose a particular problem. Local phagocytic function can be deficient, and it is often difficult to ensure adequate delivery of humeral factors (antibodies, opsonins, complement). In addition to the direct destructive effect of cell breakdown on cartilage, the pus under pressure interferes with cartilage nutrition and blood supply to the periarticular structures. At particular risk is the epiphyseal blood supply, and avascular neurosis may be the result. Antibiotics can inhibit or cure an infection only when they can reach the infecting organism in bacteriostatic or bactericidal concentrations. Infections producing pressure in a bone or joint as well as in relatively avascular tissues can impede or prevent antibiotics from reaching the primary site of infection.

B. An **acute infection of bone (hematogenous osteomyelitis)**, in its earliest phase, is a medical disease and can often be cured by prompt, appropriate antibiotic therapy. However, the time between initial infection and bone infarct is often short. If effective treatment is delayed and devascularization of the involved tissues results, then surgical treatment is a necessary adjunct to the antibiotic therapy. Even under the best of circumstances, late treatment (perhaps as early as 48 hours after the infection starts) may result in the loss or abnormal function of the joint. Thus, appropriate antibiotic therapy must be initiated as early as possible. Appropriate therapy requires knowledge of the etiologic agent and its sensitivities. Every effort should be made to obtain a bacterial culture and determine sensitivity. Once the culture specimen is obtained, it is important to institute antibiotic therapy based on a probable diagnosis using the most effective broad-spectrum antibiotics.

C. Diagnosis

1. The earliest symptom or sign that may help differentiate a bone or joint infection is usually **pain or localized tenderness in the periarticular region.** In the infant, refusal to move or use an extremity may be noted first. The cardinal signs of infection—redness, heat, and swelling—may appear later than the pain and tenderness, or not at all. When examining a child with a fever of unknown origin, note any pain or alteration of the normal range of motions of a joint and carefully palpate all metaphyseal areas to determine local tenderness. Roentgenograms are of little value in making the early diagnosis, although careful comparison with the opposite side may show abnormal soft-tissue shadows. Roentgenographic evidence of bone or joint destruction is seen during the chronic phase of the disease. Osteomyelitis should always be included in the differential diagnosis for a patient with the radiographic appearance of a bone tumor (2). Radioisotopic bone scanning, especially indium imaging, is helpful in early localization of bone infection (14). Many authorities have advocated the use of magnetic resonance imaging in the diagnosis of osteomyelitis (1,16,17,19), but we have found this technique not to be particularly useful because of the lack of specificity for the technology. Avoid overuse because of the expense involved. ESR and C-reactive protein serum levels are useful in laboratory evaluations (3,5,6,18).

2. **Identification of the infecting organism** is essential. In the early stages of the disease, particularly if there is a spiking temperature, blood cultures can often yield the organism. If acute metaphyseal tenderness is present, then the organism can frequently be obtained by inserting a needle into the site of maximum tenderness. A serrated biopsy needle is useful if subperiosteal pus is not encountered. If a joint is involved, then the

effusion should be aspirated before joint lavage. Processing the aspirates should include the following:

a. **Immediate Gram stain**
b. Inoculation of culture broth for aerobic and anaerobic **cultures**
c. **White blood cell count.** If thick, purulent material is encountered, then dilution in broth occasionally enhances the growth of organisms by decreasing the concentration of leukocytes and humeral antibacterial factors. This is done routinely in the microbiology laboratory.
d. Determination of the character of the hyaluronic precipitate, the presence of fibrin clots, and any disparity between the glucose in the aspirate and blood **glucose** may prove helpful, but the Gram stain, culture, and cell count are most valuable.

D. **Differential diagnosis. Care must be taken to differentiate soft-tissue infection, or cellulitis, from an infection occurring in a bone or joint.** This is a particularly important precaution when the infection overlies a joint, because any aspiration of a reactive sterile effusion by passing a needle through the soft-tissue infection may create a pyarthrosis. Tenderness and swelling from unrecognized trauma over a bone, particularly with some periosteal reaction, can present a confusing picture, but the absence of fever and systemic signs is helpful. Nonbacterial inflammatory arthritis, including viral and toxic synovitis and rheumatoid arthritis, must be included in a differential diagnosis, but until proved otherwise, think first of septic arthritis. Spontaneous hemorrhages in patients with hemophilia and fractures in paraplegic patients, particularly patients with meningomyelocele, are special situations that can confuse the picture.

E. **Bacterial considerations** (5,7,11)
1. **In acute hematogenous osteomyelitis,** *Staphylococcus aureus* is the most common etiologic agent in all age groups. In recent years, more than half the strains isolated have been found to be penicillin-resistant. In infants younger than 1 month, a diversity of other bacteria must also be considered. Group B streptococci and gram-negative organisms such as *Escherichia coli, Proteus* species, *Pseudomonas aeruginosa, Klebsiella pneumoniae,* and *Salmonella* species are all suspect. In infants with a complicated medical history, particularly those who have had prolonged indwelling venous catheters, extensive surgery, or intensive prior antibiotic therapy, coagulase-negative staphylococci and rarely anaerobic organisms such as *Bacteroides fragilis* and fungal agents such as *Candida albicans* (hard to diagnose) must also be considered.
2. In **septic arthritis and osteomyelitis** among infants younger than 1 month, *S. aureus* is the predominant etiologic agent. After the neonatal period and up to 4 years of age, *Haemophilus influenzae* is a major cause of septic arthritis, although *S. aureus* also is commonly found. In later childhood, the etiologic agents are the same as for adults, with *S. aureus* predominating. *Neisseria gonorrhoeae* must be seriously considered, particularly among adolescents with single (especially the knee joint) or multiple joint findings. If there has been a preceding infection or if there is a concurrent infection in another organ system, one may suspect that the etiologic agent is the same as that from the initiating focus. But, because this is not always the case, direct culture from the bone or joint infection is advised.

F. **Special considerations**
1. Infections of the intervertebral disks, or **acute diskitis,** may be encountered in children **without antecedent infection or surgery** (4). When organisms have been recovered, they have usually been staphylococcal. Infants may merely refuse to stand or walk, whereas older youngsters complain of pain in the back or lower extremity. The infection usually is low grade, particularly among children younger than 5 years of age. Roentgenograms reveal that the involved disc narrows rapidly over the first 2–3 weeks. A bone scan shows increased activity in the adjacent vertebrae. Although the process often appears self-limited, the symptoms

and course of the disease can be improved by plaster immobilization and antistaphylococcal antibiotics. The difficulty in obtaining a bacterial diagnosis, even with needle biopsy, combined with the benign course of this condition, has led many clinicians to ignore efforts at establishing a bacterial diagnosis. The condition must, however, be differentiated from vertebral osteomyelitis with secondary disc destruction; in the latter condition, it is essential to obtain the bacterial diagnosis as an integral part of treatment of what can be a severe disease. The same precaution applies to disc infections following laminectomy. In these cases, an infection should be suspected when a postsurgical patient complains of increasing back pain starting 1–2 weeks postoperatively.

2. Patients with **hemolytic disorders,** particularly those with sickle cell disease, are prone to development a subacute form of osteomyelitis. *Salmonella* infections are frequent, but other types of bacterial osteomyelitis are not uncommon (11). Because the diagnosis is usually made late, treatment is difficult and may require extensive surgical debridement and prolonged antibiotic therapy.

3. Another special problem is presented by the patient who sustains a **puncture wound** in the sole of the foot. Despite initial cleansing and occasional debridement, cellulitis, arthritis, or osteomyelitis involving the foot develops in many patients (3). This occurrence is most commonly caused by *P. aeruginosa.* Early surgical debridement of the infected including the plantar fascia, combined with preoperative and postoperative anti–*P. aeruginosa* antibiotics, has been the most effective method of management. For a serious infection, treatment is 5 days of antibiotic therapy with an aminoglycoside (e.g., tobramycin) or an antipseudomonal beta-lactam (e.g., ceftazidime) administered parenterally. Recently, ciprofloxacin has been used in gram-negative bone and joint infections (7); it must not be used in prepubertal children, however. Appropriate sensitivities guide antibiotic selection. Duration of therapy is empirical and may be guided by the clinical appearance and the CRP or ESR (3,4). Aminoglycoside doses need to be adjusted according to peak and trough serum levels and monitoring must include weekly Cr measurements and regular audiologist evaluation. Patients with human immunodeficiency virus or acquired immunodeficiency syndrome can have septic joints, which frequently may be missed because of the relatively weak immune response to the infectious agent. Joint aspiration should be performed in this setting (12).

G. **Requirements and characteristics of appropriate antibiotic treatment** (7,11,13)

1. For initial treatment of bone or joint infection, choose a **bactericidal antibiotic** effective against the suspected organism and a route of administration that ensures delivery of therapeutic levels to the infected site. The IV route is generally preferred for initial treatment (although some agents such as gentamicin and tobramycin are effective given IM). Recent studies (7) have indicated that oral antibiotics appear in therapeutic concentrations in bones and joints and, if given properly, can substitute for parenteral therapy in children. Most authorities, however, prefer the IV route.

2. The **duration of parenteral treatment** is 3–4 weeks for septic arthritis and 4–6 weeks for osteomyelitis (the longer duration for infections caused by *S. aureus).* **In adults** with selected organisms, the treatment may be completed using oral ciprofloxacin (Cipro) after the initial pain, swelling, and fever have resolved with IV antibiotics. This quinolone antibiotic has allowed oral therapy against a broad spectrum of bacteria including *Pseudomonas*(7). **In treating children** with osteomyelitis, treatment may be initiated with an IV agent such as nafcillin (Nafcil or Unipen), and the 4- to 6-week treatment course may be completed with oral dicloxacillin (Dynapen) or trimethoprim (Bactrim or Septra). **For all ages** the dosage of antibiotics (oral or parenteral) is at the

upper therapeutic level. When appropriate, adequate bactericidal drug levels for both oral as well as parenteral agents should be documented. Providing parenteral antibiotics through home health care teams greatly reduces the cost of treatment. The differentiation between a mild, well-localized infection and a localized bone tumor can sometimes require a surgical biopsy (2). The CRP or ESR is also a helpful guideline to determine the duration of treatment (3). A summary of antimicrobial agents commonly used in acute bone and joint infections is presented in Table 3-1. These agents are known to enter bone and joint sites readily when given in adequate doses. In general, bacteriostatic antibiotics should not be used in the treatment of infections of bones and joints where bactericidal antibiotics are available.

3. In an acute infection in which the organism is not immediately identified, the **choice of therapy** is determined by the organisms most commonly expected in the various age groups, along with the other factors previously listed. General guidelines are presented in Table 3-2.

4. **A local instillation or continuous irrigation with an antibiotic solution is almost never indicated.** Systemic antibiotics, properly administered, achieve adequate levels in viable tissues (7,11). In many posttraumatic conditions, delivery of local antibiotic in methylmethacrylate beads is worthwhile (13). This treatment is indicated especially when a delayed bone graft or soft-tissue muscle flap is planned. Some favorable reports have been published about an implantable pump with a reservoir for antibiotic (generally amikacin).

5. Continue antibiotics until the infection has been eliminated. A normal or declining ESR or CRP is one of the most helpful **laboratory tests** to indicate control of infection.

H. **Adjunctive treatment.** Most orthopaedists believe that the healing process is aided by **immobilizing** the infected area. There is disagreement over casting or splinting. Undoubtedly, however, patients are more comfortable when the infected area is immobilized. If damage to the bone is significant, cast immobilization may be important to prevent a pathologic fracture. If damage to articular cartilage is suspected, motion of the involved joint is recommended after a brief 1- to 2-day period of immobilization.

I. **Surgical intervention.** Appropriate antibiotic treatment instituted within the first 48 hours of acute osteomyelitis or septic arthritis is usually satisfactory. However, early diagnosis is rarely the case. **If treatment is initiated over 48 hours after onset, it is important to determine whether medical treatment alone is adequate.** Err on the side of more aggressive operative drainage. If the patient has been on an appropriate antibiotic for more than 24 hours without significant resolution of pain and temperature, then surgical intervention is indicated.

1. In a **bone infection,** metaphyseal or subperiosteal abscesses must be drained. If metaphyseal point tenderness is present, and there is doubt whether this represents significant metaphyseal or subperiosteal pus, then it is safer to err on the side of a small surgical exploration or aspiration with a biopsy needle. If pus is encountered, then open surgical drainage is indicated.

2. **Joints**
   a. In joint infections, satisfactory evacuation of pus can be achieved by **needle aspiration.** When the joint is easily visible and palpable, such as with the knee joint, repeated needle aspiration is usually adequate to keep the joint decompressed. Aspiration should be done with a 16- to 18-gauge needle. Irrigation of the joint to ensure removal of as much cellular debris as possible is helpful (5). The hip joint presents special problems (5). The blood supply to the femoral head is intraarticular; hence, any increase in pressure can deprive the entire femoral head of its circulation. Because hip joint effusions
   (*text continues on page 37*)

Table 3-1. Antimicrobial agents commonly used initially in acute bone and joint infections

Antibiotic	Usual susceptible organisms	Daily dosage (IV route)	Comment
Cefazolin (cephalosporins)	Penicillinase-producing *Staphylococcus aureus*; will also treat streptococci, pneumococci, non–penicillinase-producing staphylococci, and *Klebsiella pneumoniae*	0–7 d: 40 mg/kg divided doses q12h Infant: 60 mg/kg divided doses q8h Child: 80 mg/kg divided doses q6h Adult: 2–6 g divided doses q6h	A drug of choice; IV route preferred, but may be given IM. Adjust adult dosage according to blood urea nitrogen or, preferably, the creatinine clearance
Nafcillin	Same as cefazolin	0–7 d: 50 mg/kg divided doses q12h[a] 7 d–6 wk: 75 mg/kg divided doses q8h 6 wk–3 y: 80 mg/kg divided doses q6h Child: 150 mg/kg divided doses q6h Adult: 3–6 g divided doses q6h	A drug of choice
Methicillin	Same as cefazolin and nafcillin	No longer commonly used; too many problems	Monitor patients for proteinuria: drug has occasionally been implicated in adverse renal side effects
Clindamycin	*S. aureus*, pneumococci, streptococci (not enterococci), and many *Bacteroides fragilis* strains	Pediatric: 10–20 mg/kg PO or IV or IM in 3–4 doses Adult: 600 mg q6–8h	Considered an excellent agent for *B. fragilis* infections
Penicillin G (aqueous)	Streptococci (not enterococci), pneumococci, gonococci, and penicillin-susceptible staphylococci	0–7 d: 50,000 unit/kg divided dose q12h >7 d: 75,000–100,000 unit/kg IV or IM divided doses q8h 12 y–adult: 12–20 million units q6–8h	Useful for open fractures contaminated with barnyard waste and for treatment of clostridia infection
Ampicillin	Same as penicillin G; also *Haemophilus influenzae*, some strains of *Escherichia coli*, *Proteus*, and *Salmonella*	0–7 d: 50 mg/kg divided doses q12h 7 d–6 wk: 75 mg/kg divided doses q8h Infant: 100 mg/kg divided doses q6h Child: 150 mg/kg divided doses q6h 12 yr–adult: 8–12 g	*H. influenzae* now shows a 10%–20% ampicillin resistance in some areas. Empiric therapy must therefore be with ceftriaxone or cefuroxime

Drug	Indication	Dosage	Comments
Ceftriaxone	Select gram-negative organisms or mixed infections	0–12 yr: 50 mg/kg once daily 12 yr–adult: 2 g q24h	Generally reserved for resistant or mixed infections
Cefuroxime	Select gram-negative organisms or mixed infections	>3 mo–12 yr: 75 mg/kg divided doses q8h	Generally reserved for resistant or mixed infections
Ceftazidime	Select gram-negative organisms including *Pseudomonas* or mixed infections	12 yr–adult: 1.5 g q8h <12 yr not indicated 12 yr–adult: 1 g q8–12h	Same as cefuroxime
Gentamicin	Gram-negative infections	<12 yr: 6–7.5 mg/kg in three equal doses 12 yr–adult: 3–5 mg/kg in three equal doses (dose adjusted based on peak and trough levels)	Agent of choice for suspected gram-negative infections May be given either IV or IM. Renal function must be carefully checked, and therapy beyond 10 days must be administered cautiously because of potential nephrotoxicity and ototoxicity. May be synergistic with carbenicillin against some strains of *Pseudomonas aeruginosa*; also usually synergistic with penicillin against enterococci. Reduce dosage to 3 mg/kg/day as soon as clinically indicated. Follow with peak and trough serum levels if available
Tobramycin and mezlocillin	Same as gentamicin	0–7 d: 150 mg/kg IM or IV divided doses q12h >7 d, <2,000 g birth weight: 225 mg/kg divided doses q8h Child: 300 mg/kg IM or IV divided doses q6h Adult: 3 g q4h	Same as gentamicin Agent now used in place of carbenicillin

ᵃ Some authorities recommend that nafcillin not be used in 0 to 7-day-old infants because of poor pharmacokinetics.
Modified from Hansen BM, ed. Antimicrobial therapy, 3rd ed. Philadelphia: WB Saunders, 1980.

Table 3-2. Tentative selection of therapy when organisms are
not immediately identified

Situation	Organisms suspected	Suggested antibiotic choice
Newborn (1 mo)		
Osteomyelitis	*Staphylococcus aureus* Streptococci Gram-negative bacteria including *Escherichia coli*, *Klebsiella pneumoniae*, *Proteus* group, *Pseudomonas aeruginosa*	Nafcillin plus gentamicin or tobramycin
Septic arthritis	*S. aureus*	
1 mo–4 yr		
Osteomyelitis	*S. aureus*	Second-generation cephalosporin to cover *H. influenzae*
Septic arthritis	*Haemophilus influenzae* *S. aureus* Streptococci	Second-generation cephalosporin to cover *H. influenzae*
4 yr–12 yr		
Osteomyelitis Septic arthritis	*S. aureus*	First- or second-generation cephalosporin
12 yr–adult		
Osteomyelitis	*S. aureus*	A cephalosporin (first- or second-generation agent) or nafcillin
Septic arthritis	*S. aureus*	A cephalosporin or nafcillin (ceftriaxone if gonococcus is strongly suspected)
Special considerations Chronic hemolytic disorders Osteoarthritis Septic arthritis	*S. aureus* Pneumococci *Salmonella* group[a]	A cephalosporin (second-generation if salmonella is suspected) or nafcillin until sensitivity results are available
Infections following puncture wounds of the foot	*Pseudomonas aeruginosa*	Ceftazidime actually achieves better drug levels than aminoglycosides (gentamicin or tobramycin)
Infections following trauma or surgery	*S. aureus* Streptococci Gram-negative organisms	A first- or second-generation cephalosporin (or nafcillin) plus gentamicin or tobramycin

[a] Infections caused by *Salmonella* should be documented first by culture and sensitivity testing before empirical treatment with agents such as ampicillin (or chloramphenicol) is initiated.
Modified from Hansen ST Jr, Ray CG. Antibiotics in orthopaedics. In: Kagan BM, ed. *Antimicrobial therapy*, 3rd ed. Philadelphia: WB Saunders, 1980.

are not readily palpable, it is difficult to be certain that repeated aspirations decompress the joint. For this reason, most authorities believe that immediate surgical drainage of a septic hip is indicated, and some believe that the shoulder should be treated similarly. The possible exception is in gonococcal arthritis (15). The hip joint can be drained anteriorly between muscle planes or posteriorly with a muscle-splitting incision. The capsule and synovium are opened and drains inserted.

   b. At times, the fibrin entering the joint as a transudate forms clots and isolates segments of the joint from decompression. Hypertrophy of synovium and adhesions may also affect the ability of the surgeon to decompress the joint adequately. Under these circumstances, **it is advisable to debride the joint arthroscopically or with an open procedure.** Joints amenable to arthroscopic lavage are the knee, shoulder, and ankle.

J. **Chronic osteomyelitis** presents a different problem from acute infection. Acute infection in the earliest phase is primarily a medical disease, with surgical techniques used as an adjunct. In chronic infection, the primary problem is **surgical removal** of all dead and poorly vascularized tissue. If this removal is properly done under appropriate antibiotic therapy, it is possible to eradicate most sites of chronic osteomyelitis. The operation must be carefully planned, because it often involves significant removal of bone and surrounding tissues. In the case of chronic joint infections, it may mean complete resection of the joint with the creation of a pseudarthrosis or an arthrodesis. Rotational muscle flaps or free-tissue transfer may be required to cover areas of viable but poorly covered bone. Intravenous and oral antibiotics serve as valuable adjuncts. Patient quality of life can be profoundly impacted by chronic osteomyelitis (10); treatment leading to resolution of the infection does improve this impact.

K. **Gas gangrene**
   1. Gas gangrene can be a fatal process. **Prevention** can be achieved by thorough debridement and removal of all devitalized tissue, delayed wound closure when in doubt, and antibiotic treatment as recommended previously.
   2. *Clostridium perfringens* infections carry a 65% overall mortality rate, which increases to 75% in infants and elderly patients. The **diagnosis** should be suspected when the patient is pale, weak, perspiring, and more tachycardiac than the degree of fever warrants. The patient frequently complains of severe pain. Mental confusion and gas in the tissues are late signs, as are the characteristic mousy odor, jaundice, oliguria, and shock.
   3. Other gas-producing species in addition to *C. perfringens* (ten isolated toxins), include *E. coli, Enterobacter aerogenes,* anaerobic streptococci, *B. fragilis,* and *K. pneumoniae.* Antitoxin does not appear to help much, because it is neutralized as rapidly as it reaches muscle. **Treatment** consists of debridement and high doses of antibiotics. Penicillin is usually the best for the *C. perfringens* group; it should be given in amounts of 20–50 million units/day. Clindamycin metronidazole is a good alternative antibiotic in patients who are allergic to penicillin. Some clostridia are resistant to clindamycin, making it necessary to check sensitivities carefully. Hyperbaric oxygen is only an adjunct to surgery. Its use allows the surgeon to save more tissue than might otherwise be possible, and it does lower the mortality rate slightly. Streptococcal group A myonecrosis can have a similar course and results in death in a high percentage of cases. It must be treated with aggressive surgical debridement or amputation in addition to appropriate antibiotic therapy. Toxic shock syndrome has also been noted in orthopaedic patients and is caused by unique staphylococcal strains with unusual phage types. Toxic shock syndrome is also a surgical condition, but it carries a more favorable prognosis. Necrotizing fasciitis can be caused by several bacterial types

and often represents a debridement as well combined with appropriate antibiotic therapy. Infectious disease consultation is indicated for each of these infectious conditions.

III. **Summary**

A. Infections in the musculoskeletal system present special problems for treatment with antibiotics alone. Cartilage is avascular, tendon and ligaments are relatively hypovascular, and bone is vulnerable to situations that render it avascular. Because antibiotics can be effective only if they are delivered to the site of infection, every effort must be made to preserve a normal blood supply and normal joint fluid dynamics. The **essentials of treatment** are as follows:

1. **Prompt diagnosis,** with identification of the bacteria through culture and with sensitivity for determining the appropriate antibiotic
2. **Rapid initial treatment** with the most effective bactericidal antibiotic
3. **Constant evaluation** to assess the need for surgical drainage of pus or removal of devitalized tissue
4. **Antibiotic therapy** by a route that ensures adequate blood levels and administration until the signs of infection as manifested usually by a decreasing ESR resolve completely
5. **Judicious use of immobilization and traction** to improve patient comfort and provide the best possible environment for primary healing

B. The greatest benefit of antibiotics in musculoskeletal infection is in **preventing** the mortality and morbidity that result from chronic osteomyelitis and joint destruction from pyarthrosis. Even chronic infection can be controlled and a satisfactory functional result obtained in most patients by the use of surgery and appropriate antibiotics.

References

1. Boutin RD, Brossman J, Sartoris DJ, et al. Update on imaging of orthopedic infections. *Orthop Clin North Am* 1998;29:41–66.
2. Cottias P, Tomeno B, Anract P, et al. Subacute osteomyelitis presenting as a bone tumor: a review of 21 cases. *Int Orthop* 1997;21:243–248.
3. Crosby LA, Powell DA. The potential value of the sedimentation rate in monitoring treatment outcome in puncture wound-related *Pseudomonas* osteomyelitis. *Clin Orthop* 1984;188:168.
4. Cushing AH. Diskitis in children. *Clin Infect Dis* 1995;17:1–6.
5. Dagan R. Management of acute hematogenous osteomyelitis and septic arthritis in the pediatric patient. *Pediatri Infect Dis J* 1993;12:88–92.
6. Frederiksen B, Chritiansen P, Knudsen FU. Acute osteomyelitis and septic arthritis in the neonate, risk factors and outcome. *Eur J Pediatri* 1993;152:577–580.
7. Greenberg S, et al. Treatment of bone, joint, and soft-tissue infections with oral ciprofloxacin. *Antimicrob Agents Chemother* 1987;31:151.
8. Hendershot EF. Fluoroquinolones. *Infect Dis Clin North Am* 1995;9:715–730.
9. Henry SL, Galloway KP. Local antibacterial therapy for the management of orthopaedic infections: pharmacokinetic considerations. *Clin Pharmacokinet*, 1995;29:36–45.
10. Lerner RK, Esterhai JL Jr, Polomano RC, et al. Quality of life assessment of patients with posttraumatic fracture nonunion, chronic refractory osteomyelitis and lower extremity amputation. *Clin Orthop* 1993;295:28–36.
11. Mader JT, Landon GC, Calhoun J: Antimicrobial treatment of osteomyelitis. *Clin Orthop* 1993;295:87–95.
12. Malin JK, Patel NJ. Arthropathy and HIV infection: a muddle of mimicry. *Postgrad Med* 1993;93:143–150.
13. Ostermann PA, Seligson D, Henry SL. Local antibiotic therapy for severe open fractures: a review of 1085 consecutive cases. *J Bone Joint Surg (Br)* 1995;77:93–97.
14. Schauwecker DS. The scintigraphic diagnosis of osteomyelitis. *AJR Am J Roentgenol* 1992;158:9–18.
15. Scopelitis E, Martinez-Osuna P. Gonococcal arthritis. *Rheum Dis Clin North Am* 1993;19:363–377.

16. Tang JSH, et al. Musculoskeletal infection of the extremities: evaluation with MR imaging. *Radiology* 1988;166:205.
17. Tehranzadeh J, Wang F, Mesgarazadeh M. Magnetic resonance imaging of osteomyelitis. *Crit Rev Diagn Imaging* 1992;33:495–534.
18. Unkila-Kallio L, Kallio MJ, Eskola J, et al. Serum C-reactive protein, erythrocyte sedimentation rate and white blood cell count in acute hematogenous osteomyelitis of children. *Pediatrics* 1994;93:59–62.
19. Unger E, et al. Diagnosis of osteomyelitis by MR imaging. *AJR Am J Roentgenol* 1988;150:605.

Selected Historical Readings
Burnett JW, et al. Prophylactic antibiotics in hip fractures. *J Bone Joint Surg (Am)* 1980;62:457.
Clawson DK, Davis FJ, Hansen ST Jr. Treatment of chronic osteomyelitis with emphasis on closed suction-irrigation technique. *Clin Orthop* 1973;96:88.
Ha'eri GB, Wiley AM. The efficacy of standard surgical face masks: an investigation using "tracer particles." *Clin Orthop* 1979;141:237.
Hamilton HW, et al. Penetration of gown material by organisms from the surgical team. *Clin Orthop* 1979;141:237.
Lunseth PA, Heiple KG. Prognosis in septic arthritis of the hip in children. *Clin Orthop* 1979;129:81.
Monson TP, Nelson CL. Microbiology for orthopaedic surgeons: selected aspects. *Clin Orthop* 1984;190:14.
Patzakis MJ, Harvey P Jr, Ivler D. The role of antibiotics in the management of open fractures. *J Bone Joint Surg (Am)* 1974;56:532.
Perry CR, et al. Antibiotics delivered by an implantable drug pump: a new application for treating osteomyelitis. *Am J Med* 1986;80[Suppl]:222.
Peterson AF, Rosenberg A, Alatary SD. Comparative evaluations of surgical scrub preparations. *Surg Gynecol Obstet* 1978;146:63.
Schurman DJ, Hirshman HP, Nagel DA. Antibiotic penetration of synovial fluid in infected and normal knee joints. *Clin Orthop* 1978;136:304.

4. ACUTE NONTRAUMATIC JOINT CONDITIONS

I. **History.** Document the onset of the symptoms: Did the joint pain begin days, weeks, or months ago? Morning stiffness is important to differentiate inflammatory forms of arthritis (rheumatoid arthritis and ankylosing spondylitis) from noninflammatory forms (degenerative joint disease). The character and duration of the pain are more important. Is the pain only associated with activity or is it present even at rest? Is only one joint involved or are multiple joints affected? Are they symmetrically involved? In the hands, the proximal finger joints are often involved with rheumatoid arthritis and the distal finger joints are more often involved in osteoarthritis (1) (Table 4-1).

II. **Examination.** Check for fever because the temperature may be elevated with septic arthritis. Muscle wasting occurs more often with rheumatoid arthritis. Tenderness about the joint and increased warmth are more indicative of inflammatory conditions. The examination should determine the presence of an effusion. Severe guarding of joint motion associated with pain usually is indicative of a septic condition (Table 4-1).

III. **Roentgenographic and laboratory data**
   A. **Roentgenographic findings.** Look for evidence of periarticular soft-tissue swelling, joint effusion, osteopenia, joint space narrowing, periarticular erosions, joint subluxation, and articular cartilage or bone destruction (1). All of these findings are evidence of inflammatory (rheumatoid or septic) arthritis. In contrast, marginal osteophytes, subchondral cysts, joint space narrowing, and sclerosis are associated with osteoarthritis (Table 4-2). In the lower extremity, weight bearing radiographs increase the diagnostic value of the study.
   B. **Laboratory data** (Table 4-3)
      1. **Synovial fluid analysis involves assessing the following:**
         a. **Appearance (color)**
         b. **Clot (presence or absence)**
         c. **Viscosity**
         d. **Glucose** (compare with simultaneous serum glucose)
         e. **Cell count per cubic millimeter**
         f. **Differential cell count**
         g. The type of **crystals** that might be present in the joint fluid aspirate as evaluated under a polarizing light microscope
         h. **Gram stain and synovial fluid culture**: aerobic, fungal, Acid Fast Baccilus (AFB)
      2. Helpful **blood tests** include a complete blood count, erythrocyte sedimentation rate (ESR), C-reactive protein (CRP), uric acid, rheumatoid factor, and antinuclear antibody.

IV. **Differential diagnosis of acute nontraumatic joint conditions** (Table 4-4) (1,10,12)
   A. **Rheumatoid arthritis** (Table 4-5)
      1. **History** often reveals symmetric joint and tendon involvement, typically in a younger female patient (7).
      2. **Examination** shows synovial thickening, joint tenderness, subcutaneous nodules, weakness associated with muscle wasting, and, often, systemic disease.
      3. **Roentgenograms and laboratory data show that erosions are usually present but rheumatoid factor is present in only 75% of patients.** Roentgenograms are often normal in acute forms of rheumatoid arthritis except for signs of swelling or periarticular osteopenia. Joint fluid contains 2,000–50,000 WBC/mm³, approximately 40%–80% of which are polymorphonuclear leukocytes.
   B. **Septic arthritis**
      1. **Bacterial**
         a. The **history** may indicate drug or alcohol abuse, systemic illness (e.g., diabetes, chronic renal failure, or poor nutrition).

(text continues on page 45)

Table 4-1. History and examination

History	Rheumatoid arthritis	Septic arthritis	Degenerative joint disease
Onset	Weeks	Day(s)	Months
Morning stiffness	+ +		–
Pain duration	Hours	Constant	Minutes
Pain with activity	+ +	+ + +	±
Number of joints involved	Multiple, symmetric	One (occasionally more)	Variable
Finger joint	Proximal		Distal
Examination			
Febrile	±	+ +	0
Muscle wasting	+ +	0	+
Synovial tenderness	+	+ +	±
Increased warmth	±	+ +	0
Effusion	+	+ +	±
Joint range of motion	↓	↓ ↓ ↓	↓

+ + +, extremely important symptom or sign; + +, very important symptom or sign; +, important symptom or sign; ±, symptom or sign might or might not be present; 0, symptom or sign is not present; ↓, decreased; ↓ ↓ ↓, markedly decreased.

Table 4-2. Roentgenographic findings

Rheumatoid arthritis	Septic arthritis	Degenerative joint disease
Early		
Periarticular soft-tissue swelling	Joint effusion	Joint space narrowing
Periarticular osteoporosis		Marginal osteophytes
Late		
Joint space narrowing	Articular cartilage and bone destruction	Subchondral sclerosis
Periarticular erosions		Subcortical cysts
Articular cartilage and bone destruction		Marginal osteophytes
Joint subluxation secondary to ligamentous involvement		

Table 4-3. Synovial fluid analysis

Finding	Normal	Rheumatoid arthritis	Septic arthritis	Degenerative joint disease
Appearance	Clear	Cloudy	Turbid	Clear
Clinical viscosity test	High (fluid remains intact when slowly pulled between thumb and index finger)	Watery (fluid breaks into droplets easily)	Very watery	High
Glucose	Within 60% or more of serum glucose	Low	Very low	Normal
Cell count/mm³	200	2,000–50,000	Usually > 50,000	2,000
Differential cell count	Monos	50/50	Polys	Monos

Table 4-4. Differential diagnosis of inflammatory polyarthritis

A. **Rheumatoid arthritis (RA)**
   1. Seropositive—female, symmetric joint and tendon involvement, synovial
      thickening, joint inflammation in phase, nodules, weakness, systemic
      reaction, erosions on radiogram, rheumatoid factor present, $C'H_{50}$ level
      depressed in joint fluid that has 5,000–30,000 WBC/mm^3, approximately
      50%–80% polymorphs.
   2. Seronegative—either sex, symmetric joint and tendon involvement, joint
      inflammation in phase, little or no systemic reaction, usually no erosions
      radiographically, rheumatoid factor absent, $C'H_{50}$ not depressed in joint fluid
      that has 3,000–20,000 WBC/mm^3, approximately 20%–60% polymorphs.
B. **Collagen-vascular**
   1. Systemic lupus erythematosus—female, symmetric joint distribution identical
      to RA, hair loss, mucosal lesions, rash, systemic reaction, visceral organ or
      brain involvement, leukopenia, (false-) positive serologic test for syphilis, no
      erosions radiographically, noninflammatory joint fluid with good viscosity and
      mucin clot and 1,000–2,000 WBC/mm^3, mostly small lymphocytes. Serum
      $C'H_{50}$ often depressed, antinuclear antibody (ANA) titer elevated, anti–native-
      human DNA antibody titer increased.
   2. Scleroderma–tight skin, Raynaud's phenomenon, resorption of digits,
      dysphagia, constipation, lung, heart, or kidney involvement, symmetric
      tendon contractures, little or no synovial thickening, radiographic calcinosis
      circumscripta, positive ANA with speckled or nucleolar pattern.
   3. Polymyositis (dermatomyositis)—proximal muscle weakness, pelvic and
      pectoral girdles, tender muscles, skin changes, typical nail and knuckle pad
      erythema, symmetric joint involvement, electromyographic evidence of
      combined myopathic and denervation pattern, muscle biopsy abnormal,
      elevated creatine phosphokinase.
   4. Mixed connective tissue disease—swollen hands, Raynaud's phenomenon,
      tight skin, symmetric joint and tendon involvement, may be joint erosions
      radiographically, positive ANA speckled pattern, antiribonucleoprotein
      antibody increased, good response to corticosteroid therapy given in
      antiinflammatory doses.
   5. Polyarteritis nodosa—symmetric involvement, diverse clinical picture of
      systemic disease, histologic diagnosis.
C. **Rheumatic fever**
   Young (2–40 yr), sore throat, group A streptococci, migratory arthritis, rash,
   heart or pericardial involvement, elevated antistreptolysin O titers. Migratory
   joint inflammation responds dramatically to aspirin treatment.
D. **Juvenile rheumatoid arthritis**
   Symmetric joint involvement, rash, fever, no rheumatoid factor, radiographic
   periostitis, erosions late, can begin or recur in adult.
E. **Psoriatic arthritis**
   Asymmetric boggy joint and tendon swelling, skin or nail lesions may not be
   prominent or may follow arthritis, distal interphalangeal joints might be
   prominently involved, radiologic periostitis or erosions, no rheumatoid factor.
   $C'H_{50}$ usually not depressed in inflammatory joint fluid with polymorph
   predominance.
F. **Reiter's syndrome**
   Male, urethritis, iritis, conjunctivitis, asymmetric joints, lower extremity,
   nonpainful mucous membrane ulcerative lesion, balanitis circinata, keratosis
   blennorrhagica, weight loss. $C'H_{50}$ increased in serum and in joint fluid with
   5,000–30,000 leukocytes/mm^3. Macrophages in joint fluid with 3–5
   phagocytosed polymorphs (Reiter's cell).
G. **Gonorrheal arthritis**
   Migratory arthritis or tenosynovitis fully settling in one or more joints or
   tendons, either sex, primary focus urethra, female genitourinary tract, rectum,

(continued)

Table 4-4. (*continued*)

or oropharynx, skin lesions, vesicles, gram-negative diplococci on smear but not on culture of vesicular fluid, positive culture at primary site, blood, or joint fluid.
H. **Polymyalgia rheumatica**
  Elderly patient (>50 yr), symmetric pelvic or pectoral girdle complaints without loss of strength, morning stiffness of long duration, fatigue prominent, weight loss, joints can be involved, especially shoulders, sternoclavicular joints, knees, sedimentation rate markedly elevated, fibrinogen always elevated, alpha 2 and gamma globulin elevation, anemia, response to low-dose (10–20 mg) prednisone, serum creatine phosphokinase normal, elevated alkaline phosphatase (liver).
I. **Crystal-induced**
  1. Gout—symmetric arthritis, flexion contractures, prior history of acute attacks, tophi, joint inflammation out of phase, systemic corticosteroid treatment for RA, hyperuricemia, monosodium urate monohydrate crystals in joint fluid.
  2. Pseudogout—symmetric arthritis, flexion contractures, metacarpophalangeal, wrist, elbow, shoulder, hips, knees, and ankles, prior acute attacks (sometimes), joint inflammation out of phase, calcium pyrophosphate dihydrate crystals in joint fluid.
J. **Other**
  Amyloid arthropathy, peripheral arthritis of inflammatory bowel disease, tuberculosis, subacute bacterial endocarditis, viral arthritis.

Modified from McCarty DJ. Differential diagnosis of arthritis: analysis of signs and symptoms. In: McCarty, DJ, ed. *Arthritis and allied conditions*, 10th ed. Philadelphia: Lea & Febiger, 1985:51–52.

Table 4-5. Rheumatoid arthritis diagnostic criteria

1. Morning stiffness
2. Pain on motion or tenderness in at least one joint[a]
3. Swelling (soft tissue thickening or fluid, not bony overgrowth alone) in at least one joint[a]
4. Swelling of at least one other joint[a,b]
5. Symmetric joint swelling with simultaneous involvement of the same joint on both sides of the body[a,b]; terminal phalangeal joint involvement will not satisfy the criterion
6. Subcutaneous nodules over bony prominences, on extensor surfaces, or in juxtaarticular regions[a]
7. Roentgenographic changes typical of rheumatoid arthritis (which must include at least bony decalcification localized to or greatest around the involved joints and not just degenerative changes[b]
8. Positive tests for rheumatoid factor in serum[b]
9. Poor mucin precipitate from synovial fluid (with shreds and cloudy solution)
10. Characteristic histologic changes in synovial membrane[b]
11. Characteristic histologic changes in nodules[b]

Categories	Number of criteria required	Minimum duration of continuous symptoms	Exclusions[c]
Classic	7 of 11	6 wk (Nos. 1–5)	Any of listed
Definite	5 of 11	6 wk (Nos. 1–5)	Any of listed
Probable	3 of 11	6 wk (one of Nos. 1–5)	Any of listed

[a] Observed by a physician.
[b] Refer to original reference for further specifications.
[c] Refer to original reference for listing of exclusions.
From Medsger TA Jr, Masi AT. Epidemiology of the rheumatic diseases. In: McCarty DJ, ed. *Arthritis and allied conditions*, 10th ed. Philadelphia: Lea & Febiger, 1985:11.

b. Examination reveals severe inflammation and often a primary septic focus. Severe splinting (autoprotection by muscle spasm) of the joint is present and pain is associated with passive motion.

c. Laboratory tests show a purulent joint fluid with polymorphonuclear leukocytes predominating (WBC: 50,000–300,000/mm³). The infectious agent may be identified on smear or culture. Synovial glucose is less than 60% of a concurrent serum glucose. The ESR and CRP are elevated. Serial blood cultures obtained before antibiotic therapy often grow the infecting organism.

2. **Tubercular and fungal**

a. History may reveal a primary focus, chronic immunodeficiency (human immunodeficiency virus [HIV] or acquired immunodeficiency syndrome), drug or alcohol abuse, or poor nutrition.

b. Examination shows marked chronic joint swelling.

c. Laboratory tests reveal predominating polymorphonuclear leukocytes with acid-fast organisms present on smear and culture.

3. **Viral**

a. History often indicates antecedent or concomitant systemic viral illness.

b. Laboratory analysis of joint fluid can mimic inflammatory or noninflammatory conditions. Either mononuclear or polymorphonuclear leukocytes can predominate.

C. Osteoarthritis (nonerosive degenerative joint disease)

1. **History** reveals a middle-aged or elderly patient unless the condition follows trauma.

2. **Examination** angulatory deformities and osteophytes are frequently present in the later stages of disease (1,11,13).

3. **Roentgenograms** show narrowing of the cartilage space associated with marginal osteophytes. There is often subchondral bone sclerosis and occasionally subchondral cysts, which accompany these findings in the weight-bearing joints.

D. Crystal-induced arthritis (Table 4-6) (11)

1. **Gouty arthritis**

a. The patient complains of a **history** of acute attacks.

b. Examination can show symmetric arthritis with contractures and tophi (subcutaneous crystal deposits) in later stages. The first metatarsal-phalangeal joint is commonly affected.

c. Laboratory findings include hyperuricemia and synovial fluid containing monosodium urate monohydrate crystals. The crystals, which are seen by compensated polarized light microscopy (sometimes by ordinary light microscopy), are negatively birefringent, needle-shaped rods.

2. **Pseudogout**

a. History sometimes reveals previous acute attacks.

b. Examination discloses a symmetric arthritis with frequent contractures of the metacarpophalangeal, wrist, elbow, shoulder, hip, knee, and ankle joints. Roentgenograms may reveal the presence of calcium deposits in cartilage or, less often, in ligaments, meniscus, and joint capsule (chondrocalcinosis). The knee is the most common site. Chondrocalcinosis has been classically associated with pseudogout, but this condition is also seen with a high frequency in hyperparathyroidism, hemochromatosis, hemosiderosis, hypophosphatasia, hypomagnesemia, hypothyroidism, gout, neuropathic joints, and aging (1,11,13).

c. Laboratory analysis of the synovial fluid reveals calcium pyrophosphate dihydrate crystals that are regularly shaped and weakly positively birefringent, but have a different extinction angle compared to that of urate crystals (13).

E. Inflammatory polyarthritis other than rheumatoid arthritis (Table 4-4)

Table 4-6. Differential diagnosis of inflammatory monarthritis

A. **Crystal-induced**
   1. **Gout**—male, lower extremity, previous attack, nocturnal onset, precipitated by medical illness or surgery, response to colchicine, hyperuricemia, sodium urate crystals in joint fluid with polymorphs predominating, and WBC 10,000–60,000/mm³.
   2. **Pseudogout**—elderly, knee or other large joint, previous attack, precipitated by medical illness or surgery, flexion contractures, chondrocalcinosis on radiography, calcium pyrophosphate dihydrate crystals in joint fluid with polymorphs predominating, and WBC 5,000–60,000/mm³.
   3. **Calcific tendonitis or equivalent**—extraarticular, tendon or capsule of larger joints, previous attack same or other area, calcification on radiography, chalky or milky material aspirated from area, polymorphs with phagocytosed ovoid bodies microscopically.
B. **Palindromic rheumatism**
   Middle-aged or elderly male, very sudden onset, little systemic reaction, previous attacks, positive rheumatoid factors, little or no residual chronic joint inflammation, olecranon bursal enlargement.
C. **Infectious arthritis**
   1. **Septic**—severe inflammation, primary septic focus, drug or alcohol abuse, joint fluid with polymorphs predominating, WBC 50,000–300,000/mm³ (pus), infectious agents identified on smear and culture, or bacterial antigens identified in joint fluid.
   2. **Tubercular**—primary focus, drug or alcohol abuse, marked joint swelling for long period, joint fluid with polymorphs predominating, acid-fast organisms on smear and culture.
   3. **Fungal**—similar to tuberculosis.
   4. **Viral**—antecedent or concomitant systemic viral illness, joint fluid can be of inflammatory or noninflammatory type, either mononuclear or polymorphonuclear leukocytes may predominate.
D. **Other**
   1. **Tendonitis**—as in A.3 but without radiologic calcification, antecedent trauma, including repetitive motion.
   2. **Bursitis**—as above, but inflamed area more diffuse, antecedent trauma.
   3. **Juvenile rheumatoid arthritis**—one or both knees swollen in preteenager or teenager without systemic reaction, no erosions, mildly inflammatory joint fluid with some polymorphs, and no depression in synovial fluid $C'H_{50}$ levels.

From McCarty DJ. Differential diagnosis of arthritis: analysis of symptoms. In: McCarty DJ, ed. *Arthritis and allied conditions*, 10th ed. Philadelphia: Lea & Febiger, 1985:50.

   1. **Reiter's syndrome**
      a. **History** often reveals a sexually active man with weight loss. Patients have an equivocal response to antiinflammatory drugs. History of antecedent infectious diarrhea or urethritis should be sought.
      b. **Examination** often reveals urethritis, iritis, conjunctivitis, and nonpainful mucous membrane ulcerative lesions, with asymmetric arthritis of the joints in the lower extremities or back. Roentgenograms may show an asymmetric sacroiliitis as well as isolated involvement of the spine ("skip" areas). Heel pain can be a common associated feature of the presentation.
      c. **Laboratory data.** The joint fluid has 5,000–30,000 leukocytes/mm³ with macrophages that contain three to five phagocytosed polymorphonuclear leukocytes (so-called Reiter's cell). Measurement of HLA-B27 antigen is not very useful.

2. **Psoriatic arthritis**
   a. **Examination** shows asymmetric boggy joint and tendon sheath swelling. Skin or nail (pitting) lesions may or may not be prominent. The distal interphalangeal (DIP) joints of the hand frequently are involved (1,11).
   b. **Roentgenographic** periostitis, cortical erosions, or both can be seen along with spinal asymmetric sacroiliitis and isolated vertebral ankylosis (skip areas). The "pencil-in-cup" deformity is typically seen in the DIP joints of the hand. No rheumatoid factor is found. There is polymorphonuclear leukocytic predominance in the joint field.
3. **Systemic lupus erythematosus (SLE)**
   a. **History** reveals symmetric joint distribution identical to rheumatoid arthritis in a female patient. Hair loss and Raynaud's symptoms (vasospasm of digital arteries are common.
   b. **Examination** discloses rash (facial erythema), mucosal lesions, serositis, renal or brain involvement, and a systemic reaction.
   c. **Laboratory evaluation** shows leukopenia, prolonged partial thromboplastin time (lupus inhibitor) with anticardiolipin antibodies, a noninflammatory joint fluid with good viscosity* and mucin+, and 1,000–2,000 WBC/mm³, which are mostly lymphocytes. A depressed serum $C'H_{50}$, elevated antinuclear antibody, and an increased anti–native-human DNA antibody titer are found.
4. **Rheumatic fever**
   a. **History** reveals a sore throat, fever, rash, and migratory joint pain that responds dramatically to aspirin treatment in a young individual (2–40 years of age).
   b. **Examination** shows a rash as well as heart (murmur) or pericardial (friction rub) involvement.
   c. **Laboratory tests** result in group A streptococci isolated on throat cultures and an elevated antistreptolysin O titer.
5. **Juvenile rheumatoid arthritis (JRA)**
   a. **History** shows symmetric joint involvement. The illness can begin or recur in the adult. Short stature and limb length generally accompany the most severe forms because the physes are affected by the inflammatory process. Patients with systemic onset (10% of children with JRA) have intermittent fever with rash. Those patients (40% of total) who have involvement of five or more joints are characterized as polyarticular onset and are differentiated from pauciarticular onset patients (2). There is a very high proportion of cervical spine involvement in the patients with JRA. The prevalence of JRA has been estimated to be between 57 and 113 per 100,000 children younger than 16 years of age in the United States (2).
   b. **Examination** may reveal a rash and fever. Cardiac, renal, and ocular abnormalities may be present. Eye involvement occurs in 30%–50% of early onset JRA patients (2).
   c. **Laboratory tests** show roentgenographic periostitis with erosions later in the course of disease. Rheumatoid factor or FANA may be present. Other causes of arthritis in the child or adolescent must be excluded.
6. **Human immunodeficiency virus (HIV) infection.** Migratory arthralgia and myalgia with accompanying muscle weakness are features of this disease. Radiographic changes are nonspecific.

---

* The clinical viscosity test is considered good or high if the fluid remains intact when slowly stretched between the examiner's thumb and index finger.
+ A good mucin clot is one that occurs after a few drops of glacial acetic acid are added to a supernatant of centrifuged joint fluid and a dense, white precipitate forms.

Table 4-7. Differential diagnosis of inflammatory spondyloarthropathy[a]

A. **Ankylosing spondylitis**—man, symmetric sacroiliitis clinically and radiologically, limitation of spinal motion, uveitis, smooth symmetric spinal ligamentous calcification, ankylosis often complete, no skip areas, family history, HLA-B27 antigen often present, good response to antiinflammatory drugs.

B. **Reiter's syndrome**—man with urethritis, skin-eye-heel, asymmetric peripheral joint involvement, sacroiliitis often asymmetric and skip areas of involvement in spine, coarse asymmetric syndesmophytes in spine, ankylosis incomplete and asymmetric, HLA-B27 often positive, equivocal response to antiinflammatory drugs.

C. **Psoriatic spondylitis**—skin or peripheral joints involved, asymmetric sacroiliitis, skip areas, may be ankylosing, HLA-B27 often present.

D. **Inflammatory bowel disease**—sacroiliitis, often symmetric, ankylosing, bowel disease may be silent, spinal inflammation, unlike peripheral arthritis, does not vary with and is not responsive to treatment directed at bowel inflammation, HLA-B27 often present.

E. **Other**—infection (bacterial tuberculous, fungal), osteochondritis, multiple epiphysitis in young adult.

[a] Juvenile rheumatoid arthritis spondyloarthropathy occurs almost entirely in HLA-B27–positive boys and is regarded as juvenile ankylosing spondylitis.
Modified from McCarty DJ. Differential diagnosis of arthritis: analysis of symptoms. In: McCarty DJ, ed. *Arthritis and allied conditions*, 10th ed. Philadelphia: Lea & Febiger, 1985:52.

F. **Inflammatory spondyloarthropathy** (Table 4-7)
   1. **Ankylosing spondylitis**
      a. **History** usually reveals clinical sacroiliitis in a male patient. A positive family history often is present. A good response to antiinflammatory agents is common.
      b. **Examination** reveals limitation of spinal motion, uveitis, and diminished chest expansion. A positive Patrick's test indicative of sacroiliac involvement is typically present (1,11,13).
      c. There is **laboratory evidence** of roentgenographic sacroiliitis and smooth, symmetric spinal ligamentous calcification, often with complete ankylosis (the "bamboo spine") and no skip areas. The HLA-B27 antigen should be present.
   2. **Reiter's syndrome** (see IV.E.1)
   3. **Psoriatic arthritis** (see IV.E.2)
   4. **Spondyloarthropathy secondary to inflammatory bowel disease**
      a. The **history** may not reveal bowel disease as a prominent feature; it can be subclinical.
      b. Bowel disease is found on **examination.**
      c. **Laboratory tests** show roentgenographic evidence of sacroiliitis that is often symmetric and ankylosing.
V. **Treatment** (Table 4-8)
   A. **Rheumatoid arthritis** (3,4,8,14)
      1. **Aspirin** is inexpensive but inconvenient to take because most authorities recommend a range of 10–16 five-grain tablets per day to reach an antiinflammatory level. Some patients simply cannot tolerate the medication because of gastrointestinal side effects. Alternatively, one of the enteric-coated or time-release preparations, 650 mg PO tid or qid, may be taken with meals but not with antacids. Tinnitus must be avoided with all aspirin-containing compounds; it is an early sign of salicylate toxicity. This therapy is sufficient only for mild, nonerosive forms of rheumatoid arthritis.
      2. **Other nonsteroidal, non-aspirin antiinflammatory medications** are much more convenient, although they are more expensive. Patients who take these medications long term should have biannual laboratory

Table 4-8. Treatment

Rheumatoid arthritis	Septic arthritis	Degenerative joint disease

1. Drugs
  a. Acetylsalicylic acid
    (first)
  b. Other antiinflam-
    matory prescription
    medications
  c. Gold or
    D-penicillamine
  d. Methotrexate
  e. Sulfasalozine
  f. Chloroquine
  g. Steroids
2. Synovectomy. If done,
  usually should follow
  6 months of medical
  management. (Do not
  do a prophylactic
  synovectomy if there
  is roentgenographic
  evidence of joint
  destruction manifested
  by a severe loss of
  cartilaginous space.)
3. Joint debridement and
  synovectomy (for pain
  relief only)
4. Partial or complete
  joint replacement
5. Arthrodesis
	1. Antibiotics. Cefazolin
	  (Kefzoi) or nafcillin
	  (Nafcil or Unipen)
	  with gentamicin
	  (Garamycin) or
	  tobramycin (Nebcin)
	  until the culture and
	  sensitivity results are
	  obtained; then specific
	  antibiotic therapy
	2. Surgery. Operative
	  debridement and
	  irrigation of the joint,
	  followed by appropriate
	  drainage
		1. Antiinflammatory
		  agents
		2. Support by bracing and
		  other means
		3. Physical therapy
		  a. Heat
		  b. Exercises
		4. Surgery
		  a. Debridement
		  b. Osteotomy
		  c. Partial or complete
		    joint replacement
		  d. Occasionally,
		    arthrodesis

work to look for adverse hepatic, renal, hematopoietic, and other reactions. Physicians should educate their patients as to the potential adverse effects of any medication. One easy education tool is the patient medication instruction sheet. The treating physician may need to experiment with various antiinflammatory medications before finding which preparation is the best suited for the individual patient. Many different preparations are now marketed (7). Physicians prescribing these medications should know their cost. For example, a 1-month supply (120 tablets) of generic ibuprofen, 600 mg, (prescription or over-the-counter) costs $15–$20, whereas a 1-month supply (360 tablets) of an over-the-counter brand name form of the same drug (e.g., Advil, Medipren, Anaprox), 200 mg, costs the patient $35–$36. The dosage of any antiinflammatory drug should be the lowest possible that is effective in relieving symptoms. There are several classes of these drugs, the latest being the COX II inhibitors, which have essentially no gastrointestinal ulceration side effects and are equally effective (6,8). This therapy is sufficient only for mild arthritis.

3. **Gold** has been considered an effective treatment for rheumatoid and psoriatic arthritis; it is no longer considered to be first line therapy. Three forms of gold are available. Two are injectable in the form of water-soluble, gold sodium thiomalate (Myochrysine) and an oil-based aurothioglucose (Solganal). The usual treatment required is two test doses of 10–25 mg each followed by weekly doses of 50 mg IM for 20 weeks. A maintenance dosage of 50 mg every 4 weeks may be given for life, but

dosage is empirical and smaller doses may be effective. The third form, Auranofin, is administered orally, 3 mg PO bid. The most common toxic reaction to gold is dermatitis or albuminuria. Almost any condition can occur, and gold should be withheld if any unusual symptoms develop. Do not persist with gold if results are doubtful (4).

4. D-**Penicillamine** (Cuprimine), a derivative of penicillin, may be substituted for gold in the treatment of rheumatoid arthritis; it is also no longer considered to be first line therapy. The drug is marketed in 125- and 250-mg capsules. The starting dosage is 250 mg/day, and it can be increased by 250 mg every 3 months to a maximum of 1 g/day. This slow approach appears to lessen toxicity but retains efficacy. Because the drug is toxic, the patient must be carefully monitored, particularly for bone marrow depression, thrombocytopenia, and albuminuria (4).

5. **Methotrexate.** First line therapy.

6. **Sulfasalazine.** First line therapy.

7. **Chloroquine** is available as 250-mg chloroquine phosphate tablets. **Hydroxychloroquine** (Plaquenil), which is available in 200-mg tablets is more commonly used because it is less toxic, but it is not as effective as chloroquine phosphate (4).

   a. **Dosage**

      (1) **Chloroquine phosphate** is given in doses of 250 mg/day PO.

      (2) **Hydroxycloroquine** is given in doses of 200 mg PO bid.

      (3) It may take up to **six months to achieve a result. Attempt a dose reduction** every six months.

   b. **Precautions**

      (1) **Do not exceed the recommended dose.** This **dosage schedule** does not apply to children.

      (2) **Inform the patient of toxicity.**

      (3) Have an **ophthalmologist follow up with the patient.**

      (4) **Do not refill a prescription over the telephone; examine the patient first.**

      (5) **Stop** therapy whenever there are any complaints of visual disturbance or a question of eye toxicity.

   c. **Side effects**

      (1) The **major** side effect is blindness resulting from chloroquine combining with retinal pigment.

      (2) **Other** effects are gastrointestinal upset, skin rash, weight loss, peripheral neuritis, and convulsions.

8. **Azathioprine,** a purine analog with immunosuppressive activity, has been shown to be effective in rheumatoid arthritis; it should be prescribed by rheumatologists (3).

9. Leflunomide (Aravan)

10. Etanercept (Enbrel), a tumor necrosis factor alpha (TNF-α) inhibitor, is the first "biologic" agent for use in rheumatoid arthritis. It has been proven to be effective in controlled trials and is well tolerated; it has also been shown to be useful in combination therapy with methotrexate. It should be prescribed by rheumatologists (15,17,19).

11. **Corticosteroids** yield a dramatic effect in the treatment of rheumatic disease. Although steroids can offer dramatic relief, indiscriminate use may actually produce more harm than good. In the treatment of rheumatoid arthritis, steroids do not alter the course of the disease, and in subsequent years, the relief will probably deteriorate, because patients may have more than one disease.

    a. **Usage**

       (1) **Establish a specific diagnosis before treatment** with steroids.

       (2) **Adjust the dosage** to the situation. For rheumatoid arthritis, start with 10–20 mg to control symptoms, then taper over 2–4 weeks to the lowest tolerated dose (usually no more than

5–10 mg/day) and try not to exceed 10 mg/24 hours. For SLE crisis, one might start with 60 mg in a 24-hour period.

(3) Although more than 20 generic glucocorticosteroids are available, most rheumatologists have settled on **prednisone as the standard.**

(4) **Monitor serum electrolytes and glucose,** because steroids cause increased excretion of sodium and potassium.

(5) **Administer** the steroid **once each morning** to minimize the effect on the pituitary–adrenal axis. If there is good control of the inflammatory process, use alternate-day therapy.

(6) Obtain a **baseline eye examination** before starting long-term therapy. Steroids can cause cataracts and increased intraocular pressure.

(7) Beware of **suppressed reaction to infection** as a complicating factor, especially if the patient's general condition is deteriorating while he or she is taking steroids.

(8) With long-term therapy, be sure to recognize and manage complications of the systemic rheumatic disease as opposed to the **iatrogenic complications** of long-term steroid use, which are managed differently.

(9) Patients should always **carry information** that they are on steroids.

(10) **Supplemental increased doses** are necessary when stress occurs, even minor stress such as a tooth extraction.

b. **Undesirable effects**

(1) **Steroid diabetes** that is insulin-resistant, but without ketosis or acidosis

(2) **Muscle wasting** secondary to a negative nitrogen balance.

(3) **Buffalo hump** and **round face**

(4) Sodium retention that results in **edema** (especially important for patients with heart disease)

(5) **Hirsutism** and occasional **alterations in menstrual function** in women secondary to adrenal atrophy.

(6) **Peptic ulcer disease** with possible perforation and abscess

(7) **Suppressed wound healing**

(8) **Osteoporosis** and avascular necrosis of the femoral or humeral head. Pathologic fractures are often associated.

(9) **Lymphocytosis** and occasionally a leukemoid reaction

(10) **Subcutaneous hemorrhages and acne**

(11) **Central nervous system changes** such as psychosis, seizures, and insomnia at higher dose

(12) **Immunosuppression** with increased risk of infections, candida, herpes zoster, and so on

12. **Surgical treatment**

a. **Synovectomy**, if done, should follow at least 6 months of nonoperative management. This prophylactic procedure should not be performed if roentgenographic evidence of joint destruction manifested by a severe loss of cartilaginous space exists.

b. There is still a place for **joint debridement** and synovectomy in patients with significant joint pain, but not enough joint destruction to justify surgical joint knee replacement. Recently, arthroscopic synovectomy in the knee and shoulder has been shown to be effective.

c. **Joint replacement** may be necessary. The most common joints replaced in the patient with inflammatory arthritis are knee and hip, followed by shoulder, metacarpophalangeal, elbow, wrist, and ankle.

d. Occasionally, **arthrodesis** is indicated, especially with ankle involvement.

e. **Forefoot surgery** is frequently required and most commonly consists of first metatarsophalangeal joint arthrodesis combined with lesser metatarsophalangeal joint resection with claw toe release.

B. Septic arthritis
  1. **Antibiotics** (see Chap. 3, Table 3-2). Proper cultures must be obtained before initiating antibiotic therapy. These are obtained either as an aspirate or intraoperatively.
  2. **Drainage** of the joint is usually necessary.
     a. **Needle aspiration and irrigation** is sometimes sufficient if the joint can be easily inspected for an effusion. The joint may need decompression more than once daily. The hip joint always requires open drainage. A knee joint infection can be handled by needle de compression if the exudate is not loculated and if aspiration clearly decompresses the joint. If marked improvement is not noted within 48 hours, then the open (or arthroscopic) irrigation and debridement should be performed.
     b. **Operative irrigation and drainage** of the joint is often necessary with or without debridement. Postoperatively, wounds are usually closed over drains and judicious immobilization is used. Increasingly arthroscopic lavage is being used for knee and shoulder joint involvement.
C. Osteoarthritis
  1. Medical treatment consists of antiinflammatory doses of **aspirin** or other **nonsteroidal antiinflammatory preparations;** acetaminophen analgesia is safest (9,10). There is some evidence that the "nutricenticals" glucosamine and chondrotin sulfate have some efficacy in treating the symptoms of osteoarthritis (16). See **V.A.1** and **V.A.2** for a more complete discussion.
  2. Various **braces** are available to offer joint support (see also Chap. 6). Simple neoprene sleeves for the knee or elbow are useful. For unicompartmental knee arthritis braces that "unload" the diseased compartment are proven to be effective (12).
  3. **Physical therapy** can be helpful, especially in providing exercises to maintain muscle tone. Deep heat treatments provide symptomatic relief. The most effective therapy is patient-directed home therapy, which emphasizes maintaining strength and motion with low-impact exercise routines. Prolonged outpatient therapy is expensive and of limited value.
  4. Intraarticular steroid injections are helpful. The options available are listed in **D.2.b.** (pseudogout treatment). Recently, injection of hyaluronic acid compounds (Synvisc or Hyalgan) have been proven to be efficacious. This requires serial injections given 1 week apart over either 3 or 5 weeks. The therapy has the same effectiveness as oral antiinflammatory therapy.
  5. Various **surgical procedures** offer relief of joint pain and improved function. These include the following:
     a. **Debridement,** generally arthroscopic
     b. **Osteotomy** for varus malalignment of the knee to move the weight-bearing axis into the lateral, more normal compartment
     c. Partial or complete **joint resurfacing or replacement**
     d. Occasionally, **joint arthrodesis.** This is generally reserved for use in the previously septic joint.
     e. Autologous chondrocyte transplantation is a technique for the management of focal articular cartilage defects and is not indicated for diffuse osteoarthritis of the knee (5,18).
D. Crystal-induced arthritis (4)
  1. **Gouty arthritis**
     a. **Acute attacks** may be provoked by surgery or trauma or other systemic illness. They generally respond to the following agents:
        (1) **Colchicine,** one 0.6-mg tablet initially followed by one tablet per hour until gastrointestinal upset occurs, joint symptoms resolve, or a maximum of ten tablets has been ingested in a 24-hour period; or 2 mg IV initially (avoid injecting outside the vein by injecting into a functioning IV) followed by 1 mg q6h

until the flare symptoms resolve or a maximum of 5 mg has been injected in a 24-hour period. A suppository formulation is available for patients who cannot take oral medications. IV colchicine should be avoided in elderly patients and patients with renal disease.

(2) **Indomethacin (Indocin),** 50 mg PO qid for the first day, followed by 25 mg qid

(3) **Other antiinflammatory drugs,** which can be tried if indomethacin is ineffective or not well tolerated.

b. The **authors suggest** treatment with **colchicine,** 0.6 mg PO bid, **between acute attacks** until the patient is symptom-free for 1 year. Consultation with a rheumatologist is advised.

c. A xanthine oxidase inhibitor such as **allopurinol** (Zyloprim), 100–300 mg/day PO, works by lowering the uric acid pool of the body. The physician should be aware of the serious and possibly fatal adverse reactions to allopurinol, including agranulocytosis, exfoliative dermatitis, acute vasculitis, and hepatotoxicity. These agents should not be initiated during an acute attack, rather after resolution.

d. **Uricosuric agents:** probenecid and sulfinpyrazone. These agents increase the amount of uric acid excreted in the urine, so their use can be associated with uric acid renal calculi. As with allopurinol, the therapy should be initiated after resolution of the acute attack.

(1) **Probenecid** (Benemid), 0.5 mg PO qid up to 2 or 3 g/day

(2) **Sulfinpyrazone** (Anturane), 100 mg PO bid up to qid

e. Recommendations for **managing hyperuricemia**

(1) **Confirm** the elevated serum uric acid by repeating the test.

(2) **Determine** whether the condition is **secondary** to drugs or blood dyscrasia. One should rule out renal disease with a serum creatinine in a 24-hour serum uric acid excretion test. If uric acid excretion is greater than 1 g per 24 hours, consider treating the hyperuricemia. If renal disease is present, then allopurinol may be the drug of choice.

(3) **Generally withhold therapy** unless there has been one acute attack of gouty arthritis.

(4) **Rule out** hyperuricemia secondary to a lymphoproliferative or myeloproliferative disease.

(5) Do not treat hyperuricemia secondary to **thiazide diuretics**

2. **Pseudogout**

a. **Differentiate** pseudogout from acute gouty arthritis by joint fluid examination for specific crystals.

b. Consider **aspirating** the joint fluid or **injecting** insoluble steroids intraarticularly, using 0.1 mL for small joints and up to 1–2 mL for most large joints. The types of steroids useful for this application are as follows:

(1) **Hydrocortisone** acetate, 25–50 mg/mL

(2) **Prednisone** tertiary butyl acetate, 20 mg/mL

(3) **Triamcinolone** hexacetonide (Aristospan), 5 and 20 mg/mL

(4) **Betamethasone** acetate and sodium phosphate (Celestone), 6 mg/mL

(5) **Methylprednisolone** acetate (Depo-Medrol), 20 and 40 mg/mL

c. **Colchicine** may provide dramatic relief.

d. Many patients respond to **antiinflammatory agents,** such as indomethacin.

E. **Inflammatory polyarthritis** (assuming no coexisting chlamydia infection)

1. **Reiter's syndrome** treatment is symptomatic. The prognosis is guarded, because chronic arthritis develops in many people. Sulfasalazine, MTX may be considered for chronic moderate-to-severe disease.

2. **Psoriatic arthritis. Immunosuppressive drugs,** such as methotrexate are useful when administered in doses of 7.5–25.0 mg PO or IM once

weekly. Methotrexate can induce hair loss, cause oral ulcers, promote teratogenesis, and cause hepatitis and cirrhosis of the liver.
3. **Systemic lupus erythematosus**
   a. **Do not treat until the diagnosis is established.**
   b. **Do not overtreat.** Mild cases can be handled with reassurance, aspirin, indomethacin, or one of the many nonsteroidal antiinflammatory drugs that are available.
   c. **An occult infection** sometimes is difficult to diagnose and differentiate from an exacerbation of SLE. In these situations, be sure to rule out infections of the genitourinary tract, heart, and lungs.
   d. Advise the patient to **rest** as necessary.
   e. Avoid excessive exposure to the **sun.**
   f. **Chloroquine, hydroxychloroquine, and mepacrine** (Atabrine) usually control the skin manifestations and arthralgia. Mepacrine should be administered 100 mg/day PO. This medication can cause yellow staining of the skin, but this effect is not considered a reason to discontinue its use.
   g. **Prednisone,** less than 10 mg/day PO, may be added to the regimen if the patient does not respond to the preceding measures.
   h. **Immunosuppressive agents** are indicated as steroid-sparing agents for treatment for SLE.
   i. The treatment of this disease is empirical and must be individualized and monitored by the rheumatologist. There are no absolutes.
F. **Inflammatory spondyloarthropathy**
   1. **Ankylosing spondylitis**
      a. **The most important part of the initial therapy** is an **educational effort** by the physician or physical therapist that should cover proper sleeping position, gait, posture, breathing exercises, and "measuring up" every morning (i.e., straightening the spine every day to reach a mark placed on the wall to help prevent kyphosis or at least identify its development.
      b. **Nonsteroidal antiinflammatory drugs** are the drug of choice for milder cases. As with treatment for osteoarthritis, trial and error to identify the optimum drug is the rule. After relief is obtained, decrease the dose to the lowest possible effective dose (6).
      c. **Ophthalmologic evaluation** is indicated because anterior uveitis occurs in 10%–60% of patients.
      d. **Sulfasalazine or methotrexate** may be useful in aggressive cases.
      e. **Radiation therapy** has been abandoned because of late malignancy reports.
   2. **Treatment of Reiter's syndrome** is discussed in V.E.1.
   3. Treatment of **psoriatic arthritis** is discussed in V.E.2.
   4. **Rheumatic fever**
      a. **Rest** is recommended according to the degree of cardiac involvement (3).
      b. **Aspirin** is used for mild arthritis.
      c. **Prednisone** is used for patients with carditis and heart failure. Start with 40–60 mg/day, and adjust the dosage according to patient response.
      d. **Diuretics and digitalis** are often needed.
      e. **Penicillin** is indicated for the initial treatment as well as continued prophylaxis. See Chap. 3 for the appropriate parenteral dose.
      f. **Throat culture** family contacts.
   5. **Juvenile rheumatoid arthritis** (1,13)
      a. **Salicylates** or nonsteroidal antiinflammatory drugs are the mainstay of therapy; one third of patients can be managed with these drugs alone (2).
         (1) For **children** weighing less than 25 kg, use 100 mg/kg body weight per day in four to six divided doses.

(2) For **adults,** a total daily dose of 2.4–3.6 g of aspirin usually is sufficient.
b. Methotrexate is effective in 70%–80% of patients with JRA.
c. **Gold** is used if after 6 months of adequate salicylate and physical therapy, loss of joint function is progressive owing to active synovitis. See **V.A.3** for a discussion of gold therapy. For children, use 1 mg/kg body weight per week to a maximum of 25 mg/kg body weight per week; injectable therapy is effective in 50% of patients; oral gold therapy is ineffective.
d. **Antimalarial drugs** such as hydroxychloroquine are used as an alternative to gold. Do not exceed 200 mg/m² body surface per day. Ophthalmologic examinations are recommended every 3 months. See **V.A.7** for a more complete discussion of antimalarial drugs.
e. **D-Penicillamine** is not recommended for routine use in JRA.
f. **Corticosteroids** are rarely warranted for joint disease alone. If given, they should be administered at the lowest effective dose, preferably on alternate days for very short periods. Steroid injections into troublesome joints for synovitis may be helpful if multiple injections into the same joint are avoided.
g. **Physical and occupational therapy** is helpful to maintain function, prevent contracture, and optimize motion and muscle strength. Therapeutic maneuvers should be performed twice daily at home. Night splints to prevent deformity are usually essential.
h. **Orthopaedic surgery**
(1) **Synovectomy plays a limited role** in the early treatment of JRA.
(2) **Reconstructive surgery** (e.g., soft-tissue releases, osteotomies, and total joint replacement) is helpful.
i. **Ophthalmologic evaluation** is necessary for early diagnostic treatment of any iridocyclitis.
j. **Amyloidosis** is seen in 5% of patients and can be fatal if kidneys fail.
k. **Do not forget the whole child, the effects of this disease on other organ systems, and the child's mental health.**

References
1. American College of Rheumatology Ad Hoc Committee on Clinical Guidelines. Guidelines for the management of rheumatoid arthritis. *Arthritis Rheum* 1996; 39:713–722.
2. Arthritis Foundation. *Primer on rheumatic diseases*, 11th ed. 1999:393–398.
3. American College of Rheumatology Ad Hoc Committee on Clinical Guidelines. Guidelines for monitoring drug therapy in rheumatoid arthritis.*Arthritis Rheum* 1996;39:723–731.
4. Blackburn WD. Management of osteoarthritis and rheumatoid arthritis: Prospects and possibilities. *Am J Med* 1996;100:24S–30S.
5. Brittberg M, Lindahl A, Nilsson A, et al. Treatment of deep cartilage defects in the knee with autologous chonrocyte transplantation. *N Engl J Med* 1994;331:889–995.
6. Celecoxib for arthritis. *Med Lett Drugs Ther* 1999;41:1045.
7. Fox DA. The role of T cells in the immunopathogenesis of rheumatoid arthritis: new perspectives. *Arthritis Rheum* 1997;40:598–609.
8. Fries JF, Williams CA, Morfeld D, et al. Reduction in long-term disability in patients with rheumatoid arthritis by disease-modifying antirheumatic drug-based treatment strategies. *Arthritis Rheum* 1996;39:616–622.
9. Hochberg MC, Altman RD, Brandt KD, et al. Guidelines for the medical management of osteoarthritis: Part I. Osteoarthritis of the hip: American College of Rheumatology. *Arthritis Rheum* 1995;38:1535–1540.
10. Hochberg MC, Altman RD, Brandt KD, et al. Guidelines for the medical management of osteoarthritis: Part II. Osteoarthritis of the knee: American College of Rheumatology. *Arthritis Rheum* 1995;38:1541–1546.
Kelley WN, et al. *Textbook of rheumatology,* 4th ed. Philadelphia: WB Saunders, 1993.

11. Kirkley A, Webster-Bogaert S, Litchfield R, et al. The effect of bracing on varus gonarthrosis. *J Bone Joint Surg (Am)* 1999;81:539–548.
12. McCarty DJ. *Arthritis and allied conditions*, 12th ed. Philadelphia: Lea & Febiger, 1993.
13. Moreland LW, Heck LW Jr, Koopman WJ. Biologic agents for treating rheumatic arthritis: concepts and progress. *Arthritis Rheum* 1997;40:397–409.
14. Moreland LW, Schift MH, Banngartner SW, et al. Etanercept therapy in rheumatoid arthritis. A randomized, controlled trial. *Ann Intern Med* 1999;130:478–486.
15. Muller-Fassbender H, Bach GL, Haase W, et al. Glucosamine sulfate compared to ibuprofen in osteoarthritis of the knee. *Osteoarthritis Cartilage* 1994;2:61–69.
16. New drugs for rheumatoid arthritis. *Med Lett Drugs Ther* 1998;40:110–112.
17. Shapiro F, Koide S, Glimcher MJ. Cell origin and differentiation in the repair of full-thickness defects of articular cartilage. *J Bone Joint Surg (Am)* 1994;76:579–592.
18. Weaver A, Caldwell J, Olsen N, et al for The Leflunomide RA Investigators Group and Strand V. Treatment of active rheumatoid arthritis with leflunomide compared to placebo or methotrexate. *Arthritis Rheum* 1998;41[9 Suppl];S131(abst).
19. Weinblatt ME, Kremer JM, Bankhurst AD, et al. A trial of etanercept, a recombinant tumor necrosis factor receptor: Fc fusion protein in patients with rheumatoid arthritis receiving methotrexate. *N Engl J Med* 1999;340:253–259.

5. NONACUTE PEDIATRIC ORTHOPAEDIC CONDITIONS

I. The limping child
   A. The limping child is frequently referred to a primary physician's office or urgent/emergency care center. There is a long list of possible causes to be considered. Important components of the evaluation include a thorough history and a careful physical examination.
   B. **History.** Important features to inquire about include acuteness of onset (sudden, recent, chronic, intermittent), presence of pain, history of trauma or injury, localizing symptoms, constitutional symptoms such as fever, malaise, chills; early morning stiffness, recent illnesses and motor milestone development (walked by 15–18 months).
   C. **Past medical history** should include birth history (full term, premature, difficulties at time of delivery, neonatal intensive care unit (NICU), chronic medical conditions) and any previous surgery, injuries, or illnesses.
   D. **Physical examination.** The child should be undressed to an appropriate state. Older children and teenagers should be provided with a gown or shorts. Toddlers and small children can be examined in their diaper or underwear. Evaluation should start with careful observation of walking pattern. **Antalgic** gait is characterized by a decreased stance period on the affected limb as well as a trunk shift over the affected limb during stance. **Trendelenburg** gait (or gluteus medius lurch gait) is characterized by weak abductor muscles, resulting in the pelvis tilting in the coronal plane during stance phase on the affected limb. Patients with a history of a stroke may exhibit a **hemiplegic** style of gait affecting one half of their body. Evidence of a limb length difference should be evaluated by palpating the anterior superior iliac spine (ASIS) with the patients standing. Careful evaluation should include examination of the back, sacroiliac (SI) joints, and abdomen as well as the entire extremity involved. Gentle palpation over the entire length of the limb should be combined with gentle range of motion of the hip, knee, and ankle joints. Particular attention should be paid to any erythema, warmth, joint effusion, or focal tenderness. A thorough neurologic examination should also be completed.
   E. The differential diagnosis encompasses a broad range and is age dependent:
      1. 0–5 years old
         a. Septic arthritis
         b. Osteomyelitis
         c. Transient hip synovitis
         d. Osteochondroses (Perthes)
         e. Developmental dysplasia of the hip (DDH)
         f. Neurologic disorders (cerebral palsy, Duchenne's)
         g. Tumor (neuroblastoma, acute lymphocytic leukemia (ALL), benign tumors)
         h. Diskitis
         i. Juvenile rheumatoid arthritis
         j. Toddler's fracture
         k. Tibia vara
         l. "Growing pains"
         m. Congenital limb deficiency (femur, fibula, tibia)
         n. Nonaccidental injury
      2. 5–10 years old
         a. Septic arthritis
         b. Osteomyelitis
         c. Transient synovitis
         d. Osteochondroses (Perthes, Kohler, Osgood-Schlatter)
         e. Limb length difference
         f. Tumor (ALL, Ewing's sarcoma, benign bone tumors)
         g. Neurologic disorders (hereditary motor sensory neuropathy)
         h. Diskitis

      i. Juvenile rheumatoid arthritis
      j. Discoid meniscus
  3. 10–15 years old
      a. Osteomyelitis
      b. Slipped capital femoral epiphysis (SCFE)
      c. Osteochondroses (Perthes, Sever's)
      d. Hip dysplasia
      e. Patellofemoral pain syndrome
      f. Tumor (osteosarcoma, Ewing's sarcoma, benign bone tumors)
      g. Spondylosis
      h. Spondylolisthesis
      i. Osteochondritis desiccans
      j. Tibia vara

F. Evaluation. Plain radiographs and laboratory studies should be included. Plain radiographs should include the entire length of bony area involved, including joint above and below the area. Referred pain is common in children and frequently symptoms experienced at one site are referred from an adjacent joint. Laboratory studies should include complete blood count (CBC) with differential, erythrocyte sedimentation rate (ESR), and C-reactive protein (CRP). If rheumatologic conditions or spondyloarthropathies are being evaluated, laboratory studies should also include rheumatoid factor, antinuclear antibody (ANA), anti-streptolysin (ASO) titer, Lyme titer, and HLA B-27.

G. Additional imaging studies
  1. Three-phase bone scan. For patients with an occult source of symptoms and normal plain radiographs, a three-phase bone scan has a high sensitivity for detecting sites of abnormal bone metabolism such as fracture, infection, and benign or malignant tumor. It is relatively nonspecific.
  2. Magnetic resonance imaging. MRI is very sensitive for detecting areas of abnormal signal intensity in soft tissues as well as in the bone marrow. Marrow edema is seen early in the evolution of osteomyelitis. It frequently has a decreased signal intensity on T1-weighted images and an increased signal intensity on T2-weighted images. MRI can detect fluid collections within the soft tissues such as abscesses as well as fluid collections within the epiphysis.
  3. Ultrasound. Ultrasound has proven useful in detecting presence of joint effusions for hard to examine joints such as the hip as well as detecting the presence of a subperiosteal abscess associated with osteomyelitis. If a septic arthritis process is suspected, a **joint aspiration** should be performed without wasting time waiting for the availability of other additional imaging studies.

II. Lower extremity alignment—**intoeing**
  A. Definition. An internal foot progression angle during gait. The foot turns in relative to the line of forward progression during walking. Intoeing is a frequent cause for parental concern and an important part of the evaluation should be listening to the concerns expressed by the parents and answering their questions.
  B. Causes. Increased femoral anteversion or antetorsion (position of femoral neck relative to distal femoral condyles in the transverse plane), internal tibial torsion, metatarsus adductus.
  C. Physical examination. The patient should be undressed adequately to visualize the lower extremities. Observe child walking and running in hallway or corridor where ample room is available. Make note of the position of the feet relative to the line of forward progression (foot progression angle). Next, examine the child in the prone position on the examination table and record the lower extremity rotational profile (Fig. 5-1.) Evaluate hip internal (medial) and external (lateral) rotation. Palpate the position of rotation at which the greater trochanter is most prominent in order to estimate femoral neck anteversion. Evaluate the thigh-foot axis and bimalleolar axis in order to assess tibial torsion. Examine the plantar surface of the foot and the lateral border of the foot for evidence of metatarsus adductus.

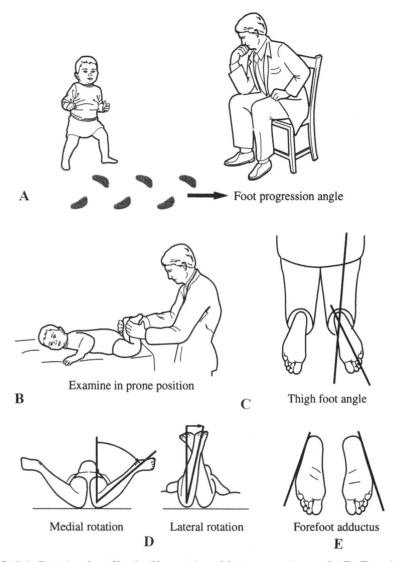

FIG. 5-1. Rotational profile. **A:** Observation of foot-progression angle. **B:** Examination of child in prone position to evaluate torsional deformity of the lower extremities. **C:** Thigh-foot angle. **D:** Hip internal (medial) rotation and external (lateral) rotation. **E:** Forefoot (metatarsus) adductus.

D. **Discussion.** Intoeing is frequently seen in young children and is a normal part of skeletal development for many. The most frequent causes **are increased femoral anteversion,** internal tibial torsion, or metatarsus adductus. Femoral anteversion in the newborn is 40–45 degrees and persists until the onset of walking age when, with growth, this gradually remodels to the adult value of approximately 10–15 degrees. Persistent femoral anteversion may be seen in children with certain neurologic conditions as well as with generalized increased ligamentous laxity. **Internal tibial torsion** is also frequently seen in infants and toddlers and also gradually corrects during the years following the onset of walking. **Metatarsus adductus** refers to a curved alignment of the foot itself in which the forefoot deviates toward the midline. The foot will have a rather curved lateral border compared with a normal foot. This is a common finding in newborn children. It is most often flexible.

E. **Treatment.** For the majority of children, treatment consists of education of the parents, reassurance, and observation. For matters of anteversion or tibial torsion, no form of bracing or night splinting is recommended. Statistically, less than 1% of children will have persistence of this condition severe enough to cause any functional or cosmetic concerns. For metatarsus adductus, simple massage and stretching can be performed by the parents for the first 6 months of age. If no improvement is seen, one may consider a course of treatment with reverse-last shoes or bracing. If the foot does not appear flexible, a course of serial casting may be considered.

III. **Lower extremity alignment—bowed legs or "knock" knees**

A. **Terminology.** In **genu varum** ("bowed legs," genu-knee, varum/varus), the distal segment is aligned toward or close to the midline. In **genu valgum** ("knock knees," genu-knee, valgum/valgus), the distal segment is aligned away from the midline.

B. **Physical examination.** The child should be undressed appropriately so that both lower extremities can be evaluated. The child should be assessed standing and again supine on the examination table. The amount of angulation at the knee can be assessed in two ways. The anatomic alignment can be measured by using a goniometer and measuring the **femoral-tibial angle.** Alternatively, one can also measure and record the distance between bony landmarks. For genu varum, one can measure the distance between the medial femoral condyles of the two knees, the **intercondylar distance.** For genu valgum, one can measure the distance between the medial malleoli of the ankles, the **intermalleolar distance.**

C. **Radiographic evaluation.** For either genu varum or genu valgum, standing anteroposterior (AP) hip to ankle radiographs of both lower extremities should be obtained.

D. **Causes.** Most children have a **physiologic basis** for their alignment. Children undergo an evolution of their lower extremity alignment. When they first start to stand and walk, they have genu varum. As they grow, this usually resolves by age 2 years old on average. Many children continue to evolve to genu valgum by age 4 years old. This continues to correct so that by age 6 years old, children have a relatively "mature" alignment of mild genu valgum anatomically. For children who do not fit this pattern, who are older, or for whom the alignment appears asymmetric, other possible causes should be explored, including **tibia vara (Blount's disease), coxa vara,** one of the skeletal dysplasias such as **chondrometaphyseal dysplasia,** or one of the forms of rickets such as familial hypophosphatemic rickets.

E. **Treatment.** For physiologic conditions, treatment usually consists of education and reassurance of the parents as well as observation. It is frequently possible to inform the patient's parents of the expected course as well as to communicate the findings and recommendations to the patient's primary physician so that continued observation can be performed during routine well-child checks. If the course of the alignment varies from what is expected, the child can return for reevaluation. Children with nonphysiologic causes for their lower extremity alignment should be referred for further evaluation. Further treatment may consist of establishing the underlying cause as well as developing an appropriate treatment plan. This may consist of observation, hemiepiphyseal stapling, hemiepiphysiodesis, or tibial and/or femoral osteotomy. These should be performed by physicians who are well experienced in planning and executing the appropriate procedures and follow-up care.

IV. **Common childhood foot conditions**
  A. **Clubfoot (talipes equinovarus)**
    1. **Description.** A congenital deformity of the foot which is comprised of ankle equinus, hindfoot varus, as well as adduction and supination of the midfoot and forefoot.
    2. **Incidence.** Clubfoot occurs in approximately 1 in 1,000 live births. Clubfoot is unilateral in 60% of patients and the ratio of incidence in boys to girls is 2:1. There may be a positive family history.
    3. **Etiology.** Multiple theories exist with the most likely cause being multifactorial. Theories include arrested fetal development, abnormal intrauterine forces, abnormal muscle fiber type, abnormal neuromuscular function, and germ plasm defects.
    4. **Prenatal considerations** include breech position, large birth weight, and oligohydramnios.
    5. **Associated conditions** include arthrogryposis, myelodysplasia, congenital limb anomalies, and various syndromes.
    6. **Physical examination.** A careful evaluation should include not only examination of the child's feet, but also the child's upper extremities, back, spine, and hips in order to look for other associated conditions. Examination of the foot should include evaluation of the ankle dorsiflexion, the hindfoot position, curvature of the lateral border of the foot, and the forefoot position as well as an assessment of the degree of flexibility of the foot.
    7. **Radiographic evaluation.** Radiographs in the newborn period are not useful because the tarsal bones are not well ossified. However, after age 3 months, radiographs are more useful. The most useful images are an AP view and a lateral view in a position of maximum dorsiflexion. **Kite's angle** is the angle subtended by the long axes of the calcaneus and the talus on the AP view. This angle is normally between 20 and 40 degrees. In the clubfoot, this angle is less than 20 degrees with relative parallel alignment. One can also assess the alignment of the talus relative to the first metatarsal to evaluate the forefoot adduction. The relationship of the talus and calcaneus should also be assessed on the lateral view. Again, in the clubfoot, this shows relative parallel alignment compared with the normal foot.
    8. **Treatment.** The goals of treatment are to achieve a plantigrade, flexible, painless foot. Initial treatment consists of serial casting, using long leg casts applied weekly with gradual correction of the foot deformity. Kite published high levels of satisfactory results with his casting technique. More recently, Ponsetti has achieved similarly impressive satisfactory results with casting and limited surgical intervention. Even though greater interest has been given to the nonoperative methods of treatment, until recently the high levels of satisfactory results were difficult to reproduce in other institutions. Therefore, an operative method of treatment of the clubfoot has also been popularized. The surgical treatment of clubfoot gained widespread acceptance with the one-stage release technique described by Turco. This has been adapted and modified by various authors since its original description. The surgical treatment essentially consists of a one-stage correction done through either a two-incision technique (Carroll) or a Cincinnati incision (Crawford). Controversies exist regarding the best age of the patient to undergo the surgery, the structures to be addressed in the surgical correction, use of internal fixation, and the duration of postoperative immobilization.

9. **Results.** Satisfactory results in surgically treated feet range from 75% to 95% based on clinical and radiographic criteria. The Ponsetti method has garnered approximately 90% satisfactory results based on patient satisfaction and clinical evaluation. Nearly all patients have some differences in the overall appearance and shape of the foot with a smaller calf circumference, a shorter foot, and a limb length difference when compared with an uninvolved foot. The amount of difference varies among patients.

B. **Flat feet (pes planus)**

1. **Definition.** A foot in which the medial longitudinal arch is absent, resulting in hindfoot valgus and forefoot supination.

2. **Presentation.** Patients with flat feet may be seen because of parental concerns regarding the appearance and shape of the foot or because of pain or difficulties with shoe wear.

3. **Patient history.** It is important to note when foot position was first noticed, whether the foot condition interferes with function, whether there is pain or history of ligamentous laxity, and whether there is positive family history.

4. **Physical examination.** Observe the foot while the patient stands and walks. Note presence or absence of medial longitudinal arch. Inspect the foot for calluses and pressure areas over bony prominences. When the patient is standing, have him or her stand on tiptoe to assess mobility of the hindfoot. If the hindfoot moves from valgus when plantigrade to varus with standing on tiptoe and the foot forms an arch, then the foot is "flexible." If not, it is "rigid." Assess the length of the Achilles tendon by examining the range of ankle dorsiflexion.

5. **Radiographic examination.** For children with a painless, flexible flat foot, no radiographs are indicated. If the flat foot is painful or rigid, then standing AP, lateral, and oblique radiographs of the foot should be obtained.

6. **Flexible flat feet.** The flexible flat foot is relatively common, although the true incidence is unknown. Most young children start with a flexible flat foot before developing a medial, longitudinal arch during the first decade of life. Most children are symptom-free and no treatment is warranted. For the older child or adolescent who experiences aching or discomfort associated with particular activities, one may wish to use an orthotic to support the arch. This does not permanently establish an arch but it may afford symptomatic relief. If the foot is flexible but there is a contracture of the Achilles tendon, one should prescribe a course of physical therapy for a heel cord stretching program and possibly a course of serial, stretching casts. If the patient with an Achilles tendon contracture remains symptomatic despite nonoperative treatment, one may occasionally consider surgical lengthening of the heel cord. For the older patient who remains symptomatic despite all conservative treatment, one may consider the calcaneus lengthening osteotomy described by Evans and popularized by Mosca.

7. **Rigid flat feet.** The most common cause for a rigid flat foot is a **tarsal coalition.** This is an incomplete separation of the tarsal bones during fetal development. The two most common types are the **calcaneonavicular** and the **talocalcaneal** coalition. The calcaneonavicular coalition may be best seen on the oblique foot radiograph. The talocalcaneal coalition may be seen on an axial (Harris) radiograph of the foot. If further radiographic imaging is required, a computed tomography (CT) scan of both feet is the study of choice. Other possible causes of a rigid flat foot include a **congenital vertical talus, juvenile rheumatoid arthritis** involving the subtalar joint, **osteochondral fractures** of the subtalar joint, and **neuromuscular** causes.

8. **Treatment** of the rigid flat foot. The goal of treatment is to achieve a pain-free, asymptomatic foot. Approximately 75% of patients with tarsal coalitions are asymptomatic. Frequently, the onset of pain coincides with

the transition of the coalition from a fibrous or cartilaginous junction to a bony bar. For the calcaneonavicular bar, this occurs around ages 8 to 12 years old; for the talocalcaneal bar, this occurs between 12 and 16 years of age. Treatment initially consists of a short-leg walking cast for 6 weeks followed by a molded orthotic. This results in a resolution of the patient's symptoms in a large number of patients. For patients who do not respond to casting treatment or for whom the symptoms recur, surgery is indicated. Operative treatment usually consists of excision of the coalition along with interposition of fat, muscle, or tendon to prevent recurrence. For patients with a talocalcaneal coalition that comprises more than 50% of the subtalar joint surface, some authors have questioned the role of resection of the coalition. For patients with severe degenerative arthrosis of the subtalar joint or persistent pain following previous resection, a triple arthrodesis should be considered.

C. Metatarsus adductus
1. **Definition.** Adduction of the forefoot in association with a neutral hindfoot and midfoot. It is usually seen in newborn children in approximately 1 in 1,000 live births. It is most often the result of intrauterine positioning.
2. **Physical examination.** A careful evaluation should include an examination of the spine, the hips, and the feet. (Orthopaedic literature cites an association of between 2% and 11% between metatarsus adductus and developmental dysplasia of the hip.) Evaluate the overall flexibility of the foot. Distinguish metatarsus adductus from other common foot conditions including clubfoot or skewfoot.
3. **Treatment.** For the newborn with a flexible foot, treatment may consist of serial stretching and massage of the foot by parents daily for the first 3 to 6 months of life. For less flexible feet or feet that do not respond to stretching, a short period of serial casting may be employed, followed by a course of reverse-last shoes. This deformity infrequently causes functional difficulties and surgery is rarely indicated.

D. Bunions (hallux valgus)
1. **Definition.** An abnormal bony prominence of the medial eminence of the first metatarsal associated with a hallux valgus deformity of the great toe. It is frequently associated with a medial deviation of the first metatarsal (**metatarsus primus varus**).
2. **Patient history.** These patients are most often adolescent or teenage girls with complaints of pain over the medial eminence, difficulty with shoe wear, or concerns regarding appearance. There may be a positive family history.
3. **Physical examination.** Clinically assess presence of hindfoot valgus and presence of a coexisting flat foot in addition to presence and severity of hallux valgus deformity. Evaluate degree of angulation as well as rotation of great toe.
4. **Radiographic evaluation.** Standing AP and lateral radiographs of the foot are recommended. On the AP radiograph, one can assess the following parameters: the first-second intermetatarsal angle, the first metatarsal-phalangeal angle, the length of the first metatarsal, and the congruency of metatarsophalangeal joint. In patients with hallux valgus, the intermetatarsal angle is greater than 10 degrees and the metatarsophalangeal angle is greater than 20 degrees.
5. **Treatment.** It is important to distinguish the functional problems that the patient is experiencing as well as the patient's and the parents' concerns. In the adolescent patient in whom the primary concern is the appearance of the foot, every effort should me made to educate and counsel the family. For patients with a symptomatic hallux valgus deformity, strong consideration should be afforded to postponing any surgical treatment until skeletal maturity is reached because there is a high recurrence rate of bunions in young adolescent patients. If surgery is considered,

careful examination of the foot is necessary to correct all of the underlying deformities, thus decreasing the risk of recurrence and increasing the likelihood of patient satisfaction.

   6. **Surgical options.** There are several surgical options. Treatment options usually consist of **soft-tissue procedures** (adductor hallucis release and medial capsule advancement) in conjunction with a **distal first metatarsal osteotomy** (Chevron, Mitchell) or a **proximal first metatarsal osteotomy.** Peterson has described a first metatarsal double (proximal and distal) osteotomy. Geissele reported that the reduction of the intermetatarsal angle is the factor that correlates most highly with both decreased risk of recurrence of angular deformity and with patient satisfaction.

V. Childhood knee disorders
A. Patellofemoral pain syndrome

   1. **Definition.** Previously termed "chondromalacia patellae" or "anterior knee pain syndrome," it describes a condition in which the pain is attributed to the patellofemoral joint. It typically is characterized by pain localized to the front of the knee.
   2. **Patient history.** Adolescent girls are usually affected more often than boys, and there is a gradual onset, most often atraumatic. There are no symptoms of locking or buckling. Pain is frequently associated with activities such as walking, running, descending stairs, and sitting for prolonged periods.
   3. **Physical examination.** One should include a thorough examination of the knee, paying particular attention to evaluate tracking of the patella, patella mobility medially and laterally, and Q-angle (alignment of extensor mechanism measured by angle of line from ASIS to patella and line from patella to tibial tubercle). Also assess the lower extremity rotational profile (see **II.C.**)
   4. **Radiographs.** AP, lateral and patella views should be obtained to evaluate for evidence of patellar tilt as well as to rule out other potential sources of knee symptoms such as osteochondritis desiccans and bony lesions.
   5. **Treatment.** Most patients with patellofemoral knee pain respond to a course of conservative treatment consisting of hamstring stretching in addition to closed-chain quadriceps (specifically vastus medialis obliquus [VMO]) strengthening. This may be augmented by use of a patellar-taping program or a patella-stabilizing neoprene knee sleeve in some patients.

B. Acute patella dislocation

   1. **Patient history.** Patients may have experienced a traumatic or a nontraumatic patella subluxation or dislocation. The patella dislocates laterally. The patient may be tender over the medial retinaculum and a joint effusion may be present.
   2. **Radiographic evaluation.** AP/lateral/patella views of the knee should be closely evaluated for any evidence of osteochondral fragments. The patella may knock off an osteochondral fragment from the lateral femoral condyle within the process of dislocating or relocating.
   3. **Treatment.** If osteochondral fragments are present, the knee should be evaluated arthroscopically. Very large fragments may need to be replaced and internally fixed; smaller fragments may simply be removed. If no osteochondral fracture is identified, treatment may consist of a short period of immobilization with a soft-sided knee immobilized followed by a program of quadriceps strengthening exercises.

C. Chronic patella instability

   1. **Patient history.** Some patients may have recurrent patella subluxation/relocation episodes. The initial course of treatment should consist of physical therapy and quadriceps strengthening exercises. If these are not successful in achieving improvement of the instability, surgical stabilization may be indicated. In the skeletally immature patient, this may consist of

a proximal realignment procedure such as an advancement of the VMO or a medial capsular plication as well as a lateral retinacular release. In the skeletally mature patient in whom the tibial apophysis is closed and there is an increased Q-angle, these procedures may be combined with a medialization of the tibial tubercle.

D. Congenital dislocation of the patella
1. **Presentation.** This condition usually presents in newborn or infant patients as a knee flexion contracture in conjunction with an external rotation deformity of the lower leg. Inspection reveals an "empty" femoral trochlea. The patella is unossified and does not appear on radiographs. It is found tethered laterally at the level of the femoral condyle. The patella, the trochlea, and the lateral femoral condyle are hypoplastic.
2. **Treatment.** Surgical correction should be performed before walking age. Correction consists of an extensive lateral release of the quadriceps and iliotibial band, a medial capsular plication and VMO advancement, stabilization of the patella with a semitendinosus tenodesis, and a patellar tendon centralization.

E. Discoid meniscus
1. **Presentation.** Patients with a discoid meniscus may have knee pain as early as age 4 years. Most patients are first seen between ages 6 and 12 years or older. The incidence varies and is estimated to be from 3% to 5% in Anglo Saxons and as much as 20% in Japanese. The majority of cases involve the lateral meniscus. Patients usually have complaints of snapping or popping of the knee.
2. **Physical examination.** Examination of the knee may reveal snapping with flexion of the knee. Unstable menisci may snap or pop in extension.
3. **Classification.** There are three principle types. Type I is stable, complete. Type II is stable, incomplete. Type III is unstable because of the absence of the meniscotibial ligament.
4. **Treatment.** For stable discoid lateral meniscus, arthroscopic sculpting of the meniscus to a normal configuration is indicated. If it is unstable, stabilization with a capsular suture is recommended.

F. Referred pain
1. **Definition.** Pain originating in one location but localized by the patient as arising from a nearby, different location.
2. Many children complain of lower extremity pain and the clinician's challenge is to determine the source of the symptoms. Children and adolescents (as well as adults) may have referred pain in which disorders occurring at one site present with pain at a distal location. A classic example is the overweight adolescent boy with knee pain. An exhaustive evaluation of the knee reveals no obvious cause of his symptoms. However, a careful and thorough examination of the entire lower extremity reveals a slipped capital femoral epiphysis. To avoid the common pitfalls, one must consider all of the diagnostic possibilities and complete a thorough evaluation.

2. Common childhood hip disorders
A. Developmental dysplasia of the hip
1. **Definition.** A spectrum of disorders ranging from complete dislocation of the femoral head to a reduced hip joint with acetabular dysplasia.
2. **Incidence.** DDH occurs in approximately 1 in 1,000 live births.
3. **Risk factors** include being first born and female, being in breech position in utero, having oligohydramnios, and having a positive family history. It has also been associated with other congenital conditions including congenital muscular torticollis, metatarsus adductus, and clubfeet.
4. **Physical examination.** In the newborn child or young infant, physical examination should start with a careful evaluation of the other parts of the child other than the hips, including the spine, neck, and upper and lower extremities. Then, focus examination on the hips, trying to detect any evidence of instability. The clinical tests performed include the Barlow/Ortolani and Galeazzi tests. The **Barlow** and **Ortolani**

tests are performed with the clinician stabilizing the pelvis with one hand and grasping the child's femur with the other, placing the thumb over the medial femoral condyle and the long finger over the greater trochanter. The hip is flexed to 90 degrees and held in neutral abduction. The Ortolani maneuver consists of abducting the hip and trying to detect the "clunking" sensation of the dislocated femoral head relocating into the acetabulum. Likewise, the Barlow test consists of two maneuvers. The first consists of adducting the hip with gentle longitudinal pressure to provoke the hip to dislocate or subluxate. The second maneuver is the same as that described for the Ortolani maneuver to achieve reduction of the dislocated hip. The **Galeazzi** test is comprised of comparing the height of the knees with the hips flexed to discern any apparent femoral shortening. One should also check for symmetric degrees of hip abduction as well as for asymmetry of the perineal skin folds. Finally, DDH can be bilateral, which can be easily missed because there is no apparent asymmetry. These children may first come to attention after walking age, with increased lumbar lordosis, limb length difference, or waddling gait caused by abductor weakness.

5. **Radiographic evaluation.** In the young infant, ultrasound is the modality of choice to detect any evidence of hip abnormality. The ultrasound allows a static assessment of acetabular development (alpha and beta angles) and percentage of femoral head coverage as well as dynamic assessment of femoral head stability with stress maneuvers. In children older than 6 months, plain AP radiographs are sufficient.

6. **Treatment**

   a. **Age 0 to 6 months.** In the newborn child up to 6 months of age, treatment consists of abduction bracing, usually performed with a **Pavlik harness.** This is usually applied at the time the instability is noted. It may also be used for children with a clinically stable hip but who have significant acetabular dysplasia noted on ultrasound. Moreover, the adequacy of the reduction or positioning in the Pavlik harness can be evaluated with ultrasound. There have been several reports in the literature of "Pavlik harness disease" in which the femoral head was not adequately reduced in the acetabulum while in the harness, leading to progressive deformation of the posterior wall of the acetabulum and exacerbation of the dysplasia. If an adequate, concentric reduction of the femoral head cannot be achieved by 4 weeks after the harness has been applied, it should be abandoned.

   b. **Age 6–18 months or the child who fails Pavlik harness treatment.** Treatment for this group is aimed at achieving a satisfactory, congruent, stable reduction. This is achieved by performing either a **closed** or an **open** reduction. Historically, traction has been employed preoperatively in order to decrease the risk of avascular necrosis of the femoral head after closed reduction. An arthrogram is frequently performed at the time of the closed reduction. If the hip is noted to have a narrow "stable zone," a limited adductor release may be performed to improve stability. If a concentric reduction is not achievable or if excessive force is required to maintain the reduction, then an open reduction may be performed. Popular methods for performing the open reduction include an anterolateral approach and the medial approach.

   c. **Age older than 18 months.** Some authors still advocate a trial of preoperative skin traction followed by attempted closed reduction. Alternatively, one can consider open reduction performed in conjunction with femoral shortening to reduce soft-tissue tension and thereby decrease risk of avascular necrosis. If significant acetabular dysplasia is present, a pelvic osteotomy may also be performed.

   d. **Secondary procedures.** For older children with persistent acetabular dysplasia or persistent hip subluxation, secondary procedures may take the form of femoral or pelvic osteotomies. Adolescents or young adults may have hip pain and previously undiagnosed dysplasia. They may be candidates for a redirectional pelvic osteotomy.

B. Legg-Calve-Perthes Disease
1. **Definition.** A condition that affects the hip joint in children; it results from a compromise of the vascular supply to the femoral head, resulting in osteonecrosis.
2. **Presentation.** Most often, Legg-Calve-Perthes disease affects children age 4 to 8 years old; however, it may affect children as young as 2 or as old as 12 years. The ratio of incidence in boys to girls is 4:1. The disease may be bilateral in 10% of patients. Patients frequently have younger skeletal age than cohorts. Frequently, the disease presents as a painless limp (Fig. 5-2.).
3. **Etiology: idiopathic.** It has been associated with abnormalities of thrombolysis as well as deficiencies of protein C, protein S, or thrombolysin.
4. **Differential diagnosis.** If bilateral hip involvement is present on radiograph, then other etiologies should be excluded, including renal disease, hypothyroidism, multiple epiphyseal dysplasia or spondyloepiphyseal dysplasia, systemic corticosteroid use, storage disorders, and hemoglobinopathies.
5. **Stages.** Waldenström originally described evolutionary stages that the disease course follows. These have been modified from the original description to include the following:
   a. **Initial stage.** Femoral head appears sclerotic early in the course of the disease.
   b. **Fragmentation stage.** Presence of subchondral fracture (Salter sign) is hallmark of onset. The femoral head assumes "fragmented" appearance as necrotic bone undergoes resorption.
   c. **Reossification stage.** There is evidence of healing; coalescence of femoral head fragmentation begins to occur.
   d. **Healed stage.** Reossification is complete. Femoral head returns to predisease density. Any remaining deformity is permanent.
6. **Classification systems.** To describe and to compare the results of treatment, various classification systems have been described.
   a. **Catterall.** Four-part system (I-IV) based on the amount of femoral head involvement
   b. **Salter-Thompson.** Two part system (A, B) simplified to <50% or >50% involvement of femoral head.
   c. **Herring:** Three-part system (A, B, C) based on height of lateral "pillar" (lateral one third of femoral epiphysis).
7. **Treatment.** For patients with Legg-Calve-Perthes disease, it is important to determine which patients to treat as well as how to treat them. Thus, one must determine which children have a poor prognosis and are at risk for having a poor outcome, therefore requiring treatment. Children who are younger than 6 years old or who have Herring group A head involvement have a good prognosis. Treatment for this group consists of primarily symptomatic treatment as well as an effort to maintain good hip range of motion. In contrast, children who are older than 6 years and who have Herring group B or group C involvement have a worse prognosis. Therefore, treatment is recommended for this group of patients. Treatment is aimed at achieving and maintaining femoral head containment within the acetabulum. Historically, **abduction bracing** was recommended. However, recent studies have questioned how effectively the brace is able to achieve containment of the femoral head, and they are now used less frequently. Surgical options include a **femoral varus osteotomy, innominate osteotomy,** or a combination of the two. Salvage procedures for patients with significant residual deformity consist of a Chiari pelvic osteotomy or a shelf procedure with or without a valgus femoral osteotomy.

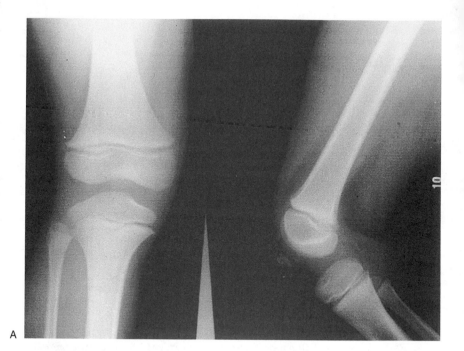

A

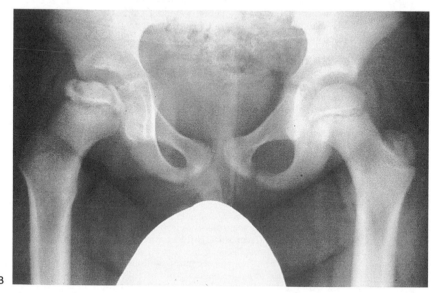

B

FIG. 5-2. A 6-year-old boy with a 1- to 2-month history of limping and right knee pain. **A:** Radiographs of the knee are normal. **B:** An anteroposterior pelvis radiograph reveals changes in the right hip consistent with Legg-Calve-Perthes disease.

C. Slipped capital femoral epiphysis
1. **Definition.** A disorder of the upper femur in which there is a separation (acutely or chronically) of the femoral epiphysis from the femoral neck through the region of the physis (growth plate). The femoral head becomes positioned posterior and inferior relative to the femoral neck.
2. **Incidence.** Approximately 3 in 100,000 children are affected, boys more frequently than girls. Bilateral involvement occurs in between 20% and 60% of cases. SCFE is seen most frequently in boys (ages 9–16 years) and in girls (ages 8–15 years). SCFE is associated with obesity with more then half of affected individuals weighing greater than the 95% percentile. Patients with an underlying hormonal or endocrine disorder have an associated increased risk for development of SCFE. A careful evaluation for endocrine disorders should be considered, including hypothyroidism, hypopituitarism, hypogonadism, parathyroid adenoma, pituitary tumor, and growth hormone abnormality for patients with bilateral involvement or who are an atypical age at presentation.
3. **Classification**
   a. **Temporal.** One method of classification is based on duration of symptoms. Acute is less than 3 weeks, chronic is greater than 3 weeks and acute-on-chronic is a sudden exacerbation of subclinical symptoms of longstanding duration.
   b. **Stability.** This classification system has gained greater popularity because it appears to be clinically more useful. A **stable SCFE** enables the patient to walk without assistance, with mild pain or discomfort. Patients with an **unstable SCFE** are unable to walk or to bear weight. Unstable SCFEs are associated with a higher rate of complications.
   c. **Displacement.** Classified according to the amount of displacement of the femoral head. This may be represented as a percentage of the femoral neck width or as an angular value measured by the lateral head-shaft angle.
4. **Treatment.** The most widely recommended form of treatment is surgical stabilization with **percutaneous pinning** *in situ*. For a stable SCFE, this can usually be accomplished with a single, cannulated screw inserted under fluoroscopic control. The aim of the procedure is to insert the screw perpendicular to the femoral head in both the AP and lateral planes with close attention to avoid penetrating the femoral head and entering the hip joint. In cases of an unstable SCFE, a second screw may be inserted to further stabilize the femoral head (Fig. 5-3.) Patients who have a severe amount of displacement may experience discomfort as a result of the distortion of the hip range of motion. For symptomatic cases, a redirectional osteotomy of the proximal femur may be performed. This can be performed at one of several levels from the femoral neck to the subtrochanteric level. The closer to the femoral neck this is performed, the greater the amount of correction can be accomplished; however, the risk of complications is greater. These are technically challenging procedures and should be performed by someone who performs them with frequency.
5. **Complications.** The primary complications associated with SCFE are **avascular necrosis** and **chondrolysis**. Avascular necrosis is uncommon with stable SCFE treated with pinning *in situ*. There is a greater incidence of avascular necrosis associated with unstable SCFE. A vigorous attempt at reduction of an unstable SCFE should not be performed. Chondrolysis is a gradual loss of the joint space. It has been associated with treatment with one or more pins as well as with a spica cast in which no internal fixation was used.

VII. Infectious and inflammatory conditions
   A. **Osteomyelitis**
   1. **Definition.** An inflammatory condition caused by an infection in bone and the medullary canal. This discussion refers to bacterial infections.

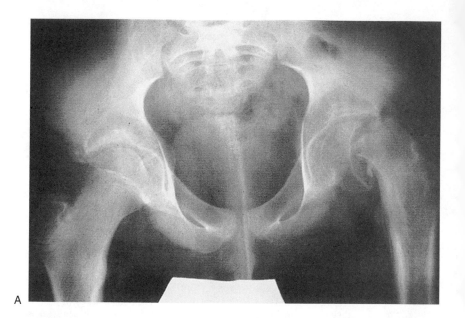

A

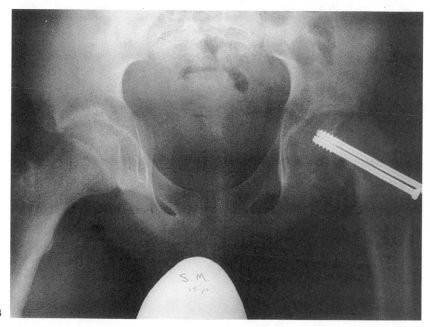

B

FIG. 5-3. Slipped capital femoral epiphysis. **A:** A 13-year-old boy with a severe, unstable left slipped capital femoral epiphysis. **B:** Two cannulated screws were inserted for stabilization.

2. **Etiology.** Bacterial seeding can occur through several methods: direct inoculation (open fractures, penetrating wounds), local extension from adjacent sites, or hematogenous spread from distant sites. Children are skeletally immature and have physes at the ends of their long bones. In the metaphyseal region of the bone just below the physis, the blood vessels form a venous sinusoid, which results in sluggish blood flow and a region of relatively low oxygen partial pressure (pO_2). This creates a hospitable environment for bacterial proliferation.
3. **Presentation.** Patients may have pain, limp, and refuse to walk or bear weight on the affected lower extremity. Constitutional symptoms of fever, malaise, and flu may or may not be present. One should inquire about immunization status as well as history of recent illnesses (e.g., otitis media, chicken pox, strep pharyngitis, upper respiratory tract illness (URTI).
4. **Physical examination.** Site of involvement may or may not be easy to identify, particularly in younger patients. Careful palpation of entire extremity and the metaphyseal regions in particular is important. All joints should be placed through a range of motion. Inspect for sites of redness, swelling, or warmth.
5. **Laboratory studies.** CBC with differential, ESR, CRP, and blood cultures are helpful in making the diagnosis. The CRP has been recognized as a more rapidly responsive test than the ESR, increasing more quickly early in the evolution of the condition and declining more rapidly in response to treatment. If the diagnosis remains unclear, consider other diagnostic possibilities such as JRA, Lyme arthritis, and poststreptococcal arthritis.
6. **Radiographic studies.** Plain radiographs of the affected area should be obtained. In osteomyelitis they may frequently be normal for the first 7 to 14 days. However, the radiographs may also be useful to rule out other diagnostic possibilities. In patients with normal radiographs in whom the diagnosis is still unclear, a technetium bone scan is a sensitive test for acute osteomyelitis. It is particularly helpful in cases involving the pelvis, proximal femur, and spine. MRI is also very sensitive and has the added benefit of having greater soft-tissue detail allowing assessment of marrow involvement, soft-tissue extension or abscess formation, and presence of joint effusions. However, MRI is expensive and frequently requires significant sedation or anesthesia for younger patients.
7. **Aspiration.** In patients with an identified focus of infection, an attempt at aspiration is recommended by many authors to identify the organism. This may be done with sedation in the emergency department or the fluoroscopic suite or alternatively under anesthesia in the operating room.
8. **Organisms.** Based on patient age:
    a. **Younger than 1 year old**
        (1) *Staphylococcus aureus*
        (2) Group B *Streptococcus*
        (3) *Escherichia coli*
    b. **1–4 years old**
        (1) *S. aureus*
        (2) *Haemophilus influenzae*
    c. **Older than 4 years old**
        (1) *S. aureus*
    d. **Adolescent**
        (1) *S. aureus*
        (2) *Neisseria gonorrhoeae*
9. **Treatment.** Appropriate intravenous antibiotic based on culture or most likely organism. Duration of antibiotic coverage is typically 6 weeks. After 2–3 weeks of intravenous treatment, the patient may be switched to oral antibiotics if the following criteria are met: (1) organism has been identified, (2) there is a satisfactory oral antibiotic to which the organism is sensitive, (3) child will take the oral antibiotic, and (4) satisfactory serum levels can be achieved with oral therapy.

10. **Surgical treatment.** If the patient does not respond to antibiotic treatment after the first 24–48 hours, consider the possibility of subperiosteal abscess or other diagnostic possibilities. Consider surgical drainage of abscess and intramedullary canal if necessary.

B. **Septic arthritis**
   1. **Definition.** An infectious arthritis of a joint, usually bacterial in nature.
   2. **Etiology.** Most frequently, it occurs as a result from adjacent osteomyelitis in which the metaphyseal portion of the bone is intraarticular (e.g., hip, shoulder, elbow, ankle). When pus from metaphysis decompresses itself through cortex, joints can become infected. Infection is also possible through hematogenous spread or direct inoculation as well.
   3. **Joints most commonly involved are the** knee (41%), hip (23%), ankle (14%), elbow (12%), wrist (4%), and shoulder (4%).
   4. **Presentation.** Young children usually refuse to walk or bear weight on the lower extremity. If infection is in the upper extremity, children simply refuse to use the affected extremity. Septic arthritis may also occur in the newborn child, particularly babies in the NICU in whom indwelling catheters are frequently present. These children may have pseudoparalysis of the affected limb with failure or refusal to move it.
   5. **Physical examination.** If the joint involved is superficial, classic signs of joint redness, swelling, and warmth are present. However, if the joint is not superficial (hip, shoulder), no visible abnormality may be detectable. However, the patient will hold the affected limb in a position of maximum comfort (e.g., keep the hip in flexion and external rotation). Any attempt at passive range of motion is painful and restricted because of guarding.
   6. **Laboratory studies** include CBC with differential, ESR, and CRP.
   7. **Radiographic studies.** Plain radiographs of the affected joint should be obtained to look for any evidence of bony destruction or erosions. For patients with suspected hip pain, an ultrasound of the hip may confirm the presence of a hip joint effusion. In some institutions, aspiration is performed under ultrasound guidance.
   8. **Joint aspiration** is mandatory to confirm the diagnosis. Joint fluid should be sent for cell count, Gram stain, and culture, and if quantity permits glucose and total protein. If the patient is a teenager in whom gonococcal infection is suspected, the laboratory should be notified in order to perform cultures on chocolate agar in addition to the routine media. The Gram stain may be positive for bacteria in only approximately 50% of patients. The cell count most often has greater than 50,000 white blood cells (WBCs) and/or greater than 90% polymorphonuclear neutrophils (PMNs).
   9. **Organisms.** Based on patient age:
      a. **Younger than 1 year old**
         (1) *S. aureus*
         (2) Group B *Streptococcus*
         (3) *E. coli*
      b. **1–4 years old**
         (1) *S. aureus*
         (2) *H. influenzae*
         (3) Group A *Streptococcus*
         (4) *Streptococcus pneumoniae*
      c. **Older than 4 years old**
         (1) *S. aureus*
         (2) Group A *Streptococcus*
      d. **Adolescent**
         (1) *S. aureus*
         (2) *N. gonorrhoeae*
      e. **Less common** organisms include *Kingella kingae, Salmonella, Neisseria meningitidis*, and anaerobes.
   10. **Treatment.** In patients suspected of septic arthritis, treatment consists of surgical incision and drainage of the affected joint. Intravenous anti-

biotics should be administered once intraoperative cultures have been obtained. Empiric coverage should be started initially based on the most likely organism involved. Once culture and sensitivities have been identified, antibiotic coverage can be tailored accordingly. The duration of antibiotics is usually 4–6 weeks. An initial course of intravenous antibiotics is followed by oral therapy until the patient's symptoms and laboratory studies have returned to normal.

C. **Transient synovitis**
   1. **Definition.** An inflammatory, noninfectious process resulting in joint swelling and pain.
   2. **Presentation.** Transient synovitis most frequently occurs in young children ages 3–8 years old. Patients often may have had a recent upper respiratory tract illness or other viral illness in the 2–3 weeks before onset of symptoms. Patients are usually afebrile with a history of several days of pain or limping. The physician must differentiate between transient synovitis and a truly infectious process such as septic arthritis or osteomyelitis.
   3. **Laboratory studies.** CBC with differential, ESR, and CRP are usually within the normal range.
   4. **Radiographic studies.** Plain radiographs are usually normal or may show evidence of a joint effusion. Ultrasound is helpful for confirming the presence of a joint effusion.
   5. **Aspiration.** Because the clinician is often confronted with having to exclude septic arthritis, joint aspiration can be helpful in order to examine the joint fluid. A Gram stain, cell count, and culture should be obtained. The Gram stain should be negative and the cell count should have between 5,000 and 15,000 WBCs with less than 25% PMNs.
   6. **Treatment.** The primary treatment objective in the treatment of transient synovitis is to ensure that septic arthritis has been excluded. Once septic arthritis is excluded, then the condition can be treated expectantly with reduction in activity, nonsteroidal antiinflammatory medications, and careful observation.

VIII. **Scoliosis and kyphosis**
   A. **Idiopathic adolescent scoliosis**
      1. **Definition.** A deformity of the spine consisting of a lateral curvature measuring greater than 10 degrees on a spine radiograph and which also has a rotational component. The word "idiopathic" suggests no identifiable, underlying cause. There may be a genetic component.
      2. **Presentation.** Most often patients are adolescent girls who have been detected either on school screening examination or by an observant primary physician. Boys are affected less often and have a lower incidence of progressive curves. The deformity may occasionally be seen in younger children. Family history is usually positive. Idiopathic scoliosis should be painless. The examiner should inquire about any neurologic symptoms including weakness, numbness, radicular symptoms, or bowel or bladder changes.
      3. **Incidence.** For curves greater than 10 degrees, the overall incidence is 2%. However, for curves measuring greater than 20 degrees and requiring treatment, the incidence is 0.2%.
      4. **Physical examination.** All patients should be examined in a gown so that the back can be well visualized. Inspect pelvic height for evidence of limb length difference. Examine shoulder height and trunk position for evidence of asymmetry. With the patient standing, have the patient bend forward at the waist. Observe the patient's back for evidence of rib cage deformity. This is the **Adam's forward bending test.** Finally, complete a thorough neurologic examination, including abdominal reflexes and tests, for evidence of long tract or upper motor neuron lesions.
      5. **Radiographic evaluation.** Radiographs should include a standing posteroanterior (PA) and lateral spine study on a long cassette to include

the thoracic, lumbar, and sacral regions of the spine. The curvature of the spine can be measured using the Cobb method.

6. **Characteristics.** For true idiopathic scoliosis, the spine is most often a painless curve that is convex to the right in the thoracic spine, the curve is not associated with any neurologic changes, and it is at risk for progression during periods of accelerated skeletal growth. If a curve does not fit this pattern, one must exclude other possible causes. If the curve is convex to the left, painful, has associated neurologic changes, or is rapidly progressive, one should consider obtaining an MRI scan in order to rule out possible underlying spinal cord abnormalities such as syringomyelia, tethered cord, diastematomyelia, or spinal cord tumor.

7. **Risk factors for progression** include young age, female gender, prepubertal status, and curve greater than 11 degrees.

8. The **goal of treatment** is to prevent further progression of the curve.

9. **Treatment** of idiopathic scoliosis depends on the size of the curve as well as the age of the patient at the time of detection. Typically, for curves greater than 11 degrees and less than 20 degrees, treatment consists of **observation** with repeat spine radiographs obtained in 4 to 6 months. The younger the child at the time of curve detection, the greater the risk for future progression of the curve. If the curve is greater than 20–25 degrees in a skeletally immature patient, **brace treatment** is indicated. Brace treatment is most effective in moderate-sized and flexible curves in growing adolescents. The goal of brace treatment is to arrest any further progression of the curve. For patients in whom a large curve of greater than 45 to 50 degrees is already present or for whom the curve progresses despite brace treatment, treatment is **surgical spinal fusion with instrumentation.**

B. **Kyphosis**

1. **Definition.** An increased curvature of the spine seen on the lateral radiograph as involving the thoracic spine, producing a rounded-back appearance.

2. **Characteristics.** Normal thoracic kyphosis is 20–45 degrees. **Scheuermann's disease** is a condition in which the curve is greater than 45 degrees and associated with wedging of three adjacent central vertebral bodies of 5 degrees or more. It may be associated with end plate changes of the vertebral bodies such as Schmorl's nodes. It should be distinguished from postural kyphosis in which the vertebral bodies do not exhibit changes and the curvature resolves with improvement of the patient's posture.

3. **Presentation.** Patients usually have one of two complaints: pain or concerns regarding appearance.

4. **Physical examination.** Careful examination of the back with the patient standing, on forward bending, and with hyperextension in the prone position can help determine the flexibility of the kyphosis. Increased thoracic kyphosis is frequently associated with increased lumbar lordosis. The possibility of hip flexion contractures should be assessed. A careful neurologic examination should also be performed.

5. **Radiographs.** Standing PA and lateral thoracolumbar spine radiographs should be obtained.

6. **Treatment.** Options include observation, bracing, and surgery. For patients who are asymptomatic with a relatively small curve, one may consider continued observation. For symptomatic patients who are skeletally immature with curves greater than 45–50 degrees, one may consider brace treatment. For symptomatic patients who are approaching skeletal maturity with curves greater than 70–75 degrees, one may consider spinal fusion surgery, which frequently consists of a combined anterior release and posterior instrumentation.

C. **Lordosis**

1. **Definition.** An increase in "swayback" appearance of the lower lumbar spine.

2. **Presentation.** The patient may complain of low back pain, concern regarding appearance, or both.
3. **Etiology.** Possible causes include posture (especially in younger patients), bilateral congenital dislocation of the hip, hip flexion contracture, hamstring weakness, increased thoracic kyphosis, spondylolysis/spondylolisthesis, and congenital spinal deformity.
4. **Physical examination** should include careful evaluation of the back, hips, and lower extremities and should also include a thorough neurologic evaluation.
5. **Radiographs.** PA and lateral thoracolumbar spine radiographs should be obtained.
6. **Treatment.** Careful exclusion of underlying abnormalities should be undertaken. If other underlying causes have been excluded and the cause is thought to be postural, then treatment may consist of further observation.

IX. **Neuromuscular disorders**
  A. **Cerebral palsy**
    1. **Definition.** A nonprogressive disorder resulting from an injury to the brain, usually within the first year of life, and resulting in impairment in motor function.
    2. **Classification** can be geographic (part of body most affected) or by type of motor dysfunction.
      a. **Geographic**
        (1) **Hemiplegia.** Arm and leg on one side only affected
        (2) **Diplegia.** Major spasticity in lower limbs, less in upper
        (3) **Triplegia.** Three-limb involvement
        (4) **Quadriplegia.** All four limbs, "total body involved"
      b. **Motor type**
        (1) **Spastic.** Increased stretch reflexes (pyramidal)
        (2) **Athetoid.** Fluctuating motor tone, often with spontaneous, involuntary rhythmic motor movements (extrapyramidal)
        (3) **Dystonia.** Similar to athetoid, intermittent, inconsistent tone
        (4) **Mixed.** A combination of spasticity and dystonia
    3. **Causes**
      a. **Prenatal.** Intrauterine infection, for example, TORCH (toxoplasmosis, rubella, cytomegalovirus, and herpes simplex), genetic
      b. **Perinatal.** Premature birth, low birth weight, asphyxia, erythroblastosis fetalis
      c. **Postnatal.** Infection, stroke, cardiac arrest, near-drowning
    4. **Hierarchical approach to problems**
      a. **Primary problems** include abnormal muscle tone, poor selective muscle control, and poor balance.
      b. **Secondary problems** include muscle and joint contractures, bony deformities (increased femoral anteversion, tibial torsion, and foot deformities).
      c. **Tertiary problems** include compensatory mechanisms for primary and secondary problems.
    5. **Treatment**
      a. **Physical therapy**
      b. **Orthotics**
      c. **Assistive devices:** wheelchair, walker, crutches
      d. **Tone-reducing agents or medications:** oral (e.g., baclofen, Valium, dantrolene) or local (e.g., Botox, phenol)
      e. **Neurosurgical options:** selective dorsal rhizotomy, intrathecal baclofen pump
      f. **Orthopaedic surgery:** soft-tissue lengthening procedures, bony realignment procedures
    6. **Nonambulatory patients.** The principle difficulties that affect patients with total body involvement are hip dislocation and scoliosis. These are

important issues for these patients because they are wheelchair-bound and frequently mentally handicapped. Painful sitting or difficulty with sitting balance resulting from scoliosis or pelvic obliquity can interfere significantly with their activities of daily living, personal care, and activity level. Patients should be monitored regularly for early detection of either hip dislocation or scoliosis.

7. **Ambulatory patients.** If children have independent sitting balance by age 2 years old, then there is approximately a 95% chance that they will eventually be able to ambulate. Children with cerebral palsy who can ambulate usually have difficulty because of increased motor tone, poor selective motor control, which results in co-contracture of muscle groups, and poor balance. Frequently, muscle contractures and bony deformities develop over time. Three-dimensional gait analysis is an invaluable tool used to assess walking in these children. Orthopaedic surgery usually consists of muscle lengthening or transfer procedures combined with bony realignment procedures for underlying torsional deformities of the lower extremities. Most often, these are combined in one surgical setting to minimize recovery time and to speed the child's return to activities. The **selective dorsal rhizotomy** is a procedure to decrease lower extremity tone by cutting approximately 30% to 40% of the dorsal afferent nerve rootlets. It is indicated for children with spastic diplegia, who have pure spasticity, no contractures, and good balance. It is usually performed in children between the ages of 4 and 8 years old. For children with cerebral palsy, optimum treatment consists of a combined approach involving the physiatrist, the neurosurgeon, the orthopaedic surgeon, the physical and occupational therapists, and the orthotist.

B. **Spina bifida**
   1. **Definition.** A malformation at the base of the spine, resulting from incomplete closure of the neural tube in which the meninges and neural elements are exposed.
   2. **Etiology** is multifactorial. There is a genetic component in that there is increased risk for first-degree relatives of patients with spina bifida. There is also an environmental role linked to insufficient dietary folic acid for childbearing age women.
   3. **Classification** is based on the level of neurologic deficit.
   4. **Associated disorders** include hydrocephalus requiring ventriculoperitoneal shunting, tethered spinal cord, Arnold-Chiari malformations, syringomyelia, and urologic problems.
   5. **Orthopaedic conditions** include scoliosis for patients with high thoracic level deficits, excessive spinal kyphosis, hip dislocation, and foot deformities.
   6. **Ambulatory function** is determined primarily by level of deficit. Patients who ambulate are usually patients who maintain active control of knee flexion and extension. Many children ambulate when young, but as they get older, it takes greater energy and oxygen consumption, and many resort to using a wheelchair.

Suggested Readings
1. Bleck EE. *Orthopaedic management in cerebral palsy. Clinics in developmental medicine Nos 99 / 100.* Philadelphia: JB Lippincott, 1987.
2. Broughton NS, Menelaus MB, eds. *Menelaus' orthopaedic management of spina bifida cystica.* Philadelphia: WB Saunders, 1998.
3. Dagan R. Management of acute hematogenous osteomyelitis and septic arthritis in the pediatric patient. *Pediatr Infect Dis J* 1993;12:88–92.
4. Fulkerson JP, Shea KP. Disorders of patellofemoral alignment. *J Bone Joint Surg* 1990;72A:1424–1429.
5. Gage JR. *Gait analysis in cerebral palsy. Clinics in developmental medicine No. 121.* New York: Mac Keith Press, 1991.
6. Geissele AE, Stanton RP. Surgical treatment of adolescent hallux valgus. *J Pediatr Orthop* 1990;10:38–44.

7. Haueisen D, Weisner D, Weiner S. The characterization of transient synovitis of the hip in children. *J Pediatr Orthop* 1986;6:11–17.
8. Heath DH, Staheli LT. Normal limits of knee angle in children, genu varum and genu valgum. *J Pediatr Orthop* 1993;13:259–262.
9. Herring JA. Legg-Calve-Perthes disease: a review of current knowledge. In: Barr JS Jr, ed. *Instructional course lectures XXXVIII*. Park Ridge, IL: American Academy of Orthopaedic Surgeons, 1989:309–315.
10. Loder RT, Richards BS, Shapiro PS, et al. Acute slipped capital femoral epiphysis: the importance of physeal stability. *J Bone Joint Surg* 1993;75A:1134–1140.
11. Lonstein JE, Carlson JM. The prediction of curve progression in untreated scoliosis during growth. *J Bone Joint Surg* 1984;66A:1061–1071.
12. Morrisy RT, Haynes DW. Acute hematogenous osteomyelitis: a model with trauma as an etiology. *J Pediatr Orthop* 1989;9:447–456.
13. Mosca VS. Calcaneal lengthening for valgus deformity of the hindfoot. *J Bone Joint Surg* 1995;77-A:500–512.
14. Murray PM, Weinstein SL, Spratt KF. The natural history and long-term follow-up of Scheuermann's kyphosis. *J Bone Joint Surg* 1993;75A:236–248.
15. Phillips WA. The child with a limp. *Orthop Clin North Am* 1987;18:489–501.
16. Staheli LT. Rotational problems in children. *J Bone Joint Surg* 1993;75A:939.
17. Stanitski CL. Meniscal lesions. In: Stanitski CL, DeLee AB, Drez CD, eds. *Pediatric and adolescent sports medicine*. Philadelphia: WB Saunders, 1994:382–384.
18. Swiontkowski MF, Scranton PE, Hansen S. Tarsal coalitions: long-term results of surgical treatment. *J Pediatr Orthop* 1983;3:287–292.
19. Viere RG, Birch JG, Herring JA, et al. Use of the Pavlik harness in congenital dislocation of the hip, an analysis of failures of treatment. *J Bone Joint Surg* 1990;72A:238–244.
20. Ward WT, Stefko J, Wood KB, et al. Fixation with a single screw for slipped capital femoral epiphysis. *J Bone Joint Surg* 1992;74A:799–809.

Selected Historical Readings

Blount WP, Clarke GR. Control of bone growth by epiphyseal stapling. A preliminary report. *J Bone Joint Surg* 1949;31:464.

Coleman SS. Diagnosis of congenital dysplasia of the hip in the newborn infant. *J Bone Joint Surg* 1956;162:548.

Gage JR, Winter RB. Avascular necrosis of the capital femoral epiphysis as a complication of closed reduction of congenital dislocation of the hip: a critical review of twenty years' experience at Gillette Children's Hospital. *J Bone Joint Surg* 1972; 54:373–388.

Langenskiold A. Tibia vara (osteochondrosis deformans tibiae). A survey of 23 cases. *Acta Chir Scand* 1952;103:1.

Moseley CF. A straight-line graph for leg-length discrepancies. *J Bone Joint Surg* 1977;59A:174–179.

Stulberg SD, Salter RB. The natural course of Legg-Perthes disease and its relationship to degenerative arthritis of the hip: long-term follow-up study. *Orthop Trans* 1977;1:105.

Turco VJ. Resistant congenital clubfoot: one-stage posteromedial release with internal fixation. A follow-up report of a fifteen-year experience. *J Bone Joint Surg* 1979; 61A:805–814.

6. COMMON TYPES OF EMERGENCY SPLINTS

I. **Emergency splinting of the spine**
   A. Patients with spinal injuries should be splinted with a **backboard** before they are moved, as shown in Fig. 6-1. Immobilize cervical spine injuries by placing sandbags, rolled towels, or rolled blankets on each side of the head. Then put a cravat through or around the backboard and over the forehead. **In this way, the head, neck, and backboard can be moved as one unit.** Commercial foam as well as plastic neck collars are available in different sizes. One can also make an adequate neck collar by placing foam or felt of the appropriate width, thickness, and length inside a tubular stockinet and then fastening the stockinet about the patient's neck. This method is particularly useful for immobilizing the neck of injured children. The only emergency indication for moving an individual with an injured cervical spine is to improve an inadequate airway.
   B. Be aware of possible **neurogenic shock,** which is treated by elevating the lower end of the backboard to improve venous return.
   C. If complete evaluation identifies a cervical spine fracture, then the patient is usually placed in **traction.** The direction of traction depends on the injury. If there is no dislocation, then a neutral or slightly extended position is preferred (see Chap. 9).

II. **Upper extremity splinting**
   A. **Remember to remove rings from an involved hand!** Swelling can make them impossible to remove without cutting them off and they obscure x-rays.
   B. Figure-of-8 splint
      1. The **principal use** is for **clavicular fractures** (see Chap. 13).
      2. **Application.** The factory-made figure-of-8 clavicular strap is recommended because it is a webbed fabric and does not stretch. If a properly fitting factory-made strap is not available for children younger than 10 years, make a figure-of-8 strap with a tubular stockinet filled with felt or cotton padding, as shown in Fig. 6-2. These should be used if they make the patient more comfortable. A sling is generally more effective in this regard.
      3. **Precautions**
         a. **Prevent skin maceration** with a **powdered pad** in the axilla.
         b. In the adult, restrict the use of the sling and encourage glenohumeral motion after 2 weeks to **prevent shoulder stiffness.**
         c. Do not tighten the figure-of-8 strap to the point that the **axillary artery or brachial plexus is compressed.**
   C. **Velpeau and sling-and-swathe bandages**
      1. These bandages are **used for shoulder dislocations, proximal humerus fractures, and humeral fractures.**
      2. One **application** of Velpeau's bandage using bias-cut stockinet is seen in Fig. 6-3. The common application of the typical sling-and-swathe bandage is shown in Fig. 6-4. Either type of bandage can be covered with a light layer of plaster to prevent unraveling of the material.
      3. **Precautions**
         a. **Prevent skin maceration** with a **powdered pad** in the axilla and between the arm and chest.
         b. **Prevent wrist and finger stiffness** with active exercise.
      4. A number of commercial **shoulder immobilizers** are available. Although they provide less secure immobilization than the Velpeau and sling-and-swathe bandages, these ready-made items have proved satisfactory. Commercial straps for acromioclavicular separations are also available.

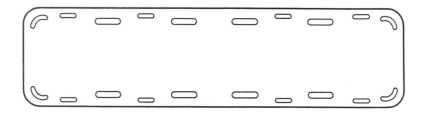

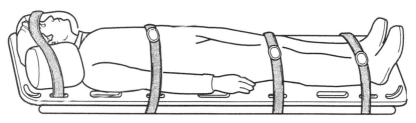

FIG. 6-1. A backboard may be used in an emergency to transport a patient with a spinal injury.

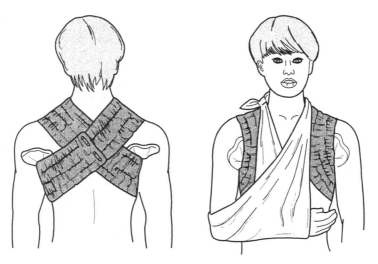

FIG. 6-2. Typical figure-of-8 splint made for a child younger than 10 years with a fractured clavicle. In adults, use a factory-made splint when possible.

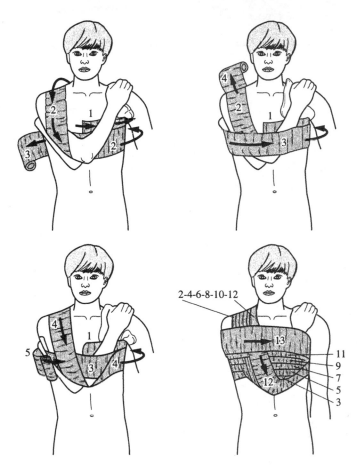

FIG. 6-3. Method for applying Velpeau's bandage.

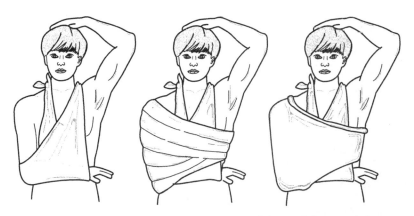

FIG. 6-4. Sling-and-swathe bandage, covered by a single layer of plaster to help prevent unraveling of the material.

D. Use **air splints** in emergency situations for the distal extremities. The air splint is closed over the extremity by its zipper and inflated by flowing air into the mouth tube. A mechanical pump can produce circulatory embarrassment and should not be used. Skin maceration occurs if air splints are used for any extended period. Cardboard or magazines can be used with tape of any sort to achieve immobilization.

II. Lower extremity splinting

A. Thomas splint

1. Use for **femoral shaft fractures** and, **occasionally, knee injuries.** The following description is for the emergency situation. The Thomas splint may also be used as fixed skeletal traction, as described in Chap. 9 **(VII.F.3).**

2. The ideal Thomas splint **application** uses a full ring splint that measures 2 inches greater than the circumference of the proximal thigh. If a full ring splint is not available, use a half ring splint with a strap placed anteriorly. The ring engages the ischial tuberosity for countertraction, and traction is applied to the end of the splint with an ankle hitch, as shown in Fig. 6-5. A Spanish windlass is made by taping several tongue blades together. These twist the material used to secure the ankle hitch to the end of the splint, producing a traction force. The half ring splint still engages the ischial tuberosity, and the strap buckles down across the anterior thigh. Towels or a tubular stockinet placed on the Thomas splint with safety pins support the leg, as shown in Fig. 6-6.

3. **Hare splints and Roller splints** are also commercially available. They differ from the Thomas splint only by the foot attachments and leg supports. They are in widespread use by emergency medical technicians.

4. Most **precautions** relate to complications of fixed skeletal traction and are discussed in Chap. 9 **(VII).** Do not leave the temporary splint on for more than 2 hours, however, because the ankle hitch places significant pressure on the skin and may produce necrosis.

B. Jones compression splint

1. Use in **acute knee trauma** (patellar, knee, and some tibial fractures) and **acute ankle injuries.**

2. Apply by wrapping the injured leg from the toes to the groin in cotton. Next, add a single layer of elastic bandage. Apply 5- × 30-inch plaster splints posteriorly, medially, and laterally to keep the ankle in a neutral position. Medial and lateral splints support the knee in the desired degree of flexion. Do not overlap the splints, or a circumferential plaster will be created about the extremity. The splints are then overwrapped with bias-cut stockinet in a herringbone fashion.

3. **Precautions**

   a. Do not apply **wraps too tightly.**

   b. Do not make **upper wraps tighter than lower wraps** or venous return will be impeded, causing swelling and circulatory problems.

4. Although they provide less satisfactory compression, commercial **knee immobilizers** are acceptable in most cases.

C. Short leg or modified Jones compression splint

1. Use in **acute ankle and foot trauma** such as ankle sprains, calcaneal fractures, and other foot injuries.

2. The splint is **applied** in a fashion similar to that described for the Jones splint except that it does not extend above the tibial tubercle.

3. **Precautions** are the same as those for the Jones compression splint.

D. Commercial leg and ankle braces

1. **Short leg walkers** constructed of a rigid foot piece and double uprights and secured with Velcro fasteners are available for conditions not requiring rigid cast immobilization.

2. **Lace-up canvas ankle supports** with removable aluminum stays are also often convenient and useful.

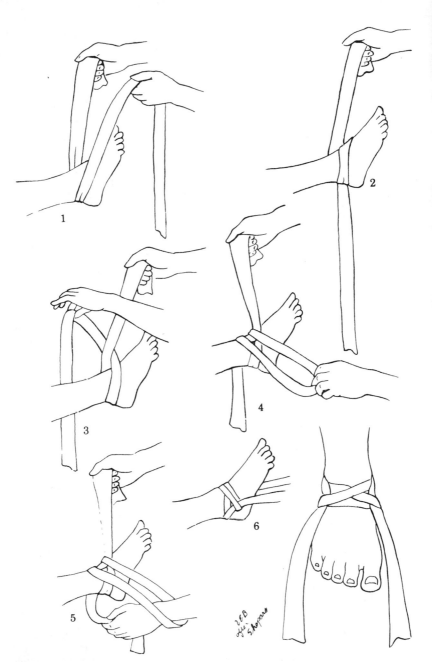

FIG. 6-5. A Collins hitch is a means of applying traction from the ankle to the end of the Thomas splint, but it is used only in emergency situations.

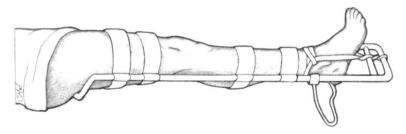

FIG. 6-6. A Thomas splint may be used at the scene of the accident for a fracture of the femur.

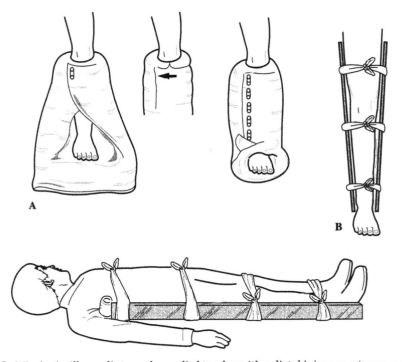

FIG. 6-7. A. A pillow splint may be applied to a leg with a distal injury as a temporary measure. **B.** Board splints may be used for lower-extremity fractures in emergency situations.

3. Air splints with inflatable radial and lateral supports have recently proven extremely useful as supports for ankle sprains and stable fractures that are well along in the healing process.

E. Other emergency splints

1. Make-do splints may be used as a temporary measure. One may apply a pillow splint, rigid cardboard, magazine, or a wooden splint to the upper or lower extremity. A pillow splint for the ankle is shown in Fig. 6-7.

2. Precautions

a. **Avoid circulatory embarrassment** by applying splint straps or wraps in such a way as to prevent pressure on the skin over a bony prominence or a tourniquet effect to the extremity.

b. **Splint**

(1) For **closed fractures,** restore gross angulation into better alignment before the splint is applied by using gentle traction first in the direction of the angulation and then in the long axis of the limb.

(2) Restore alignment in the same manner if there is **tenting of the skin** over the injury.

(3) For **open fractures,** gross alignment should be restored, the wound inspected and dressed with sterile technique, and a splint applied.

c. Cover **exposed bone** with a saline-moistened sterile dressing as first aid treatment.

7. CAST AND BANDAGING TECHNIQUES

I. Materials and equipment
A. Plaster (2,7)
1. Plaster bandages and splints are made by **impregnating crinoline with plaster of Paris**—($[CaSO_4]_2H_2O$). When this material is dipped into water, the powdery plaster of paris is transformed into a solid crystalline form of gypsum, and heat is given off:

$$(CaSO_4)_2H_2O + 3H_2O \quad \underset{\longrightarrow}{\longleftarrow} \quad 2(CaSO_4 \times 2H_2O) + heat$$

Anhydrous calcium sulfate: Hydrated calcium sulfate:
plaster of paris   gypsum

2. The amount of heat given off is determined by the amount of plaster applied and the temperature of the water (3,5). The more plaster and the hotter the water, the more heat is generated. The interlocking of the crystals formed is essential to the strength and rigidity of the cast. Motion during the **critical setting period** interferes with this interlocking process and reduces the ultimate strength by as much as 77%. The interlocking of crystals (the critical setting period) begins when the plaster reaches the thick creamy stage, becomes a little rubbery, and starts losing its wet, shiny appearance. Cast drying occurs by the evaporation of the water not required for crystallization. The evaporation from the cast surface is influenced by air temperature, humidity, and circulation about the cast. Thick casts take longer to dry than thin ones. Strength increases as drying occurs.
3. Plaster is available as bandage **rolls** in widths of 8, 6, 3, and 2 inches and **splints** in 5- × 45-inch, 5- × 30-inch, 4- × 15-inch, and 3- × 15-inch sizes. Additives are used to alter the setting time. Three variations are available. Extra-fast setting takes 2–4 minutes, fast setting takes 5–6 minutes, and slow setting takes 10–18 minutes.
B. Fiberglass cast. In recent years, a number of companies have marketed materials to replace plaster of paris as a cast. Most of these are a fiberglass fabric impregnated with polyurethane resin. The prepolymer is methylene bisphenyl diisolynate, which converts to a nontoxic polymeric urea substitute. The exothermic reaction does not place the patient's skin at risk for thermal injury (4,6,8). These materials are preferred for most orthopaedic applications except in acute fractures in which reduction maintenance is critical.
1. **Advantages.** These materials are strong, lightweight, and resist breakdown in water; they are also available in multiple colors and patterns.
2. **Disadvantages.** They are harder to contour than plaster of paris, and the polyurethane may irritate the skin. Fiberglass is harder to apply, although the newer bias stretch material is an improvement. Review in detail the instructions from each manufacturer before using the casting materials. Patients are commonly under the impression that fiberglass casts can be gotten wet. This is incorrect; if submerged, they need to be changed to avoid significant skin maceration.
C. The water. Warm water causes more heat to be given off and affords faster setting. Cold water allows for less heat and for slower setting. Plaster of paris in the water bucket from previously dipped plaster accelerates the setting time. The water used for dipping should be deep enough to cover the material rolls standing on end.
D. Cast padding
1. **Webril** has a smooth surface and less tendency for motion within the thickness of the padding than some of the other padding materials. It requires the most practice to achieve a smooth application, however.

2. **Specialist** is softer than Webril and contains wood fiber. It has a corrugated appearance, and there is more tendency for sliding to occur within the material. It is easier to apply without wrinkles than Webril, but it becomes very hard if caked with blood.
3. **Sof-Roll** is a soft padding similar in appearance to Webril but slightly thicker, and it has different tearing and stretching characteristics.
4. **Stockinet**
   a. **Bias-cut** stockinet may be used under a cast as a single layer. It is easy to apply without wrinkles and is better than tubular stockinet if there is a large difference in the maximum and minimum diameters of the extremity. Bias-cut stockinet can be made snug throughout, in contrast to tubular stockinet, which can be snug in the large diameter of the extremity but very loose in the narrow diameter. Plaster sticks to the stockinet, so there is no sliding between the cast and the stockinet padding.
   b. **Tubular** stockinet is made of the same material as the bias-cut type and is available in varying tube sizes from 2 to 12 inches.
5. **Felt or Reston** should be used to pad bony prominences and for cast margins. When padding over bony prominences, such as the anterior superior iliac spine, make a cruciate incision in the felt.
6. **Moleskin adhesive** can be used to trim cast margins.
E. **Adherent materials.** Adherent substances (such as Dow Corning medical adhesive B) are applied to prevent slipping and chafing between the skin and the padding. They can contribute, however, to an increased amount of itching inside the cast. Tincture of benzoin compound should not be used in this situation because of fairly frequent skin reactions. Commercial adhesive removers are available.
F. **Equipment**
1. Use a clean **bucket.** Plaster residue and other particles in the water can alter the setting time.
2. **Gloves** keep hands clean and prevent dry skin if one applies many casts. They also make a smoother finish than is achieved by bare hands. They are mandatory for working with fiberglass materials.
3. **Shoe covers and aprons or gowns** keep shoes and clothes clean to prevent one from appearing sloppy in plaster-covered attire.
4. Use appropriate **draping** to maintain the dignity of the patient as well as to keep plaster off all areas not casted.
5. **Cast cutters**
   a. **The cast-cutting electric saw** has an oscillating circular blade that cuts firm rigid surfaces, such as casts or bony prominences. When lightly touched, the skin vibrates with the blade but the blade does not cut. If the blade is firmly pressed against the skin or dragged along it, then it will cut. The saw is noisy and causes considerable anxiety, especially in children. Therefore, it is wise to show younger patients that cast saws are safe by touching the blade to the palm of the hand. The cast saw causes dust to fly; consequently, use of this tool is best avoided in clean operating rooms. In addition, cast saws can cut skin if applied with excessive force, so it is unwise to use them on anesthetized patients.
   b. **Hand cutters** are useful when a saw is not available or to avoid frightening a child with the noise of the saw, to lessen the amount of plaster dust in the operating room, and to remove damp plaster.
6. **Cast spreaders** are used to open the cut edges of a cast for access to underlying cast padding, which is then cut with scissors. Spreaders come in various sizes for large and small casts.
7. **Cast knives** have sharp blades and preferably large handles for better control. Sharp blades are essential; therefore, most practitioners prefer to use No. 22 disposable surgical blades.

8. **Cast benders** adjust cast edges to relieve skin binding and pressure.
9. **Cast dryers** blow warm to hot air around a plaster cast. They are generally not necessary. An exposed cast and a fan work just as well and are safer. Cast dryers can burn skin and tend to hasten the drying time of the outer layers only.

II. **Basic principles of cast application**
  A. **Casts are used** for the following **purposes:**
   1. **To immobilize** fractures, dislocations, injured ligaments, and joints, to provide relief from pain caused by infections and inflammatory processes, and to facilitate healing
   2. **To allow earlier ambulation** by stabilizing fractures of the spine or lower extremities
   3. **To improve function** by stabilizing or positioning a joint, such as for wrist drop after a radial nerve injury, which also allows more useful hand function
   4. **To correct deformities,** as in serial casting for clubfoot or joint contractures
   5. **To prevent deformity** resulting from a neuromuscular imbalance or from scoliosis
  B. **Principles.** Although plaster of paris has been used extensively in the treatment of fractures for more than 100 years, there is no unanimity of opinion as to the best technique for application. It can be safely concluded that even the tightest of skintight casts allows some motion at the fracture site, whereas a loosely fitted, well-padded cast with proper three-point fixation can provide satisfactory immobilization. Three points of force are produced by the practitioner, who molds the cast firmly against the proximal and distal portions of the extremity (two of the points) and locates the third point directly opposite the apex of the cast, as shown in Fig. 7-1. Periosteal or other soft-tissue attachments usually are required on the convex side of the cast to provide stability. In this way, a curved cast can provide straight alignment of the extremity within it. Charnley has stated, "If a fracture slips in a well-applied plaster, then the fracture was mechanically unsuitable for treatment by plaster, and another mechanical principle should have been chosen." Another method for providing immobilization by plaster is based on hydraulics. Fractures of the tibia do not shorten significantly when placed in a "total contact" cast. The leg is a cylinder containing mostly fluid, and when this water column is encased in rigid plaster, the cylinder does not shorten in height because tissue fluid is not compressible.

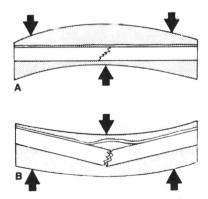

FIG. 7-1. A. Three-point plaster fixation will stabilize a fracture when the soft tissue bridging the fracture acts as a hinge under tension. **B.** If the three forces are applied in the wrong direction, the fracture displaces.

C. The following **application techniques** have been satisfactory in our hands:
1. The patient is **informed** of the procedure and instructed in whatever cooperation is necessary.
2. The surgeon or cast technician must have clearly in mind **what to do and what will be required** (the position of the patient and assistants, how many rolls of plaster will be needed, and so forth). All material and equipment required to do the job properly should be assembled. (Once cast application starts, it is difficult to stop and obtain something that was forgotten.) The patient's position must be comfortable and must allow the surgeon and assistant to apply the cast expeditiously. Special maneuvers required to perform and hold the reduction are rehearsed.
3. **A circular cast should not be used in fresh trauma or postoperatively** when one anticipates swelling, **unless** the cast is bivalved or split initially and provisions are made for adequate observation.
   a. **Adequate observation** means an examination by a competent observer at least once hourly until any swelling begins to recede. Signs of compartmental syndrome, in order of importance, are the following: increasing pain and discomfort in the extremity, increasing tenseness or tenderness in the involved compartment, pain with passive range of motion of the muscle in the involved compartment, decreasing sensation—especially to two-point discrimination and light touch—in the distribution of the nerves that travel through the involved compartment, increasing peripheral edema, and, finally, decreasing capillary filling. **Good peripheral circulation with distal arterial pulses is no assurance that a compartmental syndrome is not developing** (see Chap. 2, **III**).
   b. An excellent alternative to plaster casts in this situation is a Jones compression splint, as described in Chap. 6, **III.B.** and **C.**
4. **If unexpected swelling occurs** in a circular cast, **bivalve or split** the cast immediately all the way to the patient's skin as described in **IV.B** and **C.**
5. Unless specifically contraindicated, **clean** the part to be casted with soap and water, then dry it with alcohol. Apply the cast over a single layer of cast padding with edges of the material minimally overlapping. Protect unusual bony prominences with a ¼-inch felt or foam rubber pad with a cruciate cut in the material.
6. **Dip the plaster or fiberglass rolls in water** by placing them on end, which allows air to escape and results in complete soaking of the plaster. The bandages are sufficiently soaked when the bubbling stops. They can be left in the water up to 4 minutes without decreasing the strength of the cast, but the setting time decreases the longer they are immersed. Therefore, for maximum working time, remove bandages soon after the bubbling stops. Lightly crimping the ends of the plaster bandages helps prevent telescoping of the roll.
7. Except for very large casts (e.g., body casts, spicas), **all plaster bandages should be dipped and removed from the water at the same time.** Thus all the plaster in the cast is at the same point in the setting process. This scheme maximizes the interlocking of the crystals between the layers of plaster, thereby maximizing the strength of the cast. In addition, delamination between the bandages is decreased.
8. Use **cool water** for larger casts when more time is needed to apply all the plaster or fiberglass, and use **warm water** for smaller casts or splints. **Never use hot water,** because enough heat can be generated to burn the patient. Similarly, do not place limbs with fresh casts onto plastic-covered pillows; these tend to hamper heat dispersion significantly and may result in burning. If the patient complains of burning, it is prudent to remove the cast immediately and reapply using cooler water.
9. Keep the plaster bandage on the cast padding, lifting it off only to tuck and change directions—that is, to push the plaster roll around the patient's

body or extremity. Use the largest bandages, usually 4-inch and 6-inch bandage rolls, that are consistent with smooth, easy applications. Using large bandages allows the fastest application of plaster and provides sufficient time for molding before the critical setting period. **Six or seven layers of plaster** or two to three layers of fiberglass usually are sufficient, except in individuals who are particularly hard on casts. The cast should be of uniform thickness (seven layers, or ¼ inch). Avoid concentrating the plaster about the fracture or the middle of the cast. Avoid placing two circumferential rolls directly on top of each other while wrapping the plaster on the patient's extremity. Reinforce casts where they cross joints by incorporating plaster or fiberglass splints longitudinally. Incorporate reinforcing plaster splints into body and spica casts as described later in this chapter (**III.B** and **C**).

10. During application of the cast, **turn the padding back at the edges of the cast and incorporate it.** Another method of finishing the edges is to turn back the padding after the cast has set and to hold the padding down with a single, narrow, plaster splint, a row of ordinary staples, or moleskin.

11. **Apply all the material rapidly** so there is time to work and mold it before the critical setting period. The cast should have a sculptured look, not only for cosmetic reasons but also for comfort. If the fracture is to be stabilized by the three-point fixation principle, it is more important to maintain the three forces of pressure on the cast during the critical setting period than to have a perfectly smooth surface on the cast. This step is more difficult for fiberglass casts.

12. Once the critical period of interlocking of crystals begins, **molding and all motion should stop** until the material becomes rigid. Otherwise, the cast is weakened considerably.

13. After the cast sets and becomes rigid, **trim the edges** using a plaster knife. Use the knife by supporting the cutting hand on the cast and pulling the portion of the plaster to be trimmed up against the knife blade rather than blindly cutting through the plaster and possibly cutting the patient. If the cast is too thick or hard, use an oscillating cast saw.

14. Apply **forearm casts** to allow full 90 degrees flexion of all metacarpophalangeal joints and opposition of the thumb to the index and little fingers.

15. Extend **leg casts** to support the metatarsal heads but not to interfere with flexion and extension of the toes. This rule is invalid when the toes need support (as with fractures of the great toe or metatarsals) or when there is a motor or sensory deficit. In these situations, the cast is extended as a platform to support and protect the toes. Place a ½-inch piece of sponge rubber beneath the toes and incorporate it into the plaster for walking casts or supply the patient with a commercial cast shoe.

16. Immobilize as few joints as possible, but as a general rule, one **immobilizes the joint above and below a fresh fracture.**

17. Instruct the patient regarding
    a. **Signs and symptoms of compression** from swelling within the cast
    b. **Elevation** of the injured part above the level of the heart for 2–3 days after the injury
    c. **How soon to walk** on the cast (never sooner than 24 hours)
    d. **Instructions for weight bearing and ambulation;** this should include crutch or walker training.
    e. **How to exercise** joints not incorporated in plaster
    f. **Date of the next appointment**
    g. **Person to call** in case of cast problems or evidence of a compression syndrome

III. **Special casting/splinting techniques**
    A. Use **plaster splints** when rigid immobilization is not required or when significant swelling of the extremity is anticipated.

1. **Upper extremity**
   a. Usually splint the **wrist** dorsally by applying a 3-inch-wide plaster splint over cast padding from the metacarpophalangeal joints to the proximal forearm. While the plaster is still wet, wrap the arm with bias-cut stockinet or a single layer of an elastic bandage so that the plaster conforms to the extremity as it hardens. A dorsal splint may be preferable to a volar splint because it allows easier finger and hand function. Combined dorsal and volar splints are frequently used together; this is preferred and gives better support of the limbs.
   b. Splint the **elbow** with 5- × 30-inch plaster wraps applied posteriorly with enough distal extension to support the wrist. The splint should not go further distally than the distal palmar crease in order to facilitate metacarpal-phalangeal motion. Apply 3-inch plaster strips medially and laterally across the elbow for reinforcement. Wrap the arm and plaster splint with bias-cut stockinet or a single layer of an elastic bandage while the plaster is wet.
2. **Lower extremity.** Usually make posterior plaster splints in the lower extremity by applying a standard cast (short-leg, long-leg, or knee cylinder cast, as described in **III. D, E, F**) and then bivalving the cast and retaining only the posterior shell. Hold the posterior splint to the leg with bias-cut stockinet or an elastic bandage wrap. Alternatively, use 5- × 30-inch posterior and medial/lateral splints, leaving the anterior aspect of the leg covered only by soft roll.

B. **Body casts**
1. Apply the **basic body jacket** over large tubular stockinet. Place ⅛- to ½-inch felt pads over the shoulders (if suspenders are used), costal margins, iliac crests including anterior iliac spine, and the dorsal spine. Make a cruciate cut in the felt placed over the crests to distribute pressure uniformly over the bony prominence. Apply a single layer of plaster snugly over the padding. Splints may be used, as shown in Fig. 7-2. If suspenders are required, make a "V" with 5- × 30-inch splints. Place the point of the "V" between the scapulae and bring the ends over the shoulders. Snugly apply rolled plaster over the splints and mold. Usually extend the jacket posteriorly from the top of the sacrum to the inferior angle of the scapulae and anteriorly from the symphysis pubis to the sternal notch. A flexion body jacket, which extends only to the nipple line anteriorly, often is applied for low back pain. Body jackets may be applied with the lumbar spine in flexion or extension as well as the neutral position. For hyperextension body jackets, often used in thoracolumbar fractures, use the Goldwaithe iron apparatus for positioning, as in Fig. 7-3.
2. The **Minerva body jacket** is named after the goddess Minerva, who sprang forth from Jupiter's head when it was cleaved by Vulcan in an attempt to relieve Jupiter's headaches. Minerva appeared chanting a triumphant song and wearing a large metal headdress. The Minerva body jacket incorporates the skull and is used to immobilize the cervical spine; its most frequent application is in children. This type of jacket is applied in the same manner as the body jacket but also calls for the following steps: Place a fluted felt pad around the entire neck, with the neck halter traction over the padding. Tie the halter straps at ear level to prevent the halter's slipping off the head. Place another felt pad along the length of the spine and the occiput. Wrap the rest of the head with 3-inch sheet cotton padding. At least two operators are necessary for even application of the plaster, one for the head and one for the body. Roll 3-inch plaster bandages about the head and neck. Apply narrow splints around the chin, neck, occiput, and forehead. Use wide splints all the way from the sacrum to the occiput, with another wide splint extending from the chest to the chin. Incorporate these splints into the cast by snugly wrapping plaster bandages over them. Then mold together the plaster about the head, neck, and body at the same time. Carefully mold beneath the mandible. Cut the

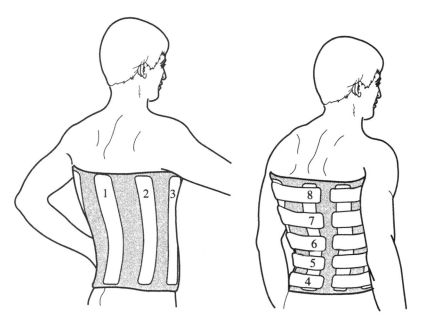

FIG. 7-2. Typical application of plaster splints for a body jacket. The splints are placed closer together in the lower aspect of the body jacket. The splints are numbered in order of application.

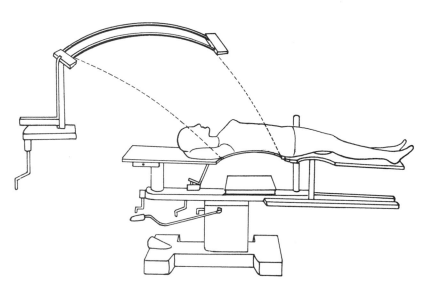

FIG. 7-3. Goldwaithe irons, used to make a hyperextension plaster body jacket. The irons are removed after the cast is set.

plaster in a "V" to release the chin and also cut out about the ears and the
face (Fig. 7-4, inset). Trim the plaster above the jaw line and leave the
eyebrows exposed. A Minerva body jacket is useful in children and when
cervical orthoses are not appropriate. This type of plaster body jacket is
shown in Fig. 7-4.

3. **Other types of body jackets**

   a. A **Risser localizer cast** is occasionally used for scoliotic spines or for
   patients with thoracolumbar fractures. Apply a pelvic plaster mold
   first; then attach pelvic and head halter traction. Make a pressure
   pad with felt backed by four to six layers of plaster. Produce or hold
   correction of the scoliosis by applying this pad against the apical ribs
   and incorporating it into the body jacket that incorporates the jaw,
   neck, and occiput, but not the head. Make the surface of the pressure
   area large enough to avoid local necrosis of the skin.

   b. **Halo traction** can be incorporated into a plaster or fiberglass body
   jacket with suspenders, and it provides continuous or fixed cervical
   traction (Fig. 7-5). The halo traction is more commonly incorporated
   into a sheepskin-lined plastic body jacket, which is more lightweight
   and comfortable (Fig. 7-6).

C. **Spica** is a Latin word that means "ear of wheat," because a spica wrap was
used to wrap sheaves of wheat in the fields. The same type of wrap is used to
immobilize proximal joints with the **spica cast.** Various types of spica casts
are described here (2).

   1. Pad a **bilateral short-leg** (panty) **spica** in much the same way as for the
   body jacket but include the legs. Use tubular or bias-cut stockinet. Pad
   bony prominences with ⅛- to ½-inch felt with cruciate incisions. Apply
   plaster or fiberglass to the upper portion of the cast as is done with the
   body jacket. Reinforce the hips with splints as shown in Fig. 7-7. Apply

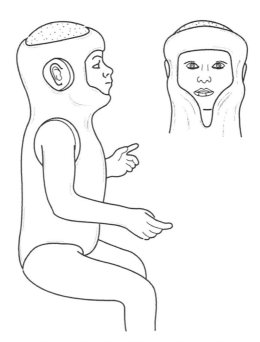

FIG. 7-4. Completed Minerva body jacket.

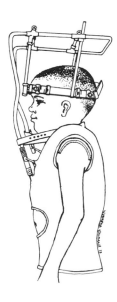

FIG. 7-5. Halo traction cast. (From Bleck EE, Duckworth L, Hunter N. *Atlas of plaster cast techniques,* 2nd ed. Chicago: Year Book, 1978. With permission.)

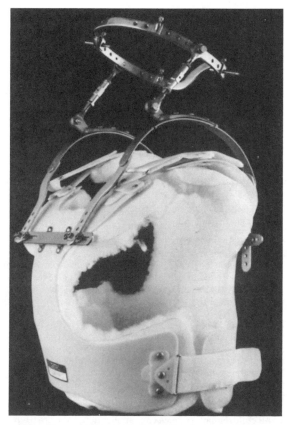

FIG. 7-6. A commercially available malleable polyethylene jacket may be substituted for the plaster cast for use with the halo apparatus. Patients report this is significantly more comfortable than the plaster jacket.

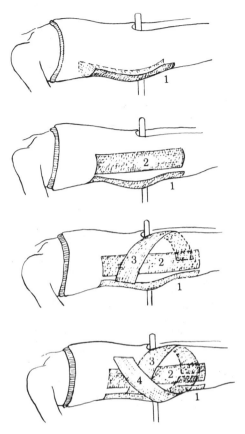

FIG. 7-7. Plaster splints to reinforce hip spicas, in addition to those used in the body jackets.

plaster or fiberglass well next to the perineal post under the sacrum to avoid weakness in the area (the intern's triangle). Snugly tie the splints in with plaster or fiberglass bandage rolls extending to the supracondylar portion of the femurs. Mold the material well over the iliac crests. The patient may be lifted from the table with the sacral rest still in the plaster. Turn the patient on his or her abdomen and cut out the sacral rest. Trim the edges of the cast in the usual manner.

2. Examples of long-leg hip spicas are shown in Fig. 7-8. Apply the leg portion of the cast like any other long-leg cast, using the special splints about the hips as described for the short-leg spica. Support the casted extremities with struts. These are usually made of wooden stakes (¼ × 2 inch or ¾ × ½ inch) or dowels. Cover with plaster or fiberglass and attach them to the casted extremity by wrapping a bandage in a cordlike figure-of-8 fashion about the strut and cast; then roll the bandage around the strut and cast to create a well-molded cast. Sedate or anesthetize infants and small children before spica cast application; they are frequently applied in the operating suite.

3. Apply the **shoulder spica** with the patient standing or supine on a spica table that has a metallic backrest. The arm may be supported with finger

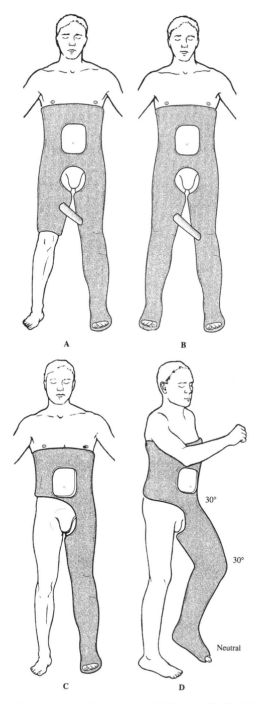

FIG. 7-8. Long-leg hip spicas. **A.** One and one-half spica. **B.** Double spica. **C.** Single spica. For all long-leg spica casts, it is important to keep the hip and knee gently flexed for patient comfort and ease of positioning. The ankle must be kept in neutral dorsiflexion (**D**). In children, it is often advisable to stop the cast at the malleoli distally, leaving the foot free.

traps, or, with a cooperative patient in the sitting or standing position, the cast may be applied while an assistant holds the arm. The principles of padding and cast application for body jackets and long-arm casts are combined to produce a shoulder spica. In addition to the splints normally used for body and long-arm casts, apply a wide splint from the lateral chest, up under the axilla, to the medial side of the arm. Place other splints across the posterior aspect of the arm, over the shoulder, to the opposite side. Tie in the splints with rolled plaster or fiberglass and place a strut between the arm and trunk.

D. **Knee cylinder casts.** Remove all hair from the medial and lateral aspects of the lower leg. Spray the leg with a nonallergenic adhesive. Place medial and lateral strips of self-adhering foam, moleskin adhesive, or adhesive tape on the skin with 6–12 inches of the material extending distal to the ankle. Then place a cuff of ¼-inch sponge rubber or felt padding measuring 1 inch in width over the strips just above the malleoli. When the strips are turned back and incorporated into the fiberglass or plaster, they suspend the cast, and with the thick padding, they prevent pressure on the malleoli. Wrap the leg with a single layer of cast padding and apply the plaster with the knee flexed 5 degrees. Extend the cast proximally as far as possible and distally to just above the flare of the malleoli; the length of the cast provides for lateral and medial stability. Mold the plaster or fiberglass medially and laterally above the femoral condyles to help prevent the cast from sliding distally.

E. **Short-leg casts**
   1. Apply the **short-leg cast** with the patient sitting on the end of a table with the knee flexed 90 degrees. Alternatively, apply it with the patient supine, the hip and knee flexed 90 degrees, and the leg supported by an assistant. The type of padding matters little, except that Webril and stockinet tend to shear less and therefore may allow for a tighter cast over a longer period of time. Use only one layer of padding except of the malleoli, where extra padding frequently is required. For most casts, have the ankle in a neutral position. Two plaster bandages usually are required, and the width selected (3, 4, or 6 inch) varies with the size of the patient. Fold 4-inch splints longitudinally in half, and place one splint on all four sides of the ankle for reinforcement before applying the second plaster bandage. Extend the cast distally from the metatarsophalangeal joints and proximally to one finger breadth below the tibial tubercle. Trim the edges as previously described.
   2. If desired, a **walking cast** may be made with either a rubber rocker walker or a stirrup walker. Place either one in the midportion of the longitudinal arch of the foot in line with the anterior border of the tibia. With a rocker walker, the medial longitudinal arch is filled with plaster splints to make a flat base. Then the walker is secured with a third plaster bandage. Commercially available walking shoes (or boots), which fit over the casted foot, are more widely used. A flat plaster base on the plantar aspect of the cast is required for these shoes. If the ankle must be held in equinus, a stirrup walker is advantageous, and the patient's opposite shoe should be adjusted to the appropriate height for walking. All walking casts should dry for at least 24 hours prior to weight bearing.

F. **Long-leg casts**
   1. First apply a short-leg **cast** as described earlier (**III.E**). Then extend the knee to the position desired and continue the cast padding to the groin. Two 6-inch plaster or fiberglass bandages usually are required for the upper portion of this cast except in patients with heavy thighs. After the first bandage is applied, fold 4- or 5-inch splints longitudinally and place them medially and laterally across the knee joint for reinforcement. After the second plaster or fiberglass bandage is applied, mold the cast medially and laterally in the supracondylar area to help prevent the cast from slipping distally when the patient begins to stand.

2. The long-leg **walking cast** is made as described in **III.E.2,** but the knee must be flexed no more than 5 degrees.
G. **Casting techniques of Dehne and Sarmiento**
   1. The cast treatment programs made popular by Dehne and Sarmiento (see historical readings) are designed to allow early weight bearing of a fractured tibia. The affected leg is placed in a very snug cast that maintains the tissue and fluids of the leg within a rigid container. Shortening is prevented by the **hydraulic principle** that fluids are not compressible. Thus, the patient can bear weight soon after a fracture without excessive further shortening, and fracture healing is benefitted by the improved vascularity derived from ambulation. The advocates of these casting techniques describe a "total contact cast." The authors believe, however, that all casts to the lower extremities should be total contact casts.
   2. The **long-leg total contact cast** as described by Dehne is applied like a long-leg walking cast with only minor modifications.
      a. **Cast the knee in extension.** Some patients, however, find this position uncomfortable and may require a position with a 3 to 5 degrees of flexion.
      b. This cast may need to be **wedged** to correct angular deformities of the fracture site. For this reason, apply one or two extra layers of the cotton roll at the fracture site.
   3. The **below-the-knee total contact,** or patellar tendon-bearing, **cast** is applied much as a regular short-leg walking cast is, with the following modifications (Fig. 7-9):
      a. Keep the affected limb in a long-leg cast or a Jones compression splint until the **swelling subsides** (2–4 weeks).
      b. Apply the **cast padding to the lower leg and extend** to 2 inch proximal to the superior pole of the patella.
      c. First apply a short-leg cast and extend it to just inferior to the tibial tubercle. Sarmiento suggests molding the cast into a **triangular shape,** with the sides of the triangle formed by the anterior tibial surface, the lateral peroneal muscle mass, and the posterior aspect of the leg.
      d. Then have the assistant position the knee in 40–45 degrees of flexion. The quadriceps muscles must be completely relaxed. Use a 4-inch bandage of plaster to extend the cast to the superior pole of the patella. Mold carefully over the medial tibial flare as well as into the patellar tendon and the popliteal fossa. The lateral wings should be as high as possible. Trim the posterior portion of the cast to one fingerbreadth or ½ inch below the level of the cast indentation that was made anteriorly into the patellar tendon. The posterior wall of the cast should be low enough to allow 90 degrees of knee flexion without having the cast edge rub on the hamstring tendons. These casts generally require the use of plaster because of the critical molding involved, which is difficult with fiberglass.
      e. If **angulation** occurs at the fracture site with this cast, replace rather than wedge the cast. If the patient ambulates well enough to maintain muscle bulk, the original cast may not need to be replaced.
      f. **Do not switch from a below-the-knee total contact cast to a regular short-leg cast** at some point midway in the healing phase of the fracture, because a regular short-leg cast offers no rotational stability.
   4. **The authors believe that a long-leg weight-bearing cast is easier and safer (in regards to skin and fracture complications) for most individuals to apply than the below-the-knee total contact cast.** Comparing the treatment results published in the literature provides no evidence that one technique is superior to the other. The theoretic advantage of providing knee motion with the Sarmiento technique is offset by the expertise required to apply this cast properly.

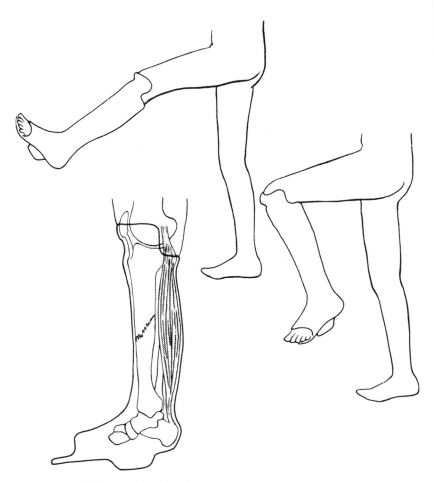

FIG. 7-9. Completed below-the-knee total contact cast.

   5. Begin **weight bearing** at 24-36 hours after plaster cast application when the patient can tolerate it; patients with fiberglass casts can be encouraged to weight bear 3-6 hours after casting.
H. Knee cast-brace
   1. A **cast-brace** is a casting device for the treatment of fractures of the distal femur or tibial plateau, which are not considered appropriate for operative management. Occasionally a cast-brace is applied after 1–3 weeks of traction, with the patient remaining in the hospital for a short period after the brace is applied. Thus, the hospital stay can be as long as 2–4 weeks. In addition, this technique allows mobility of the knee during the healing phase, so less physical therapy is needed to regain knee motion when the fracture is healed.
   2. Technique
      a. Two people are required for **application.** After the patient is lightly sedated, roll an elastic tubular stockinet over the leg. While an assistant holds the leg, apply plaster over the thigh to within 2½ cm of the ischial tuberosity and the perineum. Extend the plaster distally

to the superior pole of the patella but with enough clearance for full knee extension and flexion to 70 degrees. Then apply a short-leg cast. Make the plantar aspect of the cast flat for ambulation in a walking shoe.

b. Position **two polycentric or cable knee hinge joints** 2 cm posterior to the midline of the limb at the level of the abductor tubercle. Use large hose clamps to secure the hinge joints to the cast temporarily. A jig is helpful to keep these joints parallel. Evaluate knee motion and make adjustments before securing the uprights with plaster.

   (1) If the roentgenograms show **satisfactory alignment** of the fracture, start the patient on progressive ambulation with "touch down" weight bearing. If a knee effusion develops, instruct the patient to elevate the limb for 15 minutes of every hour. Once adequate fracture consolidation is demonstrated, the patient can be encouraged to bear weight.

   (2) If the **alignment** of the fracture is **not satisfactory,** remove the cast-brace and temporarily reinstitute traction treatment. Consider continuing standard traction therapy, reattempting a cast-brace again in 2–3 weeks, or performing internal fixation.

IV. **Cutting, bivalving, and splitting casts**
  A. **General techniques**
    1. In removing or splitting casts, use the **oscillating saw.** Reassure the patient by giving a cast saw demonstration before actually cutting the cast. Stabilize the hand holding the electric saw on the cast, and push the blade through just the plaster with short repetitive strokes, as shown in Fig. 7-10. Avoid bony prominences as the cast saw can cut into the skin over them.
    2. **Windows** may be cut from the cast to expose wounds. The windows must be replaced, however, and rewrapped with either a new plaster or an elastic bandage to prevent window edema.
  B. Should unexpected swelling occur, **bivalve the cast. Bivalving is superior to simply splitting the cast.** The technique consists of cutting the plaster as well as the cast padding on both sides of the extremity. The anterior and posterior parts of the cast can be held in place with bias-cut stockinet or an elastic bandage. Advantages of this technique are that the anterior half of the cast may be removed to inspect the compartments and that complete anterior, posterior, and circumferential compression is relieved.
  C. **Splitting** a cast requires cutting a ½-inch strip of plaster from the full length of the cast; otherwise, the proximal aspect of the plaster may act as

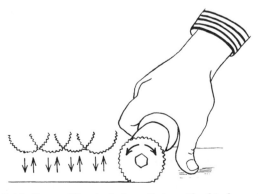

FIG. 7-10. Saw-cutting technique that avoids skin laceration.

a circumferential tourniquet (1). Again, divide the plaster and padding down to the skin, because soft dressing might also cause constriction. In the case of the lower extremity, the cast is split anteriorly with a diamond-shaped section of plaster removed from the anterior aspect of the ankle. Spread the cast for relief of the symptoms. Pad the area with felt where the strip of plaster was removed and overwrap with a rubber elastic bandage to avoid window edema. **This technique is not as satisfactory as bivalving a cast, but is often appropriate for managing postoperative swelling.**

V. Adhesive strapping and bandaging
    A. Terminology
        1. Use **adhesive strapping** (taping) for the possible prevention and treatment of athletic injuries. Use strips of adhesive tape instead of one continuous winding.
        2. Bandaging (wrapping) uses nonadhesive materials (gauze, cotton cloth, and elastic wrapping) in the treatment of athletic injuries. Employ one continuous unwinding of material.
    B. Adhesive strapping
        1. Purposes of strapping
            a. To protect and secure protective devices
            b. To hold dressings in place
            c. To limit motion
            d. To support and stabilize
        2. Construction factors
            a. Tape grade (backing material). Heavy backing materials have 85 longitudinal fibers per square inch and 65 vertical fibers per square inch. Lighter grades have 65 longitudinal fibers per square inch and 45 vertical fibers per square inch. **Store** the tape in a cool, dry place. Keep the tape standing on end and not on its side.
            b. Adhesives. Use a rubber-based adhesive primarily with athletes because strength of backing, superior adhesion, and economy are needed. Use acrylic adhesives in surgical dressing applications because a high degree of backing and superior adhesion are not the primary requirements.
        3. Application and removal
            a. Preparation
                (1) Clean the skin with soap and water and dry.
                (2) Remove all hair to prevent irritation.
                (3) Treat all cuts and wounds.
                (4) Apply a nonallergic **skin adherent.**
                (5) Position properly.
            b. Size of tape
                (1) Use ¼- to 1-inch tape on **fingers, hands,** and **toes.**
                (2) Use 1¼- or 1½-inch tape on **ankles, lower legs, forearms,** and **elbows.**
                (3) Use 2- or 3-inch tape on **large areas, knees,** and **thighs.**
            c. Rules of application
                (1) Avoid continuous strapping because this causes constriction. Use one turn at a time and tear after overlapping the starting end of the tape by 1 inch.
                (2) Smooth and mold the tape as it is laid on the skin.
                (3) Overlap the tape at least one-half its width over the tape below.
                (4) Allow the tape to **fit the natural contour** of the skin—that is, let it fall naturally and avoid bending around acute angles.
                (5) Keep the tape roll in one hand and **tear** it with the fingers.
                (6) Keep constant and even **unwinding tension.**
                (7) For **best support,** strap directly over the skin.
            d. Techniques for removal
                (1) Remove the tape along the longitudinal axis rather than across it. If near a wound, **pull toward the wound,** not away from it.

(2) **Peel** the tape back by holding the skin taut and pushing the skin away from the tape rather than by pulling the tape from the skin.
4. **Skin reactions. Most tape reactions are mechanical,** not allergic. Allergic reactions are characterized by erythema, edema, papules, and vesicles. Test for an allergic reaction by patch testing. If the test is positive, the above signs manifest themselves within 24–48 hours.
   a. **Mechanical irritation** is produced when tape is removed from the skin. It frequently occurs as a result of shearing the skin when the tape is applied in tension or used for maintaining traction. Such application induces vasodilation and an intense reddening of the skin, which disappears shortly after tape removal. The reaction is due to simple skin stripping—that is, direct trauma to the outer skin layers resulting in loss of cells.
   b. **Chemical irritation** occurs when components in adhesive mass or the backing of the tape permeate the underlying tissues. This irritation is largely eliminated through tape construction.
   c. **Another irritative effect** is localized inhibition of sweating, which is corrected by the use of nonocclusive (porous) tape.
C. **Bandaging**
   1. **Purposes of bandaging**
      a. **To hold dressing in place** over external wounds
      b. **To apply compression pressure** over injuries and thus control hemorrhage
      c. **To secure splints** in place
      d. **To immobilize** or limit motion of injured parts
   2. **Materials**
      a. **Gauze,** which holds dressings in place over wounds or acts as a protective layer for strapping.
      b. **Cotton cloth** for support wrapping or dressing
      c. **Elastic wrapping** for compression wrapping or dressing
D. **Medicated bandage**
   1. The medicated bandage (Unna's boot) **contains** zinc oxide, calamine, glycerine, and gelatin and **usually is indicated** for lower extremity areas of skin loss that require protection and support. This type of support dressing prevents edema and allows ambulation in patients with known venous conditions at the time of cast removal.
   2. **Application**
      a. **Cleanse** the area and position the ankle at a right angle.
      b. **Make a circular turn** with the medicated bandage **around the foot** and direct the bandage **obliquely over the heel.** Then cut the bandage. This procedure ensures a flat surface.
      c. **Repeat** until the heel is adequately covered. Make the first layer snug and apply the roll in a pressure-gradient manner; that is, apply the greatest pressure distally with progressively diminishing pressure over the upper leg.
      d. **Do not reverse any turns** because the ridges formed may cause discomfort as the bandage hardens. Overlap each turn one half of a preceding turn. Avoid winding the bandage on too tightly.
      e. **Cover the leg** approximately three times and extend the bandage 1–2 inches below the knee; otherwise, the bandage may slip toward the ankle. Allow the bandage to harden. Prevent soiling of clothing with gauze or stockinet over the medicated bandage. Leave the bandage on for 3–7 days, and repeat treatment if necessary.
VI. **Joint mobilization**
   A. **Following cast removal**
      1. **While the cast is still on,** range-of-motion exercises of the adjacent joints not immobilized and isometric exercises for the immobilized muscles (e.g., weight bearing in a cast) serve both to improve nutrition and to

decrease atrophy of articular cartilage, bone, and muscle. Edema and the rehabilitation required after cast removal are also minimized.
2. **Warn the patient that after removal of any cast from a lower extremity, some swelling is normal.**
3. **Once the cast is removed,** an elastic stocking or bandage is desirable for support.
   a. Prescribe a **specific exercise program** to increase range of motion. Moist heat, such as a bath or whirlpool, may help mobilize the joint.
   b. If swelling appears to be a problem, **contrast baths** may be indicated (the 3-3-3 treatment): rest 3 minutes in cool water, exercise 3 minutes in warm water, repeat 3 times; follow with 30 minutes of elevation. Repeat the entire process 3 times daily.
   c. **Active exercise** is the key to success. Passive range-of-motion exercise too frequently becomes a repeated manipulation. Manipulation under anesthesia is occasionally necessary, but this should be followed with an aggressive inpatient therapy program.
B. It is not always true that the sooner **joints adjacent to a fracture** are mobilized, the better the range of motion obtained. The following factors must be considered:
   1. **Fractures not involving articular surfaces**
      a. Joint movement is slow to return and poor in range if attempted movement produces **pain,** associated muscle spasm, and involuntary splinting.
      b. **Early joint movement can delay fracture healing if fixation is not rigid.**
      c. **A normal joint tolerates longer periods of immobilization.** The "safe" period of immobilization coincides well with the normal time necessary for adjacent fracture healing. Only in the older patient with degenerative changes in the joint is there a likelihood of intraarticular adhesions and periarticular stiffening, even with short periods of immobilization.
      d. **Some joints may tolerate immobilization better than others,** but this presumption is not well documented.
      e. Postinjury or postcasting **edema is "glue."** This fluid is soon filled with young fibroblasts. Excessive formation of collagen causes early and frequent permanent stiffness, especially when collateral ligaments are immobilized in a shortened position (metacarpophalangeal joints, for example).
      f. **Isometric exercises** within the cast are recommended. Allow the extremity to move within the limits of the cast.
   2. **Fractures involving articular surfaces**
      a. **Reduce intraarticular fractures anatomically if possible.** If operative intervention is indicated, then a goal of internal fixation is to allow range-of-motion exercises or continuous passive motion within the first 2 or 3 days postoperatively.
      b. **If anatomic restitution cannot be achieved,** then early motion may allow mobile fragments to be molded into a better position. This motion should improve the potential of fibrocartilage resurfacing. Early movement is difficult to define, but some movement should be started within the first week.
   3. **Between these two groups** is a considerable degree of overlap. If it is anticipated that a complicated and often incomplete open reduction and internal fixation is not secure enough to allow early movement of the joint, then it may be better to treat the fracture nonoperatively. The **objective** is the **best possible final range of movement.**

References
1. Bingold AC. On splitting plasters. *J Bone Joint Surg (Br)* 1979;61:294.
2. Bleck EE, Duckworth L, Hunter N. *Atlas of plaster cast techniques*, 2nd ed. Chicago: Year Book, 1978.

3. Callahan DJ, Carney DJ, Daddario N, et al. The effect of hydration water temperature on orthopaedic plaster casting strength. *Orthopedics* 1986;9:683–985.
4. Callahan DJ, Carney DJ, Daddario N, et al. A comparative study of synthetic cast material strength. *Orthopaedics* 1986;9:679–681.
5. Lavalette R, Pope MH, Dickstein H. Setting temperature of plaster casts. *J Bone Joint Surg (Am)* 1982;64:907.
6. Pope MH, Callahan G, Lavarette R. Setting temperatures of synthetic casts. *J Bone Joint Surg (Am)* 1985;67:262–264.
7. Wehbe MA. Plaster uses and misuses. *Clin Orthop* 1982;167:242.
8. Wytch R, Mitchell C, Ritchie IK, et al. New splinting materials. *Prosthet Orthot Int* 1987;11:42–45.

Selected Historical Readings

Charnley J. *The closed treatment of common fractures*, 3rd ed. Baltimore: Williams & Wilkins, 1972:179–183.

Dehne E, et al. Nonoperative treatment of the fractured tibia by immediate weight bearing. *J Trauma* 1961;1:514.

Connolly JF, King P. Closed reduction and early cast-brace ambulation in the treatment of femoral fractures. *J Bone Joint Surg (Am)* 1973;55:1559.

Sarmiento AA. functional below-the-knee cast for tibial fractures. *J Bone Joint Surg (Am)* 1967;49:855.

8. ORTHOPAEDIC UNIT CARE

I. The following **orthopaedic unit care** advice is devised based on the early principles developed in the 1940s by J. H. Means, M.D., at Massachusetts General Hospital. Over the last decade and a half, though, a large portion of orthopaedic care has moved to the outpatient setting. The principles described pertain to the inpatient as well as outpatient or short-stay unit. The orthopaedic unit must present a warm, friendly, and quiet atmosphere as an essential part of the treatment program. Most patients who enter the hospital are frightened and need constant reassurance from everyone on the unit. The **desired atmosphere can be maintained only if all the people on the unit function as a team** and realize that the patient is an individual with a need for privacy. To have an effective team, it is necessary for each individual to understand the goals of the treatment program for each patient. Therefore, careful communication is required, as is recognition that the best run orthopaedic services are those that involve all of the personnel in the decision-making process. To maintain the best possible environment for most patients and to ease the problems of communication, it is helpful to schedule and standardize activities and procedures. This principle is even more important with the current emphasis on shortened length of hospital stay.

II. Rounds. Rounds are important in that they constitute an evaluation for the benefit of the patient and an educational experience for all of the participants. Be certain that the best interests of the patient are not sacrificed for education. All participants must be constantly mindful that significant harm can be done with innocent words. For example, the use of such words as "beautiful" when applied to a symptom or physical sign displayed by the patient may provoke resentment. If a doctor should describe as "beautiful" something that the patient knows is evidence of disease, the patient may infer that the doctor is taking satisfaction in the illness. The knowledge that any word uttered in the presence of the patient can stimulate a reaction in him or her is fundamental to the **art of healing.**

A. The **approach to the patient** must be direct and personal. The patient must be made to feel that he or she is receiving sympathetic attention as a living human being rather than being scrutinized like a specimen in a museum. This does not necessarily mean that scientific discussion is inappropriate at the bedside. Properly conducted, it can be an excellent teaching experience for those in attendance and help the patient understand his or her problems more completely. If the leader of the rounds addresses the patient with friendly words of inquiry or explanation, then the patient tolerates an abundance of clinical discussions without annoyance. Indeed, when managed along these lines, most patients, instead of resenting visitations from large groups, relish the attention they are attracting and enjoy participating in the process.

B. Do not present case histories at bedside. Devote attention to examining the patient, giving advice, or obtaining further history. Conduct debate or lengthy discussion away from the bedside and out of the patient's hearing range. The medical student, resident, and nurse who are to report on or present the case should take a position opposite that of the lead physician at the bedside. Refer to patients by name. References to age, sex, or race are out of place unless essential to the discussion and cannot be perceived by those in attendance. One is under no less temptation on rounds than elsewhere to enliven conservation with witticisms or wisecracks. The laughter that these jokes may provoke can be beneficial if the patient shares it. Laughter can be cruel when the patient thinks it is directed toward him or her.

C. The head nurse is an integral part of rounds. The nurse prepares for them as well as participates in them. When the patient is examined, the nurse should take a station at the head of the bed to promote the comfort of the patient during the examination. The doctors and students have much to learn from the nurse in charge and vice versa. Before starting rounds, the nurse or the assistant should ask visitors (except close adult members of

the family) to leave the patient's bedside. The radio or television set is lowered in volume or turned off. Each member of the team performs his or her role with dispatch so that the whole activity runs smoothly and gives an impression of efficiency and dignity to patients and visitors.
  D. **Consultations** are an important part of patient care and usually are ordered by the attending physician with a statement as to the current care, opinions, and so on. Make every effort to assist the consultant. When the consultant enters the unit, the resident or nurse assigned to the case should introduce the patient and explain the purpose of the visit. This individual should be available to the consultant during the examination and be prepared to present a lucid review of the consultant's opinions at the next session of rounds.
III. **Workup routines**
  A. Either before or as soon as possible after admission, the house officer should conduct a **complete history and physical examination** of the patient. This workup should be reviewed, corrected, amended, and signed by the chief resident and attending physician within 24 hours. The authors prefer problem-oriented medical records. An example of the initial record follows:
    1. **Database**
      a. **Chief complaint**
      b. **Patient profile** (including past medical history) and social data
      c. **Present illness**
      d. **History and systems review**
      e. **Physical examination**
      f. **Laboratory reports**
    2. **Inpatient problem list,** which should be maintained in the outpatient care record
    3. **An initial plan** keyed by number to the inpatient problem list
      a. **Diagnostic** plan
      b. **Therapeutic** plan
      c. **Patient education**
  B. Anticipate any **side effects or complications** from either the primary problems or the treatment plans and make appropriate provisions for prophylactic medications or other measures. **Plan ahead** to keep the patient comfortable and content. **Use** every moment of hospitalization to the maximum.
  C. **Write progress notes** as often as there is any change in the patient's condition or when a consultation is obtained. The patient should be seen daily and an entry made in the medical record after each visit. The authors prefer the problem-oriented style of progress notes. The note should be accompanied by a date and time of the entry.
    1. **Narrative notes** are numbered and titled according to the inpatient problem list and are organized as follows:
      a. **Subjective** data
      b. **Objective** data
      c. **Assessment**
      d. **Plan**
        (1) **Diagnostic**
        (2) **Therapeutic**
        (3) **Patient education**
    2. **Flow sheets** are used when data and time relationships are complex.
    3. **Discharge summary**
      a. **Identifying data**
      b. **Dates of admission and discharge**
      c. **Master problem list** with the appropriate dates
        (1) Use two columns, one headed **active problems** and one **inactive problems.**
        (2) **Give each problem a number. Once a problem is assigned a number, whether on an inpatient list or on a master list, do not use the number again.**
      d. List of **operations and procedures,** including the dates

   e. Description of the inpatient problems
   f. Physical examination
   g. Laboratory data
   h. Hospital course for each problem, including laboratory data, treatment, and plans when appropriate
   i. Discharge medications and disposition
IV. **Routine orders and management of inpatients**
   A. The **initial orders** should state
      1. The **condition** of the patient
      2. The type of **activity** desired
   B. Careful attention to **diet** is an important part of the overall treatment program (21,24,35). When patients are generally well and suffer boredom from hospitalization, mealtime can become a happy break in an otherwise dull routine. However, it is important to protect patients from too many calories when they are in bed. Hospitalization also provides an excellent opportunity for weight reduction education for obese patients because they can be counseled about foods that they may eat in abundance without increasing weight. It is usually not possible to reduce the weight of a patient confined to bed unless the caloric intake is restricted to between 600 and 800 calories/day; this is generally inappropriate during the hospital stay. Wound healing in patients with multiple factors or amputation for vascular disease is critically dependent on adequate nutrition. Young individuals who have sustained multiple fractures may require considerably more in the way of calorie and protein supplements (21,24,35); this is particularly true of competitive athletes. Patients who are physically active have a much lower overall complication rate; assessing the patient about their exercise habits aids in predicting those with increased risk (31). Hospitalized patients tend to eat poorly and can quickly become vitamin C–depleted. Patients should receive vitamin C supplements daily, either IV or PO. Prescribe a multivitamin preparation for most patients. If significant bleeding has occurred, use therapeutic doses of iron to bring the hemoglobin level to normal, followed by supplemental doses for a few months to replenish the iron stores. Patients often request calcium supplements "to help the fracture heal." This should be avoided, however, because high-calcium diets in active patients who are suddenly immobilized causes an excessive calcium load on the kidneys, which can lead to renal calculi (29). Patients restricted to bed rest should be encouraged to take fluids for the same reasons. Consultation with a dietitian is indicated for multiply injured, elderly, or obese patients.
   C. **Preoperative preparation**
      1. **Patient preparation.** Orthopaedic patients should have a 10-minute chlorhexidine (Hibiclens) or povidone-iodine (Betadine) scrub before surgery. If the patient is ambulatory, then the scrub is most easily accomplished by a shower with chlorhexidine or hexachlorophene soap at home the night before surgery. The authors advise that shaving of any hair from the operative field be done in the operating room. If shaving is done the evening before surgery, then small nicks or lacerations often occur that can become colonized overnight and increase the risk of a postoperative infection (16). Fracture blisters should be kept intact and dressed sterilely preoperatively. As long as they are not blood-filled, they do not predispose to an increased risk of infection (17,18,36).
      2. **Laboratory data.** Patients undergoing a surgical procedure usually have a hemoglobin test within 30 days of surgery. The erythrocyte sedimentation rate (ESR) should be determined for all patients with a history of infection. If the age of the patient (generally older than 50 years of age) or the history indicates, then a chest roentgenogram and electrocardiogram (ECG) are appropriate. Whenever blood transfusion is deemed likely, autologous blood donation should be considered. This can be set up through the local blood bank. Up to 3 units of blood can be drawn and stored over a 3-week period. Generally, a fourth week before

the scheduled procedure is allowed for recovery. Because this is not possible for acute trauma cases, the use of intraoperative suction-collection-filtering-retransfusion (Cell-Saver) should be considered.

D. **Antibiotics are used for open fractures and should be used prophylactically for many types of orthopaedic procedures.** In general, they are reserved for procedures that last longer than 2 hours, for installation of implants, and for nerve and tendon repairs (8). A detailed description of antibiotics used in trauma is found in Chaps. 1 **(III.D)** and 3 **(II.G)**, and their use with surgery is discussed in Chap. 10 **(I.B.2)**. Know well the characteristics of the antibiotics used, and obtain a careful history to ascertain possible allergies to antibiotics before administration. The use of surgical drains does not appear to decrease the risk of deep infection (26). Careful attention to skin preparation at the initiation of the procedure can limit the risk to the patient (16,32).

E. **Analgesics, sedatives, and hypnotics.** Virtually all orthopaedic patients admitted for acute problems have pain and anxiety. It is important to make the patient comfortable through adequate medication as quickly as possible. Take into consideration the size of the patient, the amount of medication received previously, and the type of orthopaedic problem or operation causing the pain. (For example, fractures of the transverse process of the spine or of the pelvis and operations about the knee, especially in well-muscled young individuals, tend to cause severe pain.)

1. Ideally, the analgesic and sedation regimen should keep the patients on a **diurnal schedule** so that they stay awake during the daytime and sleep at night. Sleeplessness is itself debilitating. Patients can tolerate considerably more pain or discomfort during the daytime, when there are distractions, than at night. For this reason, it is frequently helpful to use lighter analgesics during the daytime hours. Consider administering nonopiate analgesics during the day immediately before and after discharge from the hospital.

2. **Analgesics.** It is best if the physician can anticipate a patient's pain and its severity, because standing orders may then be written on a time-related basis to provide adequate patient comfort. This regimen helps avoid anxiety in the patient as to the timing of the next dose of analgesics and prevents reinforcing pain behavior patterns, which occurs with pain analgesic orders. Most helpful in this regard has been the development of patient-controlled, parenteral, opiate administration systems. When patients are allowed to titrate small doses of analgesia, they avoid toxicity yet keep their blood levels above the minimum effective analgesic concentration. Morphine and meperidine are the two most widely used drugs with these systems. The recommended and commonly used analgesics are listed in Tables 8-1 and 8-2 (2).

2. **Narcotics** all have similar adverse side effects and produce addiction after approximately 4 weeks. The beneficial effects (analgesia and hypnosis) as well as the adverse side effects vary among patients. Establish as quickly as possible, by trial and error, the most effective drug (the patient may be able to provide guidance through previous experience). Use this drug as generously as necessary to achieve pain relief. **Narcotics are invaluable in the control of pain but should never be used for chronic pain problems (22).** Anticipate the undesirable side effects (such as reducing the cough reflex and level of respiration, depressing bladder tone, lowering bowel motility, producing nausea and, occasionally, vomiting) and initiate measures to counteract them. Counsel the patient to relieve apprehension regarding these side effects. The patient will then require lower doses. The reduced dose, in turn, decreases the undesirable effects of the analgesics. Patients with chronic pain need the help of an anesthesia pain consultant (20).

3. **Sedatives and hypnotics**
   a. For patients with severe anxiety, it is frequently helpful to combine the analgesics with a **sedative or tranquilizing drug.** If a patient

Table 8-1. Dosing schedule of recommended commonly used nonopioid analgesics

Generic name	Appropriate adult dose (mg)	Duration of action (h)
Aspirin	325–650	4
Acetaminophen	325–650	4
Ibuprofen [a]	400–800	6–8
Naprosyn [a]	250–500	6–8
Piroxicam [a]	20	16–24

[a] Use during the first 3 or 4 days after acute trauma may allow for more bleeding, swelling, and pain.

is to undergo physical therapy, then avoid muscle relaxants during the day. Hydroxyzine (Vistaril), 50 mg PO or IM, is useful in conjunction with analgesics, such as meperidine (Demerol) or one of the codeine derivatives (e.g., Tylenol No. 3), to control the anxiety and decrease the need for large doses of analgesics.

   b. Generally provide a hospitalized patient with a **hypnotic** for sleep. Time-honored hypnotics include chloral hydrate (Noctec), 0.5–1.0 g PO; secobarbital (Seconal), 100 mg PO; or flurazepam (Dalmane), 15–30 mg PO. The dose can be repeated after at least 45-minute intervals if the patient is still awake.

   c. **When drug abuse is suspected,** use either diphenhydramine (Benadryl) or hydroxyzine PO or IM, 50–100 mg q4h for anxiety, and use 100 mg for sleep.

   4. The **"CAGE"** questionnaire is a useful tool to detect patients with alcohol abuse as an underlying problem. Medical consultants should manage these cases (28).

F. Prevention of thromboembolism

   1. Thromboembolism is a specter that stands over every surgeon. **Elderly patients and those undergoing bed rest for longer than a day** should be put on a prophylactic program. This program includes slightly elevating the foot of the bed, applying elastic bandages or stockings on the legs, applying sequential compression devices, and initiating an active muscle exercise program to stimulate circulation through the lower extremities. **High-risk patients** include those with a history of previous thromboembolic disease, previous surgery to the lower extremities, or chronic venous disease; patients on oral contraceptives; patients with a history of cancer or significant fractures of the pelvis or femur; patients who smoke; or patients undergoing a lower extremity replacement arthroplasty (14, 15,38). Spinal or epidural anesthesia may decrease the incidence of deep vein thrombosis (DVT) (37). These high-risk patients should have prophylactic therapy. Duplex ultrasound is an extremely accurate method for DVT screening (4,14).

   2. **Warfarin, aspirin, dextran, heparin, low-molecular-weight heparin and sequential compression devices have been used in prophylactic treatment.** The actual treatment selected is largely up to the surgeon, because current studies do not provide conclusive evidence to support or discredit any particular therapeutic regimen. Evidence has supported the prophylactic use of warfarin, low-molecular-weight heparin or aspirin, but as soon as any evidence of fresh thrombi was detected, all patients were switched to warfarin therapy (1,6,9,10,13,19,25,30,33). The relative risks of embolic disease versus the complications of anticoagulants (hemorrhage, subsequent infection) must be weighed for each patient undergoing treatment.

   3. A **therapeutic regimen** for antithromboemboli therapy in trauma is presented in Table 8-3.

Table 8-2. Dosing schedule of recommended commonly used opioid analgesics

Generic name	Onset (min)	Peak action (min)	Duration (h)	Equivalent to 10 mg MS intramuscular	
				PO form	IM form
Morphine	60	60–90	4, 5	60	10
Slow-release morphine	60	180	8	45	NA
Hydromorphine	15–30	30	3–4	7.5	1.5
Meperidine	40–60	60–120	2–4	300	100
Methadone	60	120	6–8	200	130
Codeine	45	60	3–4	200	130
Oxycodone	45	60	3–4	30	15

MS, morphine sulfate.

Table 8-3. Antithromboembolic therapy in trauma

Condition	Qualifier	Treatment recommendation
Normal patient (No high risk history)	Early mobilization with cast	Extremity elevation and exercise
Normal patient (No high-risk history)	Lower extremity surgery or cast	Aspirin, exercises, early mobilization
High risk patient	Previous deep vein thrombosis pelvic/ femur fracture	Subcutaneous heparin preoperatively, coumadin 1.2–1.5 pro time control postoperatively
Positive duplex ultrasound		Heparin IV Coumadin
Positive duplex ultrasound	Pelvic procedure planned	Vena cava filter
Pulmonary emboli	Pulmonary angiogram diagnostic	Heparin IV Coumadin
Recurrent embolization (or pulmonary embolism with planned pelvic surgery)	Pulmonary angiogram diagnostic	Vena cava filter

   a. If **warfarin** is chosen for DVT prophylaxis for elective surgery, then give 10 mg the night before the operation and 5 mg the night after. Thereafter, alter the dose to maintain the prothrombin time, as determined by International Normalized Ratio at roughly two times the normal control (1). Although this time is difficult to regulate, when properly managed it gives the best results in prevention of fatal pulmonary embolism.
   b. If **aspirin** is chosen, then give 600 mg the night before the operation, 1200 mg bid rectally until oral intake is tolerated, and then use 600 mg bid PO.
   c. If **low-molecular-weight dextran** is selected, then give 50 mL/ hour during and after the operation up to 500 mL. Consider repeating daily for 3 days. Aspirin and dextran have been used in combination, but the rate of complications is high.
   d. If **heparin** is selected, then the usual dosage is 5,000 IU SQ q8h. It has also been given in combination with dihydroergotamine, 0.5 mg IM. The treatment is started at operation. For patients who have pelvic or femoral fractures, use subcutaneous heparin preoperatively and warfarin to maintain the prothrombin time at 1.5 times control level postoperatively.
   e. If low-molecular weight heparin is chosen the usual starting dose is 30 mg SQ Q12'. The advantage of this therapy is no monitoring of hematologic parameters is necessary.
   4. **Whatever drug regimen is selected, continue it until the patient is ambulatory or ready for discharge from the hospital; then discontinue the drug. The usual duration for use is 4 weeks after surgery.**
   G. Posttraumatic and postoperative **urinary retention** is not uncommon. If the bladder has been overdistended, it takes several days to regain normal tone. For this reason, if the patient requires catheterization, it should be done with

a small catheter that has a 5-mL balloon. Leave the catheter in the bladder and attached to closed gravity drainage. The catheter should be left in place until the patient is ambulatory or is off narcotics during the daytime (11).

H. Bowel. Make every effort to ensure that the patient's bowel habits are not disturbed. Changes in diet and analgesics are frequent causes of constipation. Prescribe bulk producers or stool softeners routinely for every patient. Docusate sodium (Colace), 100 mg bid, usually is satisfactory, but it may be necessary to supplement this with 30–60 mL of milk of magnesia at bedtime. Mineral oil is a useful stool softener, but it should be administered with caution because it interferes with vitamin absorption.

I. Skin. Pressure sores are prevented by good nursing care (23). Patients who are unable to change position frequently following surgery or trauma must be turned by the staff. Skin checks for redness are critical, especially in paraplegic and quadriplegic patients or in patients with concomitant head injury. If the orthopaedic condition does not allow frequent change in position, consider using special flotation mattresses or rotating beds (3).

J. Activities and physical therapy. The postoperative activity/physical therapy plan should be recorded in the written operative note. Each morning on rounds the staff decides what activity or therapy the patient should have that day. Activities may take diverse forms from minor diversions to a full-scale physical therapy program. Barbells and pulleys can be used to toughen the hands and strengthen triceps and shoulder muscles in preparation for crutch ambulation. Barbells are also useful in increasing chest muscle activity and improving cardiopulmonary exchange. All muscles, except those immediate to the injured or operative area, should be exercised in a set daily program. This exercise provides excellent distraction as well as a general sense of improved well-being. In addition, it may help prevent a thromboembolic episode. Regularly scheduled turning, the use of an incentive spirometer, coughing, deep breathing, and leg exercises are integral to any early physical therapy program. It is essential to turn all patients and inspect any areas of potential pressure at least once every 4 hours (27).

K. Preoperative check sheet for a general orthopaedic procedure

1. **Diagnosis**
2. **Condition**
3. **Diet**—nothing by mouth before surgery
4. **Activity**
5. **Vital signs**
6. **Enema** (optional for hip and back surgeries)
7. **Chlorhexidine, povidone-iodine, or hexachlorophene shower or scrub** two or three times, especially after any enema
8. **Laboratory data**
   a. Hematocrit/hemoglobin
   b. Urinalysis for joint replacement patients
   c. Chest roentgenogram if patient is older than 50 years
   d. ECG if patient is older than 50 years and no recent ECG results are available
   e. ESR if there is history of infection
   f. **Roentgenogram of operative area**
   g. **Blood gases** if there is history of significant trauma, the patient is older than 60 years, or there is history of pulmonary problems
   h. **Blood typed and cross-matched if significant loss is anticipated.** The use of an intraoperative suction, collection, and transfusion system such as the "cell saver" should be anticipated and used when blood loss is anticipated to be more than 500–600 mL (5). Similarly, the efficient use of a tourniquet can limit blood loss and should be planned for (7).
9. **Antibiotics** if indicated
10. **Analgesics** if indicated
11. **Hypnotic**
12. **Instruction in physical therapy** that may be required postoperatively

L. **Postoperative check sheet** for a general orthopaedic procedure
1. **Operation performed**
2. **Patient condition**
3. **Diet or IV orders**
4. **Activity or position**
5. **Vital signs**—record intake and output if indicated
6. **Patient turned, coughing, incentive spirometry, and deep breathing encouraged** q1–4h
7. Small urinary catheter inserted **if no urine** is produced within 8 hours postoperatively
8. Appropriate **analgesic** prescribed on a time-related basis or patient-controlled system
9. **Hypnotic**
10. **Multivitamin and vitamin C** supplements IV or PO
11. **Postoperative hematocrit/hemoglobin** (if indicated, preferably at least 8 hours postoperatively)
12. **Postoperative roentgenogram** if indicated
13. **Physical therapy orders**
14. **Physician notified** if blood pressure is less than 90/60, pulse is greater than 100, or temperature is greater than 38 degrees C
15. **When a diet is tolerated**
    a. Therapeutic doses of **iron if anemic**
    b. Anticoagulation therapy if indicated
    c. **Docusate sodium** and **milk of magnesia** as needed
16. **Social service consultation** if needed for disposition

References

1. Abelseth G, Buckley RE, Pinco GE, et al. Incidence of deep-vein thrombosis in patients with fractures of the lower extremity distal to the hip. *J Orthop Trauma* 1996;10:230–235.
2. Abramon CZ, et al. Drugs for pain. *Med Lett Drugs Ther* 1993;35:1.
3. Allman RM, et al. Air-fluidized beds or conventional therapy for pressure sores: a randomized trial. *Ann Intern Med* 1987;107:641.
4. Anard SS, Wells PS, Hunt D, et al. Does this patient have deep vein thrombosis? *JAMA,* 1998;279:1094–1099.
5. Benli IT, Akalin S, Duman E, et al. The results of intraoperative autotransfusion in orthopaedic surgery. *Bull Hosp J Dis* 1999;58:184–187.
6. Bergquist D, Benoni G, Bjorgell O, et al. Low-molecular weight heparin (enoxaparin) as prophylaxis against venous thromboembolism after total hip arthroplasty. *N Engl J Med* 1996;335:696–700.
7. Bono JV, Carl AL, Schneider JM. Exsanguination: gravity vs. esmarch. *Contemp Orthop* 1995;30:117–119.
8. Boxma H, Braekhuizen T, Patka P, et al. Randomized controlled trial of single-dose antibiotic prophylaxis in surgical treatment of closed fractures: the Dutch trauma trial. *Lancet* 1996;347:1133–1137.
9. Brandjes DPM, Buller HR, Heijboer H, et al. Randomized trial of effect of compression stockings in patients with symptomatic proximal vein thrombosis. *Lancet* 1997; 349:759–762.
10. Brasel KJ, Borgstrom DC, Weigelt JA. Cost-effective prevention of pulmonary embolus in high-risk trauma patients. *J Trauma* 1997;42:456–462.
11. Carpiniello VL, et al. Treatment of urinary complications after total joint replacement in elderly females. *Urology* 1988;32:186.
12. Ewing JA. Detecting alcoholism; the CAGE questionnaire. *JAMA* 1984;252: 1905–1907.
13. Fordyce MJF, Ling RSM. A venous foot pump reduces thrombosis after total hip replacement. *J Bone Joint Surg (Br)* 1992;74:45–49.
14. Froehlich JA, et al. Efficacy of compression ultrasound for detection of deep venous thrombosis in orthopaedic patients with hip fractures: a prospective study. *J Bone Joint Surg (Am)* 1989;71:249.

15. Geerts WH, Jay RM, Code KI, et al. A comparison of low-dose heparin with low-molecular weight heparin as prophylaxis against venous thromboembolism after major trauma. *N Engl J Med* 1996;335:701–707.
16. Gillam DL, Nelson CL. Comparison of a one-step iodophor skin preparation vs. traditional preparation in total joint surgery. *Clin Orthop* 1990;250:258–260.
17. Giordano CP, Koral KJ, Zuckerman JD, et al. Fracture blisters. *Clin Orthop* 1994; 307:214–221.
18. Giordano CP, Scott D, Kovel K, et al. Fracture blister formation: a laboratory study. *J Trauma,* 1995;38:907–909.
19. Gould MK, Dembitzer AD, Doyle RL, et al. Low molecular weight heparins compared with unfractionated heparin for treatment of acute deep venous thrombosis: a meta-analysis of randomized, controlled trials. *Arch Intern Med* 1999;130: 800–809.
20. Haddox JD, Joranson D, Angasola RT, et al. The use of opioids for the treatment of chronic pain: a consensus statement from the American Academy of Pain Medicine and the American Pain Society. *Clin J Pain* 1997;13:6–8.
21. Herrman FR, Safran C, Levkoff SE, et al. Serum albumin level on admission as a predictor of death, length of stay and readmission. *Arch Intern Med* 1992;152: 125–130.
22. Jamison RN, Ross MJ, Hoopman P, et al. Assessment of postoperative pain management: patient satisfaction and perceived helpfulness. *Clin J Pain* 1997;13: 229–236.
23. Khan FM, Moran CG, Pinder IM, et al. The incidence of fatal pulmonary embolism after knee replacement with no prophylactic anthoagulation. *J Bone Joint Surg* 1993;75:940–941.
24. Klein JD, Hey LA, Ya CS, et al. Perioperative nutrition and postoperative complications in patients undergoing spinal surgery. *Spine* 1996;22:2676–2682.
25. Knudson MM, Morabito O, Paiement GD, et al. Use of low molecular weight heparin in preventing thromboembolism in trauma patients. *J Trauma-Injury Infect Crit Care* 1996;41:446–459.
26. Lange GJ, Richardson M, Busse MJ, et al. Efficacy of surgical wound drainage in orthopaedic trauma patients: a randomized prospective trial. *J Orthop Trauma* 1998;12:348–350.
27. Maklebust J. Pressure ulcers: etiology and prevention. *Nurs Clin North Am* 1987; 22:359.
28. O'Connor PG, Schottenfeld RS. Patients with alcohol problems. *N Engl J Med* 1998;338:592–602.
29. O'Donnell D, Gunn J. Hypercedeemic and nephrolithiasis following multiple fractures. *J Bone Joint Surg* 1991;73:174.
30. Paiement GD, et al. Advances in the prevention of venous thromboembolic disease after hip and knee surgery. *Orthop Rev* 1989;18(Suppl):1.
31. Reilly DE, McNeely MJ, Doerner D, et al. Self reported exercise tolerance and the risk of serious perioperative complications. *Arch Intern Med* 1999;159:2185–2192.
32. Ritter MA, Campbell ED. Retrospective evaluation of an iodophor-incorporated antimicrobial plastic adhesive wound drape. *Clin Orthop* 1988;228:307–308.
33. Rodrigues JL, Lopez JM, Proctor ME, et al. Early placement of prophylactic vena cava filters in injured patients at high risk for pulmonary embolism. *J Trauma* 1996;40:797–804.
34. Sasso RC, Williams JF, Dismasi N, et al. Postoperative drains at the donor sites of iliac crest bone graft: a prospective, randomized study of morbidity at the donor site in patients who had a traumatic injury of the spine. *J Bone Joint Surg (Am)* 1998; 80:631–635.
35. Smith TK. Prevention of complications in orthopaedic surgery secondary to nutritional depletion. *Clin Orthop* 1987;222:91.
36. Varela CD, Vanghan TK, Carr JB, et al. Fracture blisters: clinical and pathological aspects. *J Orthop Trauma* 1993;7:417–427.
37. Wiklund RA, Rosenbaum SH. Anesthesiology. *N Engl J Med* 1997;337:1132–1141.
38. Williams-Russo P, Sharrock NE, Mattis S, et al. Cognitive effects after epidural vs. general anesthesia in older adults. *JAMA* 1995;274:44–50.

Selected Historical Readings

Harris WH, Athanasoulis CA, Waltron AC, et al. Prophylaxis of deep-vein thrombosis after total hip replacement, dextran and external pneumatic compression compared with 1.2 or 1.3 grams of aspirin daily. *J Bone Joint Surg (Am)* 1985;67:57.

Henry CP, et al. Effects of extradural bupivacaine on the haemostatic system. *Br J Anaesth* 1986;58:301.

Jensen JE, et al. Nutrition in orthopaedic surgery. *J Bone Joint Surg (Am)* 1982; 64:1263.

Kay SP, Moreland JR, Schmitter E. Nutritional status and wound healing in lower extremity amputations. *Clin Orthop* 1987;217:253.

McKenzie PJ, Wishart HY, Smith G. Long-term outcome after repair of fractured neck of femur: comparison of subarachnoid and general anaesthesia. *Br J Anaesth* 1984; 56:581.

Means JH. *The amenities of ward rounds and related matters.* Boston: Massachusetts General Hospital Print Shop, 1942.

Michelson JD, Lotke PA, Steinberg ME. Urinary bladder management after total joint replacement surgery. *N Engl J Med* 1988;319:321.

Schaeffer J. Catheter-associated bacteriuria. *Urol Clin North Am* 1986;13:735.

Thorburn J, Louden JR, Vallance R. Spinal and general anaesthesia in total hip replacement: frequency of deep vein thrombosis. *Br J Anaesth* 1980;52:1117.

Weed LL. *Medical records, medical education, and patient care,* 3rd ed. Chicago: Year Book, 1970.

9. TRACTION

I. **Objectives.** Although traction is being used with decreasing frequency for fracture care in the Western world, a knowledge of these effective principles is necessary for special indications or situations in which equipment or expertise is not available.

  A. Traction maintains the **length** of a limb as well as **alignment and stability** at the fracture site. Treating femoral fractures with fixed skeletal traction is an example.

  B. Traction can **allow joint motion** while maintaining alignment of the fracture. For example, the Pearson attachment on a Thomas splint allows knee movement during traction treatment of a femoral fracture; overbody or lateral skeletal traction allows elbow motion while maintaining alignment of a humeral fracture.

  C. Traction can **overcome muscle spasm** associated with bone or joint disease. An example is Buck's traction, which is used with hip injuries.

  D. **Edema is reduced** in an extremity by a traction unit that elevates the affected part above the heart.

II. **Essential materials.** The bed must have a firm mattress or a bed board. Elevate the head or the foot of the bed by using either shock blocks or the bed's intrinsic elevation system. Attach an overhead frame, trapeze, and side rails to the bed so the patient can shift position. Traction equipment includes bars, pulleys, ropes, weight hangers, skeletal traction apparatus, and, in some instances, plaster cast materials. Various figures in this chapter show the type and placement of equipment about the bed.

III. **Skin traction**

  A. Skin traction may be used as a definitive method of treatment as well as a first aid or temporary measure. The **traction force** applied to the skin is transmitted to bone via the superficial fascia, deep fascia, and intermuscular septa. Skin damage can result from too much traction force. The maximum weight recommended for skin traction is 10 lb or less, depending on the size and age of the patient. If this much weight is used, then discontinue the skin traction after 1 week. If less weight is used and if the skin is inspected biweekly, then skin traction may be safely used for 4–6 weeks. Pediatric patients need skin inspection on a more frequent basis.

  B. **Application**

    1. **Carefully prepare the skin** by removing the hair as well as washing and drying the area.

    2. **Avoid placing adhesive straps over bony prominences.** If bony prominences are in the area of strap application, cover them well with cast padding before the adhesive straps are applied. Always use a spreader bar to avoid pressure on bony prominences or at least relieve pressure on them.

    3. Make the **adhesive straps** from adhesive tape, moleskin adhesive, or a commercial skin traction unit consisting of foam boots with Velcro straps. Place the straps longitudinally on opposite sides of the extremity, with free skin left between the straps to prevent any tourniquet effect. Attach the free ends of these straps to the spreader bar. Hold the straps in place by encircling the extremity with an adhesive or elastic wrap. Then apply the traction rope to the spreader bar.

    4. Support the leg in traction to **prevent edema and irritation of the heel.**

IV. **Skeletal traction**

  A. **Definition.** Skeletal traction is applied through direct fixation to bone.

  B. **Equipment**

    1. **Kirschner wire** is a thin, smooth wire, that is 0.0360—0.0625 inches in diameter. The advantages of Kirschner wire are that it is easy to in-

sert and that it minimizes the chance of soft-tissue damage or infection. The disadvantage is that it rotates within an improper bow and can cut through osteoporotic bone. These complications are minimized by using the proper traction bow. Even though Kirschner wire is small in diameter and flexible, it can withstand a large traction force when the proper traction bow is used. This special bow provides the wire with rigidity by applying a longitudinal tension force. If properly placed and not improperly stressed, the wire does not break, causing less bone damage than the larger Steinmann pins.

2. **Steinmann pins** vary from 0.078 to 0.19 inches in diameter and come in smooth and threaded forms. Because they are large enough to have inherent stability, the Steinmann pin bow (Böhler bow), which attaches to these pins, does not exert tension along the pin as does the Kirschner traction bow. The two types of pins should be readily recognized and used with the appropriate bow (Fig. 9-1).

3. **Factors to be considered**

   a. A **nonthreaded wire or pin** is smaller, more uniform, less easily broken, more easily inserted, and removed with less twisting than the threaded type. A disadvantage is that it can slide laterally through the skin and bone. Even with careful attention, it can move enough to disturb the traction or predispose to a pin tract infection.

   b. The **threaded wire or pin** has stress risers at each thread, breaks more easily, must be larger in diameter to gain the same strength, and takes a longer time to insert. In inserting a threaded pin, one is tempted to go rapidly with the hand drill, which creates an undue amount of heat. On the other hand, because the threads prevent lateral slippage of the pin, this type is preferable to the nonthreaded variety for long-term traction.

4. The wires and pins are available with two types of points. One is a **trocar**, a blunted point that tends to grind through the bone with relatively little cutting ability. The other is a **diamond-shaped point**, a modified type of drill that passes through bone more easily and with less heating. Wires and pins that are dull, sharpened off-center, or bent should not be used. These wander during insertion and create a hole that is too large.

5. Note that pins and wires are frequently used as **internal fixation** devices for fractures; such use is discussed in other chapters.

C. Pin and wire insertion guidelines

1. Pin or wire insertion is a surgical procedure, so **some form of consent** is needed, at least with a witness in attendance who signs a note in the chart attesting that informed consent was obtained. A signed, witnessed surgical consent is preferred.

2. Establish the **status of neurovascular structures** before inserting the pins. Placement of the pins requires a knowledge of the specific anatomy and the location of vital structures. **Rule:** Always start the pin on the side where the vital structures are located. This gives better control and better avoidance of these structures. For instance, start an olecranon pin on the medial side to avoid the ulnar nerve.

3. **Skin preparation.** The skin should be free of signs of infection. Follow aseptic procedures, using a topical germicidal antiseptic, drapes, mask, and gloves.

4. It is difficult to obtain enough **anesthesia** to block the periosteum completely. Anesthetize the skin and subcutaneous tissue with 1% lidocaine on the starting side of the bone. Go down to the periosteum with the needle tip and insert enough lidocaine around this area to produce some anesthesia. If there is pain as the pin is inserted and approaches bone, then inject more anesthetic. Drill the pin approximately halfway through the bone, get an idea where it will come out, and then anesthetize the opposite side. In a case in which the wire penetrates two bones, such as the tibia and fibula, it is impossible to anesthetize the area between the two

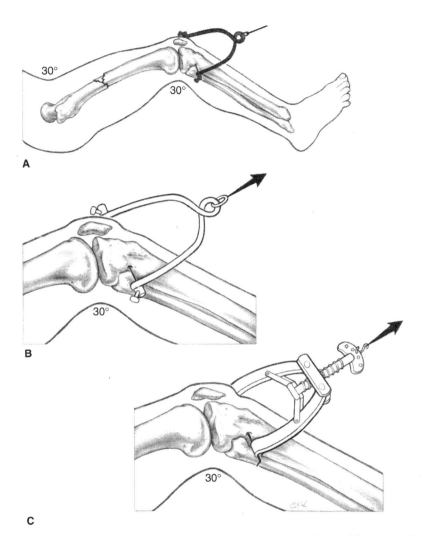

FIG. 9-1. Traction bows. When using skeletal traction to treat femoral fractures, the knee is kept in slight flexion **(A)**. Proximal tibial traction is reserved for adults. To avoid physeal injury in children with resultant recurvation deformity, distal femoral traction proximal to the distal femoral physis is used. For larger Steinmann pins, a Böhler bow is used **(B)**. The tensioning capabilities of the Kirschner bow allows the use of smaller Kirschner wires **(C)**.

bones. Tell the patient ahead of time that this may be painful for a few seconds but that as soon as the drilling stops, the pain will cease.

5. **Skin incision.** When starting the procedure, pass the wire or pin through a stab wound made with a No. 11 blade. If only a puncture skin wound is made by the pin, then **tight** skin adherence to the pin predisposes to an infection. If an abscess does occur, then drain it by extending the stab wound. Apply a tincture of benzoin compound to the entrance and exit wound to provide some adhesiveness between the skin and metal, thereby lessening the chance of a pin tract infection.

6. Pins and wires should be inserted using a **hand drill** rather than a power tool. When placing one or two wires, the time supposedly saved by using power equipment is expended in preparation time. There is also a tendency to use too high a speed and generate too much heat, thereby promoting development of bone necrosis around the pin insertion. A ring sequestrum can occur. The smaller the pin and the slower the twist on the hand drill, the faster the pin is inserted. Adequate support of the limb or adequate help must be available so that, as the pin is being inserted, the limb does not shift and cause the patient further pain.

7. Traction wires or pins are **best placed in the metaphysis.** Steinmann pins usually are not placed in dense cortical bone. Use caution to avoid open epiphyseal plate damage, which can result in a growth disturbance. For example, in the area of the tibial tubercle, assume in female patients younger than 14 years and in male patients younger than 16 years that the epiphyseal plate is open. Because of the risk of physeal injury in the proximal tibia, choose the distal femur for skeletal traction in such young patients if possible. Ideally, pass the pin through only skin, subcutaneous tissue, and bone. Avoid muscles and tendons.

8. **Do not violate a fracture hematoma** by skeletal wires or pins for traction or else the equivalent of an open fracture will result.

9. **Do not penetrate joints** with traction wires or pins as pyarthrosis can occur. Do not enter the suprapatellar pouch with distal femoral wires or pins.

10. **Points to remember** about wire or pin insertion:
    a. Chuck the wire or pin so that just **an inch or so is exposed** to prevent wandering and bending.
    b. **Tighten chuck sufficiently** to prevent score marks that are sources of metal corrosion and fracture.
    c. Be certain the wire **does not bend** as it is inserted.
    d. Use the proper traction bow (Fig. 9-1).

D. **Specific areas of insertion**

1. **Metacarpals.** Place the wire through the diaphysis of the index and middle metacarpals. To facilitate insertion, push the first dorsal interosseous muscle in a volar direction and palpate the subcutaneous portion of the bone. Angle the wire to pass through the index and middle metacarpals and to come out the dorsum of the hand, so as to preserve the natural arch.

2. **Distal radius and ulna.** Usually place the wire or pin through both the radius and the ulna. This site is rarely used.

3. **Olecranon.** Take care to avoid an open epiphysis. Do not place the pin too far distally because this causes elbow extension, and it is more comfortable to pull through a flexed elbow than an extended elbow. Use a moderate-sized wire or pin and insert from the medial side to avoid the ulnar nerve. Use a very small bow.

4. **Distal femur.** Start on the medial side, anterior enough to avoid the neurovascular structures. This insertion is best accomplished by placing the pin 1 inch inferior to the abductor tubercle. If the pin will be used for traction on a fracture table for delayed intramedullary nailing, make sure it is placed far anterior, off the coronal midline. Fluoroscopy should be used to help the surgeon avoid an open physis.

5. **Proximal tibia.** Place the wire or pin 1 inch inferior and ½ inch posterior to the tibial tubercle, starting on the lateral side to avoid the peroneal nerve. Take extreme care to avoid an open epiphysis; if the anterior portion of the proximal tibial epiphyseal plate is violated, genu recurvatum can occur.

6. **Distal tibia and fibula.** Start the pin 1 to 1½ fingerbreadths above the most prominent portion of the lateral malleolus to avoid the ankle mortise. Insert it parallel to the ankle joint and angulate it slightly anteriorly. The surgeon should feel the pin pass through the two fibular cortices and then the two tibial cortices. Pass the pin through both bones to avoid the tendons and neurovascular structures. If the pin is placed too far proximally, the foot rests on the bow, and a pressure sore may occur.

7. **Calcaneus.** Generally select a large diamond-point pin. The preferred insertion site is 1 inch inferior and posterior from the lateral malleolus or 1¾ inch inferior and 1½ inches posterior from the medial malleolus. Because of the position of the tibial nerve, the medial site is preferred. If the pin is placed too far posteriorly, it causes a calcaneal position of the foot. If the pin is placed too far inferiorly, it may cut out of the bone. If the pin is placed too far superiorly, it can enter the subtalar joint and also spear the flexor tendons or tibial artery. Infections that are difficult to treat often occur when the calcaneus is used for long-term traction.

V. **Cervical spine traction**
   A. **Neck halter traction** is the simplest of the different types of cervical spine traction but usually is not used in the treatment of acute cervical spine fractures or dislocations, being reserved for chronic conditions such as a cervical radiculopathy. Apply the traction to the mandible and occiput with a soft, commercially made halter.
      1. When **continuous traction** is used with the patient in the supine position, do not exceed 10 lb (5 lb is usually sufficient). With the patient sitting, approximately 8 lb may be added to the attached weight to account for the weight of the head. The total attached weight should not exceed 15 lb with the patient in the sitting position. The traction should not be strictly continuous but used for 1–3 hours followed by rest intervals to allow jaw motion and to relieve pressure on the skin.
      2. If **intermittent traction** for short periods of time is used three times daily, then up to 30 lb may be used.
      3. **Problems** associated with head halter traction are related to the weight used and the position of the neck. The optimum position is usually neutral or in slight flexion. Temporomandibular joint discomfort can ordinarily be relieved by changing the direction of traction force or decreasing the attached weight. Symptoms from local skin pressure may be relieved by the above methods or by appropriate padding.
   B. **Skull tong traction** is a form of cervical spine traction and is applied by one of the many types of skull calipers (tongs) (Fig 9-2). The most satisfactory caliper is screwed into the skull without the need for previous trephining and does not penetrate more than a preset depth. The Gardner-Wells tongs are recommended (Fig. 9-3) (3). With this type of apparatus, heavy traction can be applied to the skull for as long as required. It is especially useful for cervical spine fractures and dislocations. Perform the following procedures after the scalp is cleaned and draped; local shaving is sufficient and is not absolutely mandatory.
      1. The **Gardner-Wells skull traction tongs** are easy to insert. After preparing the skull, position the tongs below the temporal crest and tighten. A spring device within the tong points automatically sets the correct depth and tension. Then the indicator protrudes 1 mm from the knob of the tong, at which time the correct pressure (equivalent to 6–8 in-lb) is exerted. Retighten these pins in a sequential manner to the same value the next day, and then do not tighten them again unless loosening occurs.

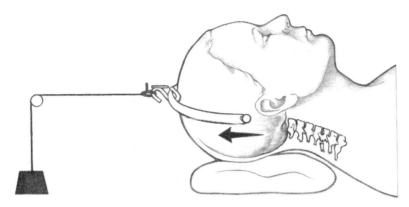

FIG. 9-2. Tong traction. This treatment is used for most cervical fractures and dislocations. The points are positioned just above the ear pinnae. Padding can be used to generate more flexion or extension of the cervical spine as is indicated for reduction based on lateral cervical roentgenograms.

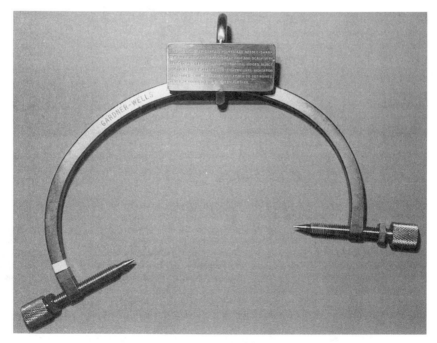

FIG. 9-3. Gardner-Wells tongs.

2. Keep the head end of the frame slightly elevated so the patient's body acts as counteraction.

3. Initiate cervical traction at 10–15 lb and incrementally increase only after checking the appropriate roentgenograms. Initiating traction at higher weights can occasionally result in marked distraction of ligamentous injuries. For definitive traction, **Crutchfield's rule of 5 lb/level** starting with 10 lb for the head allows for a maximum range of 30–40 lb for a C5-6 injury.

C. **Fixed halo skull traction.** The halo device, originally introduced by Nickel and Perry (1,4), can be used alone for traction or combined with a vest or cast.

   1. **Materials**
      a. **Halo ring** (five standard sizes available). Carbon fiber rings are preferred because radiographs and magnetic resonance imaging (MRI) scans can be obtained without distortion.
      b. **Five skull pins** (one spare included)
      c. **Two torque screwdrivers**
      d. **Four positioning pins**
      e. **A wooden board** (4 × 15 × ¼ inch)

   2. **Application** procedures are modified from those described by Young and Thomassen (6) and Botte and colleagues (1).
      a. **Shave and trim hair** around the pin sites (optional). The pin sites should be 1 cm above the lateral third of the eyebrow and the same distance above the tops of the ears in the parietal and occipital areas. Place the halo just inferior to the greatest circumference of the head (Fig. 9-4).
      b. Position the patient supine on a bed with the head extended beyond the edge. **Have the head supported** by an assistant's hands or by a 4-inch wide board placed under the head and neck.
      c. Place a **sterile towel** under the patient's head. This step is not necessary if an attendant is holding the head.
      d. Select a halo ring that allows for **1.5 cm clearance.** If MRI studies are anticipated, then an MRI-compatible ring and pins must be used (carbon fiber material).
      e. **Autoclave** the halo ring, skull pins, and positioning pins.
      f. The assistant, wearing gloves, **positions** the halo ring around the head with the raised portion of the ring over the posterior part of the skull. Use positioning pins and plates to place the ring in the proper attitude and to equalize the clearance around the head.
      g. Infiltrate the skin with an **anesthetic** at the four pin sites.
      h. The **skull pins** should be at a 90-degree angle to the skull and turned to finger tightness. The skull pins are designed so that no scalp incisions or drill holes are needed. The shape of the point draws the skin under it and does not cause bleeding. Try to avoid puckering of the skin at the pin site. If puckering does occur, then remove the pins, flatten the skin, and repenetrate.
      i. Both operators use the **torque screwdrivers** simultaneously, turning opposing skull pins. Gain increments of 2 in-lb evenly up to the maximum desired by the physician. A suggested maximum is 4 ½ in-lb for children and 6–8 in-lb for adults.
      j. **Remove the positioning pins.**
      k. Incorporate the **support rods** of the halo apparatus into the plaster body jacket, as shown in Fig. 7-5, or use a sheepskin-lined molded plastic body jacket that is commercially available or custom made by an orthotist (Fig. 7-6).
      l. **Tangential roentgenographic views** of the skull or a computed tomography (CT) scan can be ordered to check the depth of the skull pins but are not routinely necessary.

   3. **Care of pin sites**
      a. **Clean** around the pins with peroxide solution using a Q-tip twice daily.

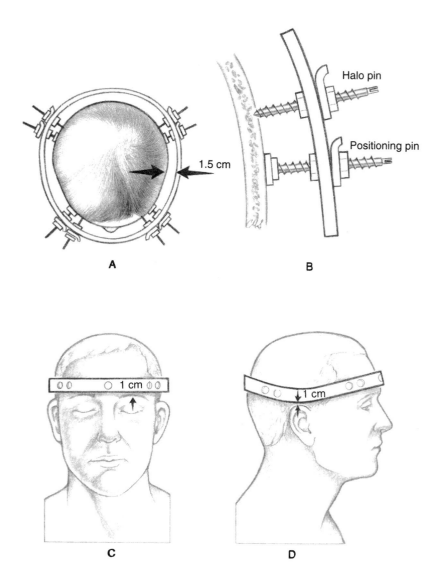

FIG. 9-4. Principles of a halo ring application. The correct ring size allows for 1.5 cm of clearance **(A)**. Positioning pins are used to stabilize the ring while the skull pins are inserted **(B)**. The proper position of the ring is 1 cm above eyebrows and ear pinnae **(C, D)**.

b. **Check the torque** of the pins for the first few days. **Note:** If the patient complains of repeated looseness or if the proper torque cannot be gained, then move the pin to another place on the ring by the aforementioned method. Do not remove a loose pin until the fifth replacement pin is inserted.

VI. **Upper extremity traction**

A. **Dunlop's or modified Dunlop's skin traction.** This type of traction is occasionally useful for the management of supracondylar humeral fractures. Place the patient supine and suspend the arm in skin traction with the shoulder abducted and slightly flexed. In addition, slightly flex the elbow. Modification of this type of traction provides counteraction on the humerus, which can be achieved with the arm over the edge of the bed and counterweight suspended from a felt cuff over the humerus, or with a felt cuff over the forearm pulling laterally with the elbow flexed (Fig. 9-5). Two disadvantages of Dunlop's traction are that it cannot be applied over skin injuries and that elevation of the humeral fracture above the level of the heart is not possible with this method.

B. **Overbody or lateral skeletal traction**

1. In the management of extraarticular humeral shaft and metaphyseal fractures, it is occasionally desirable to maintain the shoulder in flexion without abduction but with the elbow at a right angle by placing the arm over the body. Maintain this position through olecranon skeletal traction, which allows some flexion and extension of the elbow if the traction pin is properly inserted. Because the hand and wrist usually tire in this position, support the wrist with a plaster splint. Skeletal traction through the olecranon may also be used in the lateral position (Fig. 9-6).

2. A special, rarely used adaptation of upper extremity olecranon traction may be made by **placing the patient in a shoulder spica cast** that

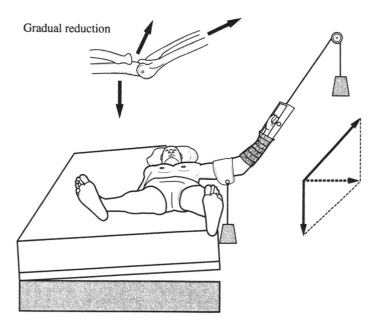

Gradual reduction

FIG. 9-5. Modified Dunlop's traction. A weight of 1–5 lb is usually required. Associated circulatory embarrassment might be aggravated by increasing elbow flexion.

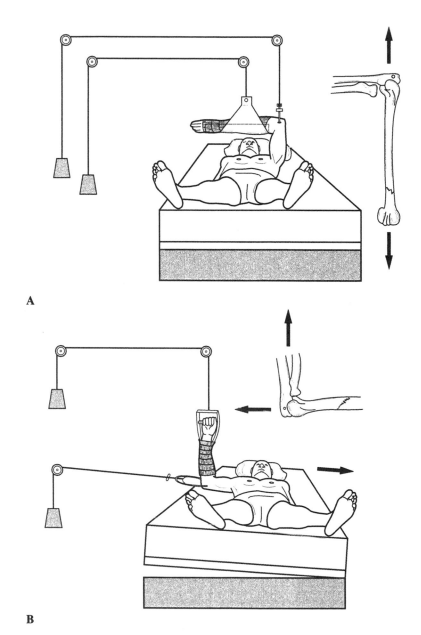

FIG. 9-6. Olecranon pin traction. **A:** Overbody traction. Note that the elbow joint can move without disturbing the fracture. The hand and wrist rest in a plaster splint. **B:** Lateral traction.

incorporates an olecranon pin into the plaster to apply fixed skeletal traction. This adaptation allows the patient to be ambulatory.

VII. **Lower extremity traction**

A. Apply **Buck's extension skin traction** (Fig. 9-7) to the lower extremity to reduce muscle spasms about the knee or hip. However, do not use this form of traction for back conditions. Control rotation to some extent by placing the leg on a pillow with sandbags on the lateral side of the ankle. Although Buck's traction is commonly recommended for hip fractures, its use should be limited in duration. For intracapsular fractures, keep the hip flexed to increase hip capsule volume and thereby limit pain. The effectiveness of this type of traction in decreasing pain has not been demonstrated (2).

B. **Hamilton-Russell's traction** (Fig. 9-8) may be used for hip or femoral fractures, especially in children weighing 40–60 lb. Accomplish the traction with either skin traction or distal tibial skeletal traction plus a sling placed beneath the posterior distal thigh (avoid pressure in the popliteal fossa). A rope is attached to the sling and goes first to an overhead pulley, then to a pulley at the foot of the bed, next to a pulley on the foot plate attached to the spreader bar, then to a fourth pulley at the end of the bed, and finally to the attached weight. Analysis of the vector forces shows that the traction applied to the leg is increased considerably by moving the overhead pulley toward the foot of the bed. If this type of traction is used on a child, one usually attaches 3 lb to the traction apparatus. Produce a counteraction with the patient's body weight by elevating the foot of the bed.

C. **Split Russell's traction** has the same indications and vector forces as Hamilton-Russell's traction. The difference is that split Russell's traction uses two separate ropes and weights, as shown in Fig. 9-9.

D. **Charnley's traction unit** (boot) is useful for applying skeletal traction to a lower limb and is recommended for routine use (Fig. 9-10). This limits rotational forces on the limb controlling alignment, maintains the ankle in neutral position, and limits the stress on the traction bow. The unit is assembled

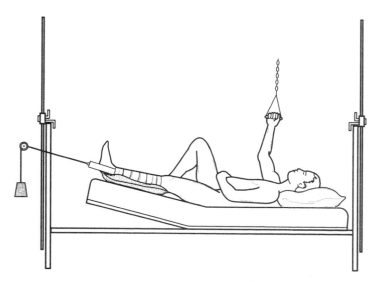

FIG. 9-7. Buck's extension skin traction. Note elevation of the foot of the bed and support under the calf. Protect the fibular head and malleoli. A weight of 5–7 lb of traction is sufficient.

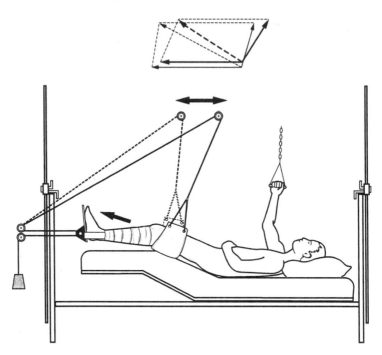

FIG. 9-8. Hamilton-Russell's traction. Note that the resultant force on the femur is a summation of vector analysis and depends on the position of the overhead pulley. Change the angulation of the distal fragment by moving the single overhead pulley.

by inserting a wire or pin through the proximal end of the tibia and then incorporating the wire or pin in a short-leg cast. The advantages are as follows:

1. The foot and ankle are maintained in a **functional position.**
2. The limb is suspended in a cast, and there is no pressure on the calf muscles or peroneal nerve.
3. **Movement** of the skeletal pin or wire is **reduced** to a minimum.

E. **Balanced suspension skeletal traction** provides a direct pull on either the tibia or the femur through a wire pin. Rest the lower extremity on a stockinet or a cloth towel stretched over a Thomas splint. The splint, with or without a Pearson attachment, is balanced with counterweights to suspend the leg in a freely floating system. Attach separate suspension ropes to both sides of the proximal full ring Thomas splint, run the ropes through overhead pulleys, and fasten weights to ropes at either end of the bed but not over the patient. Control rotation of the ring by individually adjusting the amount of attached weight. Suspend the distal end of the splint from a single rope to an overhead pulley, with the weight attached to the rope at one end of the bed. For safety reasons, place no weights over the patient. Control rotation of the extremity by a light counterweight attached to the side of the splint or by a crossbar attached to the plaster cast. The Charnley traction unit (boot) is ideally suited for both balanced suspension and fixed skeletal traction (which is discussed next) (Fig. 9-11). A **Pearson attachment** allows for flexion motion of the knee joint, which is an advantage, especially for those in traction for a long period of time or for those who have a comminuted tibial plateau fracture.

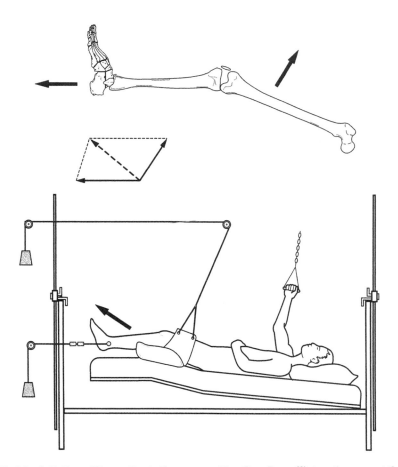

FIG. 9-9. Split Russell's traction is the same as Hamilton-Russell's traction except that two separate ropes and weights are used instead of one.

F. Use **fixed skeletal traction** in the initial treatment of femoral fractures in patients who will go on to intramedullary nailing or who need to be transported either in the hospital or to another facility.
   1. **If the fracture must be reduced,** then the apprehensive patient or the patient with a transverse fracture usually requires general or regional anesthesia.
   2. Apply the **Charnley traction unit** to the lower leg.
   3. Select a **full or half ring Thomas splint** that is 2 inches greater than the proximal thigh (5). This leeway is critical because a ring that is too tight causes distal edema and one that is too loose is ineffective. The ring must fit against the fibrofatty tissue in the perineum and the medial arch of the buttocks. The half ring is placed against the ischium and the strap tightened loosely against the anterior thigh.
   4. While the leg is supported in traction, place the ring on the limb. Attach a single **master sling** of nonextensible cloth (a double-thickness cloth towel is ideal) measuring 6–9 inches long to the splint beneath the fracture. Adjust tension to support the limb. If the sling is too tight, then it

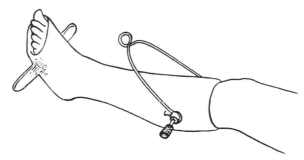

FIG. 9-10. Charnley's traction unit consisting of a skeletal wire or pin incorporated into a short-leg cast, which has a crossbar fixed to the sole. The unit is commonly employed for femoral fractures treated with skeletal traction.

causes excessive flexing of the proximal fragment; if it is too loose, then it does not control the fracture. Attach this sling to the splint with several clamps available for attaching ropes.

5. Make a supporting or master pad that is 1–1½ inches thick and 6–9 inches long from an abdominal dressing or a folded towel. Insert a safety pin into the pad to assist localization of the pad on roentgenograms. Place this pad beneath the fracture and adjust it to maintain the normal anterior bow of the femur. A single sling is placed on the Thomas splint distally to support the short-leg cast.

6. **Check the reduction.** End-on reduction for transverse fractures is ideal in the adult, but take care to avoid distraction. If the patient will have delayed intramedullary nailing, maintain some distraction. In the child,

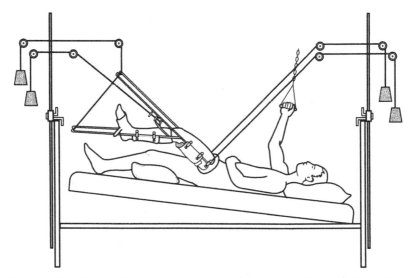

FIG. 9-11. With balanced suspension traction, the various weights are adjusted until satisfactory alignment and suspension of the femoral fracture are achieved within the Thomas splint. Note the Charnley traction unit, firm mattress, bed board, and master pad. Wrap an elastic bandage about the thigh and splint to minimize the acute swelling.

bayonet apposition is preferred. With the oblique fracture, it is important to feel bone-on-bone contact to be certain there is no soft-tissue interposition. If there is interposition, then it can usually be dislodged by manipulation. Then assess length, alignment, and rotational positions and attach traction to the end of the splint. Extend two ropes from the Steinmann pin around the sides of the splint and attach them to the splint end. Tape two tongue blades together to form a Spanish windlass to adjust tension. After the first day or two, when muscle spasm subsides, only slight traction is necessary to maintain the appropriate alignment. It might not be possible to gain full length initially because of unusual tense swelling of the thigh. Attach a second pad or C-clamp to add cross-traction if needed for better alignment, particularly in the more transverse fracture patterns.

7. **Suspend the splint** to allow patient mobility in bed and to reduce edema. Figure 9-12 depicts the completed setup.

8. **Follow-up care,** particularly in the first few weeks, is important. Wash the skin beneath the ring daily with alcohol, dry thoroughly, and powder with talc every 2 hours. The conscious patient may perform this care each hour and massage the skin to improve blood supply. If it is necessary to relieve skin pressure under the ring, then apply traction directly from the end of the splint; slight distraction is preferred when intramedullary nailing is to be delayed for more than 24 hours. Be careful, however, not to cause distraction at the fracture site when using fixed skeletal traction as the definitive treatment. Start quadriceps exercises within the first few days and continue on an around-the-clock basis. All the elements outlined earlier are essential for effective utilization of fixed skeletal traction.

VIII. **Complications of skeletal traction**

A. An **infection** of the pin tract is a common complication, but its incidence is reduced when the previously stated guidelines for pin and wire insertion are carefully followed. If an infection with a small sequestrum occurs, it is wise to

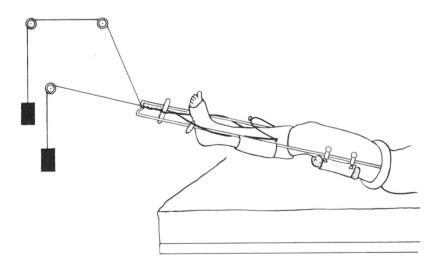

FIG. 9-12. Fixed skeletal traction. Note the Charnley traction unit, the method of adjusting traction force via the windlass, the position of the master pad, and the traction on the end of the Thomas splint to relieve skin pressure on the proximal thigh. Place an elastic bandage around the thigh and splint to help control edema.

remove the pin, curette the pin tract, and replace the pin. The infection usually subsides satisfactorily with antibiotic therapy.

B. **Distraction** of bone fragments at the fracture site is avoided by frequently measuring extremity length, by using roentgenograms to check the position of fragments, and by keeping traction to a minimum. Distraction is best assessed by lateral roentgenograms because anteroposterior roentgenograms may not be perpendicular to the fracture and may underestimate the distraction. Otherwise, distraction can predispose to a delayed union or nonunion of the fracture.

C. Use heavy traction with care and close observation to avoid **nerve palsy.** If paralysis does occur, adjust and possibly abandon the traction.

D. **Pin breakage** is unusual but can occur if very heavy traction is used for long periods, especially in a restless patient. To protect the pin, incorporate it into plaster in the manner of the Charnley traction unit. Decrease the potential of metal corrosion and fracture by using a wire or pin that is not scored.

References

1. Botte MJ, Byrne TP, Garfin SR. Application of the halo device for immobilization of the cervical spine utilizing an increased torque pressure. *J Bone Joint Surg* 1987;69A:750.
2. Finsen V, Borset M, Buvik GE, et al. Preoperative traction in patients with hip fractures. *Injury* 1992;23:242–244.
3. Gardner W. The principle of spring-loaded points for cervical traction. *J Neurosurgery* 1973;39:543–544.
4. Garfin SR, Botte MJ, Enteno RS, et al. Osteology of the skull as it effects halo pin placement. *Spine* 1985;10:696–698.
5. Henry BJ, Vrahas MS. The Thomas splint: questionable boast of an indispensable tool. *Am J Orthop* 1996;25:602–604.
6. Young R, Thomassen EH. Step-by-step procedure for applying a halo ring. *Orthop Rev* 1974;3:62.

Selected Historical Readings

Charnley J. *The closed treatment of common fractures,* 3rd ed. Baltimore: Williams & Wilkins, 1972.
Nickel VL, Perry J, Garret A, et al. The halo. *J Bone Joint Surg* 1968;50A:1400.

10. OPERATING ROOM EQUIPMENT AND TECHNIQUES

I. **Preparation for surgery**
   A. **Scheduling surgery**
      1. **Prepare the patient** so that the risks, goals, and benefits of the selected procedure are understood. Ideally, the patient or legal next of kin should know the nature of the patient's condition, the nature of the proposed treatment, the alternative treatments, the anesthetic risks, the anticipated probability for success, and the possible risks. Explain the postoperative dressings, casts or splints, exercise program, and other special requirements, When the patient has been so informed and has all questions answered, obtain a signed operative permit.
      2. **Review the technique** of the proposed operation. At the time surgery is scheduled, be confident that the patient's condition meets the appropriate indications for the proposed surgery. Know the anatomy and the surgical approaches involved in the selected surgical procedure. Carefully plan the procedure with the proper alternatives to reduce the length of time the wound is open. Be sure that all special equipment, implants, assistance, and time are available as expected. Complete any necessary templating of roentgenograms and preoperative planning drawings (11).
   B. **Before surgery**
      1. **Patient preparation.** Check to make sure the physical examination, chest roentgenogram, electrocardiogram, hematocrit, and other indicated preoperative studies do not contraindicate surgery. Obtain a preoperative consultation from a specialist in internal medicine for all patients with unstable medical conditions. Order blood, tetanus prophylaxis, and special medications as indicated. If an extremity operation is planned, be sure that the nails are properly trimmed and cleaned. Have the patient, family, and support system begin planning early for post-discharge or post-operation disposition needs, such as transportation home, wheelchairs, hospital beds, wheelchair access to the home, and commodes.
      2. **Antibiotics** (1)
         a. **Preoperative antibiotics** should be administered for surgery that is associated with a high risk of postoperative deep wound infection, that is, when any implant is inserted, the operation results in a large hematoma or dead space, the anticipated operating time is greater than 2 hours, or the surgeon is operating on bones, joints, nerves, or tendons. Various studies have shown immediate preoperative and postoperative antibiotics to be beneficial with surgery involving musculoskeletal tissues (1,14,24) . See Chap. 1 for utilization of antibiotics with open wounds and trauma or "dirty surgery." The duration of antibiotic therapy can be limited to 24 hours postoperatively without increasing the risk to infection.
         b. The **timing** of the antibiotic therapy is as important as **dosage.** Ideally, the antibiotic level should be highest when the tourniquet is inflated or the surgical hematoma (potential culture medium) is formed. Thus, the antibiotics **must be given before surgery.** Because the highest blood levels with IV administration are achieved immediately, the ideal time to give IV antibiotics is when the patient is in the preoperative area or operating room during the 10- to 15-minute period just before the tourniquet is inflated or before the surgical incision is made. Some surgeons who believe that the tissue concentration of antibiotics is more important than the blood levels administer the first dose approximately 2–6 hours before surgery. Either way, the antibiotics are readministered at the recommended intervals throughout the operative procedure except when a tourniquet is used. The surgeon must also be aware of the

effect of blood loss on the antibiotic levels. If the blood loss equals one half of the patient's volume, then approximately one half of the effective amount of the antibiotics has also been lost. The interval between the recommended doses for that patient, therefore, must be cut in half.

    c. The authors recommend using one of the **first generation cephalosporins,** which are bactericidal for bacteria usually found in wound infections following musculoskeletal surgery; staphylococcal and steptocconal specimens. The recommended antibiotics are listed in Table 10-1.

  3. Patients who have been on long-term steroid therapy need adjustments made in their **steroid dosage** when they undergo surgery or other major stress. The following is the simplest published regimen that the authors have found (5).

    a. On the **day of surgery,** order hydrocortisone sodium succinate (SoluCortef), 100 mg IV, to be given with the premedication before surgery.

    b. Use the **same dose** on the **first postoperative day.**

    c. Use 50 mg of **hydrocortisone** on the **second postoperative day.**

    d. Use 25 mg of **hydrocortisone** on the **third postoperative day,** and then continue only with the patient's normal oral daily dose.

  4. Surgery in patients with insulin-dependent diabetes mellitus

    a. In the morning before surgery, the patient should omit breakfast and take about one half of the normal insulin dose SQ.

    b. After surgery, use a **glucose measuring instrument every 4–6h** to monitor blood glucose levels. The following **sliding scale** is useful: If the glucose level is greater than 350 mg/dL, give 15 units regular insulin SQ. If the level exceeds 250 mg/dL, give 10 units regular insulin SQ.

    c. Return patients to their usual insulin dosage regimen as soon as they return to their normal activity level and to their usual American Diabetic Association diet.

  5. Surgery in patients with hemophilia (2,17)

    a. For a discussion of the **types of hemophilia** and **methods for replacing deficient factors,** see Chap. 1 **(VI.).**

    b. Medical management of a patient with hemophilia who needs surgery requires precise assays of **factor levels** and **prior survival studies** of replacement factors to learn the effect of inhibitors and the biologic half-life in a particular patient. Aim to achieve 100% plasma levels just before anesthetics for surgery are administered. Maintain the level at 60% of normal for the first 4 days and more than 40% for the next 4 days. A level of 100% is also necessary for manipulation of a joint under anesthesia and for removal of pins. A 40% level is needed for suture removal. Levels of 20% are maintained for postoperative physical therapy for as long as 4–6 weeks after major joint surgery. Forty units of factor per kilogram of body weight administered just before anesthesia (unless survival studies done before surgery show that higher doses are needed) usually achieve close to 100% plasma factor levels.

C. Day of surgery

  1. Be sure the **anesthesia** is adequate in terms of time, relaxation, and ability to position the patient properly (8,18). Supervise **positioning, preparing, and draping** so the planned procedure can be accomplished without difficulty (7). While the assistant prepares the patient, the surgeon can go to the instrument table with the scrub nurse and review each instrument and implant from start to finish, outlining the planned procedure. The surgeon can also indicate what may be needed if any complications arise. The idea is to ensure that all equipment is available, to review the procedure in the surgeon's mind, and to prepare

Table 10-1. Recommended prophylactic antibiotics for orthopaedic surgical procedures (open trauma, joint replacement, bone, joint, tendon, ligament, and nerve surgery)[a]

Bactericidal antibiotics	Dosage for adults	Notable contraindications	Possible complications
Cefazolin[b] (Kefzol or Ancef)	1–2 g q6–8h	History of an anaphylactic reaction to a penicillin drug requires careful usage; with renal insufficiency, the dose must be adjusted to the creatinine clearance	Cephalosporins occasionally cause a false-positive urine reaction with the Clinitest tablets (use test tape instead) and rarely cause blood dyscrasias, overt hemolytic anemia, or renal dysfunction; cephalothin frequently causes a positive Coombs' test
Vancomycin[c]	1 g initially, then 500 mg, q6h	With impaired renal function, dose must be adjusted to patient's creatinine clearance	Rapid IV administration can cause hypotension, which could be especially dangerous during induction of anesthesia, so administer at rate of no more than 10 mg/min

[a] Antibiotics should be given immediately postoperatively and then one dose (IV) or up to 24–48 hrs after surgery.
[b] Cefazolin can also be given IM.
[c] For hospitals in which *Staphylococcus aureus* and *Staphylococcus epidermis* frequently cause wound infection or for patients allergic to cephalosporins.

the nurse so that nurse and surgeon can work together efficiently. See App. E for the position and draping of the patient. See **3.c** for a discussion of skin preparations.

2. **Pneumatic tourniquets** (19,20,22)

a. When a tourniquet is to be used, the necessary **apparatus** includes a cuff with a smooth, wrinkle-free surface that is a proper size. Select a tourniquet so that the width of the cuff covers approximately one third of the patient's arm length. Check the tubing for leaks. The tourniquet gauge should have a safety valve release, because excessively high pressures can cause paralysis. The inflating device must allow rapid attainment of desired pressure.

b. Plan surgery to **minimize** the **operative time** and, as a consequence, the **tourniquet time.** The conventional safe maximum inflation time of the tourniquet is 2 hours. The cuff may be applied about the arm or thigh but generally not about the forearm or leg. There is no evidence that padding between the cuff and the skin is of any value, and such padding can cause skin wrinkles. Apply a plastic sheet with the adhesive edge placed on the skin distal to the tourniquet and cover the tourniquet with the plastic sheet as shown in Fig. 10-1, thereby preventing skin preparation solutions from getting underneath the cuff. Exsanguinate the limb with an Esmarch rubber bandage or with elevation of the limb above the patient's heart for 60 seconds before inflating the tourniquet. An Esmarch bandage should not be used in cases of tumors or infection. Flexing the knee or elbow before inflating the tourniquet makes positioning and closure easier and prevents the possible complication of a ruptured muscle, which can occur by forced flexion of a tourniquet-fixed muscle. Rapidly inflate to the desired pressure. This is 175–250 mm Hg in the upper extremity, depending on the arm circumference and the patient's systolic blood pressure, and 250–350 mm Hg in the lower extremity, depending on thigh circumference (10,19). Tissue pressure is always somewhat lower than tourniquet pressure, but

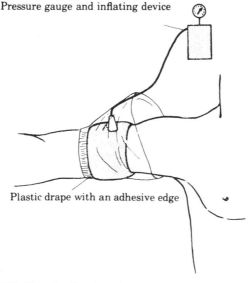

Pressure gauge and inflating device

Plastic drape with an adhesive edge

FIG. 10-1. Application of a pneumatic tourniquet.

at 30-cm circumference, it is close to 100%, declining to 70% at 60 cm circumference (9,10,19,23). The pressures should be decreased for infants and small children. Immediately after deflation, remove or loosen the cuff to prevent a venous congestion from proximal constriction of the extremity. If the tourniquet is deflated and reinflated during surgery, the time for reversal of the tourniquet-produced ischemia is proportional to the tourniquet time; that is, approximately 20 minutes is required for reversal after 2 hours of tourniquet time. In addition, tourniquet effects occur more rapidly after repeated use, and there is probably some summation of these effects. Double tourniquets are used for IV-required anesthesia (Bier blocks) (12). Individual variations such as age, vascular supply of the limb, condition of the tissues, and vascular diseases all influence the patient's tolerance to tourniquet usage. In general, avoid using tourniquets in trauma cases except where dissection around major nerves is required.

    c. **Complications** of tourniquets include blisters and chemical burns (from "prep" solutions that leak under the tourniquet) of the skin, swelling, stiffness, and paralysis. Electromyographic changes have been demonstrated following the use of a tourniquet even within the approved time ranges.

3. The following is a **summary of Occupational Safety and Health Administration (OSHA) regulation No. 1920, "Bloodborne Pathogens,"** emphasizing staff and surgeon responsibilities.

    a. **Wash hands immediately after removing gloves.**

    b. **Wash** (with soap and water) **any exposed skin** (or flush mucous membranes) **immediately** (or as soon as feasible) **after contact with blood or potentially infectious materials.**

    c. **Do not bend, cut, recap, or remove needles or other sharps.** If recapping is the only feasible method, then it must be done by using a mechanical device or the one-handed method.

    d. **Do not eat, drink, smoke, apply cosmetics or lip balm, or handle contact lenses** in work areas where there is a reasonable likelihood of occupational exposure.

    e. **Perform all procedures involving blood or potentially infectious material to minimize spraying and splattering.**

    f. If **outside contamination of transport containers** is possible (or there is a potential for puncture), place potentially infectious material in a second container to **prevent leakage during handling.**

    g. **Use personal protective equipment** such as gloves, face shields, masks, gowns, shoe covers, and so on, in situations in which there is risk of exposure to blood or potentially infectious material.

    h. **Following an exposure, complete an incident report identifying the route of exposure and source individual.** A tube of the patient's blood should be drawn, labeled "spin" and held until the patient's consent can be obtained. The employee health nurse is to be contacted for testing as indicated.

    i. **Hepatitis B virus (HBV) immunization is recommended for all employees** and is usually available by contacting the employee health nurse. The authors believe that every surgeon is responsible for knowing his or her own human immunodeficiency virus, hepatitis B, and hepatitis C serologic status.

4. **Prevention of surgical wound infections** (13)

    a. Operating room rituals are designed to **decrease infection.** Despite the best designs, wound contamination and subsequent wound infection continue. It is generally conceded that most wounds become contaminated; however, usually only those with devitalized tissue or foreign bodies become frankly infected. A study of the possible sources of coagulase-positive staphylococci that contaminated surgical wounds during 50 operations revealed that bacteria of bacteriophage types that were present only in the air were found in 68% of the wounds; 50% of wounds contained bacteria of bacteriophage types that were found in the patient's nose, throat, or skin; 14% had bacteriophage types found in the noses and throats of members of the scrubbed surgical team; and 6% of the wounds had bacteriophage types found on the hands of the scrubbed surgical team. Maximum contamination occurs early in the operative procedure when there is a considerable amount of air circulation caused by individuals moving about the room. After the air quiets, the rate of contamination is less, but an increased exposure time allows increased contamination. It is important to keep traffic in the operating room to an absolute minimum, to walk slowly, and to avoid fanning the air with quick opening of the doors, drapes, and towels.

b. Studies show considerable variation in the **filtration efficiency of different masks.** Cloth masks are only about 50% efficient in filtering bacterial organisms and are rarely used. Numerous disposable masks have a bacterial filtration efficiency greater than 94% according to the manufacturers. Fiberglass-free masks are probably safer. Prolonged use (averaging 4½ hours of operation time) and the use of moist masks do not impair ability to filter, except in the case of cloth masks. Since the surgical masks work on a filtration principle, double masking can actually increase the air contamination with bacteria, because double masking makes transportation of air through the mask pores more difficult and forces more unfiltered air to escape along the sides of the mask.

c. Although airborne contamination is by far the most important source of contamination, **skin contamination** does occur. Even with the use of 1% or 2% tincture of iodine, the deeper areas of the epidermis are not bacteria-free. With a 1% concentration, no cases of skin irritation have occurred. If a higher concentration is used, however, then the excess iodine should be removed with alcohol after 30 seconds. One 5-minute scrub with povidone-iodine is as effective as a 10-minute scrub in reducing bacterial counts on the skin and keeping them down for as long as 8 hours. A 7.5% povidone-iodine (Betadine) skin disinfectant yields 0.75% available iodine. More recent work shows that **chlorhexidine gluconate** (Hibiclens) may be the scrub detergent of choice for both the surgeon and the patient (16). A comparative study between hexachlorophene (pHisoHex), povidone-iodine, and chlorhexidine showed the latter to be probably the most effective. There was a 99.9% reduction in resident bacterial flora after a single 6-minute chlorhexidine scrub. The reduction of flora on surgically gloved hands was maintained over the 6-hour test period. In addition, the pharmacology of chlorhexidine is reportedly more effective against gram-positive and gram-negative organisms, including *Pseudomonas aeruginosa.*

d. Extremity draping. Plastic drapes do not totally eliminate the patient's skin as a possible source of infection. Drape the extremities as described in App. E.

e. Intraoperative procedures to prevent postoperative wound infection include the elimination of any large collection of blood. A hematoma is an excellent potential culture medium. Wound suction is used whenever one anticipates continued bleeding into the wound; however, their use in fracture, joint replacement, and spine surgery has not been proven to decrease the incidence of wound infection. Surgical wounds are carefully irrigated to remove any potential contaminated residue before closing. *In vitro* experiments using bacitracin 50,000 units plus polymyxin B sulfate (Aerosporin) 50 mg in a liter of saline or lactated Ringer's solution have shown that 100% of *Staphy-*

lococcus aureus, Escherichia coli, the *Klebsiella* organisms, and *P. aeruginosa* bacteria were killed by a 1-minute exposure to the antibiotic solution (21). *Staphylococcus epidermidis* organisms were also killed. Only the *Proteus* organisms showed significant resistance to this antibiotic irrigation (only 3%–22% were killed). *Proteus* organisms are uncommon as a cause of immediate postoperative infections in musculoskeletal surgery, however, when the wounds are not previously contaminated or infected. Data indicate that irrigation of surgical wounds with a solution containing bacitracin and polymyxin B sulfate or bacitracin and neomycin could potentially lower the incidence of postoperative infections (3). A large number of patients are sensitive to neomycin, so its use is generally discouraged. Polymyxin B is sometimes difficult to obtain from the manufacturer. In this situation, some surgeons use a dilute Betadine solution as a topical antibiotic irrigant; however, this solution is toxic to tissue. Splash basins are a source of bacterial contamination and should not be used.

    f. The incidence of infection increases in wounds open longer than 2 hours. Whether this is a result of the increased exposure to the air, failure of masks, skin contaminants, or more trauma in the wound is not certain. Even with lengthy surgical cases, with good surgical technique the rate of deep wound infection on "clean" orthopaedic cases should not exceed 1%.

    g. Laminar air flow systems appear to be an effective means of reducing postoperative infection rates as long as the flow of air is kept laminar or streamlined across the operative area (e.g., during hip surgeries). These systems are not effective if the air becomes turbulent across the operative area because, for example, of the position of people in the operating room (e.g., during knee replacement surgery) (6).

    h. Hooded surgical exhaust systems are effective but cumbersome and costly. They are often used to protect the operating team from infection by high-risk patients.

    i. Whenever a subsequent surgical wound infection occurs in a clean, uneventful surgical case, consider a **nasal culture** from all those present at the time of the operation.

5. Malignant hyperthermia

    a. Pathophysiology. The target organ in malignant hyperthermia is, skeletal muscle. Certain triggering events, such as the administration of halothane or succinylcholine, precipitate release of calcium from the calcium-storing membrane (sarcoplasmic reticulum) of the muscle cell. The abnormal transport of calcium results in recurrent sarcomeric contractions and consequent muscle rigidity. The metabolic rate is accelerated, causing heat and increased carbon dioxide production with accelerated oxygen consumption. Core body temperature increases.

    b. History. The potentially fatal syndrome is an autosomal dominant metabolic disease. In 40% of reported cases, an orthopaedist is the first to encounter this disorder. The incidence in the United States is approximately 1:1,000. The syndrome is associated more frequently with patients having congenital and musculoskeletal abnormalities: kyphosis, scoliosis, hernia, recurrent joint dislocations, club foot, ptosis, or strabismus. Malignant hyperthermia can occur at any age but is most likely to occur in a young individual with a large muscle mass. After exposure to an anesthetic (or other stress), body temperature rapidly increases.

    c. Examination. A rapid elevation in body temperature is noted early. Cardiac arrhythmias usually are concurrent, can progress to ventricular tachycardia, and may end in ventricular fibrillation with subsequent death. The soda lime canister may turn blue and become palpably hot. Tetanic muscle contractions occur in approximately 60% of cases. Like so many conditions in orthopaedics, early recognition is crucial. Temperature and electrocardiographic monitoring during surgery is mandatory. A rapid temperature elevation (even from an initial subnormal temperature), tachycardia, hypertonia of skeletal muscle, unexplained hyperventilation, overheated soda lime canister, dark blood, sweating, and blotchy cyanosis are all indicative of possible malignant hyperthermia.

d. Treatment

(1) Prevention

(a) Obtain a **careful past history and family history,** inquiring especially about fatal or near-fatal experiences following emotional, physical, traumatic, or surgical stress or about a relative who died of an obscure cause.

(b) Administer prophylactic **dantrolene (Dantrium) orally** in doses of 2.2 mg/kg body weight (range of 2–4 mg/kg body weight) at 12 and 4 hours before the induction of anesthesia when the history is positive.

(c) **Avoid** the use of **halothane (Fluothane)** and **succinyl-choline (Anectine)** in high-risk patients.

(2) Management of an evolving malignant hyperthermia syndrome

(a) Immediately **discontinue all anesthetic agents and muscle relaxants** and terminate the surgical procedure as quickly as possible.

(b) **Hyperventilate with oxygen.**

(c) **Use IV sodium bicarbonate,** 4 mL/kg body weight, and repeat as necessary until blood gases approach normal.

(d) Administer **mannitol,** 1 g/kg body weight and **furosemide** (Lasix), 1 mg/kg body weight, which help maintain urine output to clear myoglobin and excessive sodium.

(e) Treat hyperkalemia with approximately 50 mg of **IV glucose** with 50 units of **insulin.**

(f) Control arrhythmias with procainamide (Pronestyl).

(g) **Cool the patient** with immersion in ice water and expose to an electric fan to facilitate evaporation. Refrigerated saline or Ringer's lactate administered intravenously is helpful. Maintain cooling procedures until the body temperature is less than 38°C.

(h) **Dantrolene** (approximately 12 mg/kg body weight) used intravenously **is one of the mainstays of treatment** and probably works by reducing calcium outflow from the sarcoplasmic reticulum into the myoplasm.

(i) **Physiologic monitoring** by electrocardiography and measurement of the central venous pressure, blood gases every 10 minutes, volume and quality of renal output, serum electrolytes, glucose, serum glutamic oxaloacetic transaminase (SGOT), creatine phosphokinase (CPK), and blood urea nitrogen (BUN) is important.

(j) Good **prognostic signs** are lightening of the coma (often heralded by restlessness), return of reflexes, return to normal temperature, reduced heart rate, improved renal output, and return of consciousness.

e. Complications

(1) Weakness and easy fatigability persist for several months.

(2) Death owing to ventricular fibrillation can occur within 1 or 2 hours from the onset of the condition. If death occurs later, then it is usually a result of pulmonary edema, coagulopathy, or massive electrolyte and acid-base imbalance. If the patient dies after several days in a coma, then the cause is usually renal failure or brain damage.

II. Orthopaedic operating room instruments and their usage

A. Introduction. Much of the remaining discussion is modified from a psychomotor skills course originally organized for the University of Washington Department of Orthopaedic Surgery residents by F. G. Lippert III, M.D.

B. Techniques for checking the function of grasping type surgical instruments (15) . The breakdown of high-quality instruments is often the direct result of their misuse. Forceps, hemostats, needle holders, and clamps frequently are misused in orthopaedic surgery. They can be misapplied to various pins, nails, screws, and plates when pliers are not readily available. They are also misused to clamp large sponges, tubing, and needles.

1. It is annoying to a surgeon and hazardous to the patient when **forceps or a hemostat** springs open. This mishap is caused by forceps malalignment, worn ratchet teeth, or lack of tension at the shanks.

   a. Start the equipment check by visually checking **jaw alignment** by closing the jaws of the forceps lightly. If the jaws overlap, they are out of alignment. Then, determine whether the teeth are meshing properly on forceps with serrated jaws. In addition, try to wiggle the instrument with the forceps open and holding one shank in each hand. If the box has considerable play or is very loose, then the jaws are usually malaligned and the forceps need repair.

   b. To check the **ratchet teeth** on instruments, clamp the forceps to the first tooth only. A resounding snap should be produced. Then hold the instrument by the box lock and tap the ratchet teeth portion of the instrument lightly against a solid object. If the instrument springs open, then it is faulty and needs repair.

   c. Test the **tension between the shanks** by closing the jaws of the forceps lightly until they barely touch. At this point there should be clearance of $\frac{1}{16}$ or $\frac{1}{8}$ inch between the ratchet teeth on each shank.

2. To test the function of the **needle holder,** first clamp the needle in the jaws of the holder, then lock the instrument on the second ratchet tooth. If the needle can be turned easily by hand, then set aside the instrument for repair. When the instrument is new, it holds a needle securely on the first ratchet tooth for a considerable time. Needle holders such as a Crile, Wood, Derf, or Halsey, used in plastic surgery, should hold at least a 6-0 suture. Needle holders such as Castroviejo or Kalt should hold a 7-0 suture.

C. Surgical exposure instruments. There are various methods for testing the efficiency of **surgical scissors.** The Mayo and Metzenbaum dissecting scissors should cut four layers of gauze with the tips of their blades. Smaller scissors (less than 4 inches long) should be able to cut two layers of gauze at the tips. All scissors should have a fine, smooth feel and require only minimum pressure by the blades to cut properly. The scissors action should not be too loose or too tight. Check the tips of the scissors for burrs or for excessive sharpness. Closed tips of the scissors should not be separated or loose. The precise setting of the blade is very important. Sharpening surgical scissors is a skilled procedure, usually requiring an exceptional craftsman to properly grind and set the blades.

2. **Periosteal elevators**

   a. Periosteal elevators are instruments designed to **strip (or elevate) periosteum from bone.** As the instrument is pushed along the surface of the bone, the soft tissue is lifted from the underlying bone. Periosteal elevators are thus instruments for blunt dissection and are designed to follow bony surfaces without digging into the bone or wandering off into the soft tissues. They are also useful in blunt separation of other tissue planes such as in the exposure of the hip joint capsule. The use of periosteal elevators is most satisfactory in areas where tissue planes are not too firmly adherent. At bony attachments of a ligament or capsule, collagen fibers plunge deeply into the bone so that the elevator does not slide on a tissue interspace; sharp dissection with a scalpel is more appropriate here. In fracture fixation, periosteal stripping, which can adversely affect blood supply and bone healing, should be minimized, if possible.

b. Elevators are made in **different sizes and shapes.** They may be narrow or wide. Sharp corners allow insertion of the instrument into a tissue plane or beneath the periosteum. On the other hand, most blade corners are rounded to avoid producing damage when pressure is applied to the central portion of the blade.

c. The **technique** of making a periosteal incision with a scalpel before the elevator is used helps form well-defined edges. When periosteum is being elevated from bone, the first rule of safety is to always keep the blade against bone. If the instrument is allowed to slip off into the soft tissues, then vessels and nerves can be damaged. It is important to use two hands whenever possible to have a stable grasp on the instrument and to maintain fine control. A gentle rocking motion while advancing the blade produces more even results (Fig. 10-2). Although periosteal elevators need not be honed to the same sharp edge required for bone-cutting osteotomes, they do require some tissue-penetrating ability to be most effective. Nevertheless, they should not be so sharp as to incise soft tissue instead of stripping it.

d. **Important guidelines for tool selection and usage**
   (1) Select the **correct size.** Generally, use a small elevator for small bones and a large elevator for large bones.
   (2) Select the **correct shape.** Usually, a sharp elevator is used to elevate periosteum and a rounded elevator to dissect soft tissue.
   (3) The **periosteum is incised with a scalpel.**
   (4) The **corner of the elevator** is used to reflect a periosteal edge.
   (5) The **periosteum is elevated evenly** without tearing.
   (6) The elevator is **kept on the bone.**
   (7) The **bone is not engaged** by the elevator.
   (8) A **rocking motion** is used while advancing the elevator.
   (9) **Two hands** are used, one for power and one for stability and dissecting.

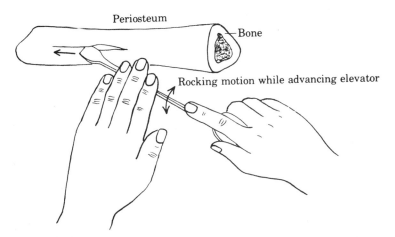

Periosteum

Bone

Rocking motion while advancing elevator

FIG. 10-2. Proper use of a sharp-edged periosteal elevator. (Modified from G. Spolek, unpublished data, 1974.)

(10) **Overpenetration** into the soft tissues by the elevator **should be avoided.**

(11) A **gentle technique** must be used.

D. **Bone cutting instruments: osteotomes, gouges, and mallets**

1. The **major difference** between an osteotome and a chisel is that an osteotome bevels on both sides to a point, whereas the chisel has a bevel on only one side (Fig. 10-3). The term **osteotome** is made up of **osteo,** which means "bone", and **tome,** which means "to cut"; the purpose of the tool is to cut bone. The cut should be produced under excellent control; otherwise, the bone can be split. Osteotomes come in different shapes and sizes. There are different types of handles that make for differences in holding and striking surface capabilities.

2. **Selection of instruments**

   a. **Chisels** are used to remove bone from around screws and plates instead of osteotomes because they can be easily sharpened when the edges are nicked from being hit against the metal. It is better to keep a set of chisels specifically for removing metal implants.

   b. **Osteotomes** are used to cut bone and to shave off osteoperiosteal grafts. In fusion procedures, they are used to remove the cartilage and subchondral bone as well as to perform "fish scaling" of the surface of bone for bone graft union.

   c. **Gouges** are used to provide strips of cancellous bone graft from the iliac crest. They are also used to clean out the cartilage and subchondral bone from concave joint surfaces.

   d. **Mallets** are used to produce power to drive the aforementioned tools through bone and cartilage.

3. **Proper technique**

   a. The dominant hand is used to grasp the mallet, which strikes the back of the instrument and drives it through bone. **While hitting the osteotome through bone of increasing density,** notice that the sound becomes high-pitched and the osteotome moves a shorter distance with each blow. In addition, there is a tightening or holding quality about the osteotome so that it moves less freely. This tightness is an indication that bone is coming under more tension and that a split of the bone is about to occur. Decrease the tension by working the osteotome back and forth through the bone. Occasionally,

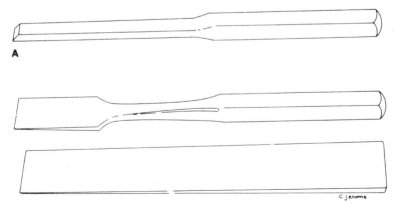

FIG. 10-3. Differences between an osteotome and a chisel. **A:** A chisel. **B:** Two types of osteotome.

it is necessary to remove the osteotome to take a different direction or a slightly different angle. It is frequently important to prescore the bone so that the cutting goes directly toward it instead of splitting the bone in an unwanted area.

    b. Precautions include preventing the osteotome from sliding off the bone or from cutting through the bone rapidly and then plunging into soft tissue. The nondominant hand merely supports and directs the osteotome against bone until it gets started but does not apply any major pressure on the tool. Starting the cut is best accomplished by placing the osteotome at right angles to the bone, then angling the tool only after the initial score and cut have begun. These precautions protect both the patient and the hands of the assistant.

    4. Specific **maintenance** is necessary in the handling and sharpening of the tools. The sharpening of an osteotome or a gouge is a difficult and critical procedure that must be undertaken with great caution. If the tool is overheated during sharpening, then the temper is lost. The loss can be recognized by the bluish-gray color of the metal in contrast to the silvery color usually associated with stainless steel. In addition, care must be taken in cleaning and handling the tools while they are on a surgical table so that the ends do not become damaged by other instruments. Keep them in a rack during the sterilization process, not in a basin with other tools.

E. Bone saws and files. In general, the operator must control the amplitude, direction, and length of force applied to the saw. The use of lactated Ringer's (or saline) irrigation to disperse heat is always recommended.

    1. The proper use of **Gigli's saw** includes making a scribe mark at the start of the technique if possible. The surgeon must be careful not to drop or tangle the saw cable, to keep the cable at approximately 90 degrees, and to use the middle two thirds of the saw while applying a constant, steady tension. Excess body movement should be avoided. The use of saline coolant is recommended.

    2. A **bone file** or rasp is usually used to round the edge of a bone cut. Both hands should be used to control the direction of the tool and only a forward force should be applied.

F. General bone screw biomechanics

    1. Holes are generally drilled in bone for the purpose of inserting screws to hold orthopaedic implants. Careful, even compulsive, attention to detail in selecting equipment and in drilling holes properly is vital to the performance of an implanted fixation device. The interlocking threads of screw and bone overlap by less than 0.02 inch. Any failure of equipment or technique that decreases this margin drastically reduces the holding power of the screw. Given the severe loading environment in which most orthopaedic implants operate, the holding power of a screw is an important matter. Force concentrations that occur when a screw fails to hold properly can result in a rapid failure of the implant.

    2. Drill bits (11)

        a. Common defects in equipment. Since hole drilling is frequently taken for granted (the major attention being paid to the implant itself), drill bits come to the operating room in various stages of disrepair.

            (1) A **dull point** is one of the most serious and least noticed defects. When the point is sharp, virtually all heat generated in drilling is carried away in the bone chips that are formed. Even slight dullness drastically increases friction between the point and the bone. This friction causes excessive heating and can affect the strength of the bone around the hole as well as cause inefficient cutting, which results in an oversized hole.

            (2) The flutes should be examined for **nicks and gouges** that score the walls of the hole, causing excessive heating and oversized holes.

(3) A drill with a **scored shank** does not sit straight in the chuck and causes the same trouble as a drill sharpened off center.

(4) Drill bits of the **wrong size** are sometimes selected. A difference of just 1/100th of an inch is enough to diminish the holding power of a screw severely, even though insertion of the screw appears normal.

(5) A **bent drill bit** causes the same difficulty as a drill bit sharpened off center. One cannot tell whether a drill bit is bent by simply looking at it; it must be rotated in the fingers. Even small **bends** create holes that are irregular, and the drill bit is very susceptible to breakage.

b. **Technique**

(1) Prevent the drill point from **wandering off center.**

(a) To keep the point from **wandering on penetration** and to protect surrounding soft tissues, use an appropriate-sized **drill guide.** Start the hole perpendicular to the surface. When bone penetration begins, shift to the desired direction. Always use saline to cool the drill bit.

(b) Thin surgical drill bits are flexible, and if the drill is inadvertently held **slightly off perpendicular,** then the point may bend the opposite way, making the point wander.

(c) If the drill bit is **not positioned properly in the chuck** or if debris is present in the chuck or on the shank, then the drill bit may wander off center. Another error involves insertion of the drill bit too deeply into the chuck, which causes damage to the flutes when the drill is tightened. Check the drill for these problems before proceeding.

(2) **Tighten the chuck down.** If the chuck is loose, then it can rotate relative to the drill and score the shank.

(3) **Too little force** (not too much force) is a common defect in technique. Push hard enough to cause a constant progression of the drill bit; otherwise, too much energy is being dissipated as friction rather than as cutting, causing excessive heating.

(4) **Avoid overpenetration.** Slow the drill motor when the drill bit tip begins penetrating (noted by a change in resistance) and finish with care. With care, the surgeon will note that the frequency of the sound made by the drill drops just before penetration of the cortex. The tip should not penetrate more than one eighth of an inch through the opposite cortex.

(5) When the drill bit breaks through the opposite cortex, **keep it rotating in the same direction as you back it out.** The chips are thus carried out with the drill bit instead of being left in the hole.

(6) Drill motors should be **lubricated frequently.** Special surgical lubricants are available. Do not use mineral oil or ordinary oil, because they are not permeable by steam and can harbor bacteria and spores even after autoclaving.

c. **Adhere to the following points when using drills:**

(1) **Choose the correct drill bit.** Reject dull, scored, bent, oversized, and incorrectly pointed drill bits. In general, use new drill bits for each case.

(2) **Insert the drill bit correctly in the chuck** with the drill bit centered and the chuck tightened on the shank only. Use quick release systems to avoid potential problems.

(3) **Tighten the chuck sufficiently.**

(4) **Start the drill hole perpendicular to the surface;** then change to the desired direction.

(5) **Maintain adequate pressure** on the drill to promote cutting and lessen heat production.

(6) **Maintain the proper direction** of the hole and penetrate the far cortical wall carefully, with the drill bit minimally penetrating.

(7) **Keep the drill rotating while backing it out** in order to clear the hole of bone chips.

3. **Screws** (11)

    a. Cortical bone screws are fully threaded and come in a variety of sizes for different sized bones. Non–self-tapping screws require a tap to cut the threads into the bone before insertion (Fig. 10-4).

    b. Cancellous bone screws have a thinner core diameter plus wider and deeper threads to better grip the "spongy" bone. They are fully or partially threaded. Tapping is required only through the bone surface.

    c. Lag screw fixation can be achieved with either a partially threaded cancellous screw or by drilling a "gliding hole'' (of the same size as the outer thread diameter) for the near cortex, allowing a cortical screw to produce lag compression.

    d. Large and small **cannulated cancellous bone screws** are designed to pass over a guidewire. With this type of system the surgeon can place a guidewire exactly where desired so that the cannulated drill, tap, and screw passes over this wire for precise placement.

    e. Length of screw. Drilling the proper hole is only the first step in firmly fixing the screw into the bone. The second part is selecting a screw that is of adequate length (4).

        (1) To use a **depth gauge** properly, do not insert the gauge any farther than necessary. Be sure to have hooked the far end of the hole and not an intermediate point. Consider allowing additional length (usually 2 mm) over the scale reading on the depth gauge when choosing the screw length.

        (2) A **self-tapping screw** has a tapered point whose holding power is further reduced by the flutes cut for tapping purposes. The **distal 2 mm of the self-tapping screw has no holding power at all, and the next 2 mm has very little. Screw lengths are measured from the proximal edge of**

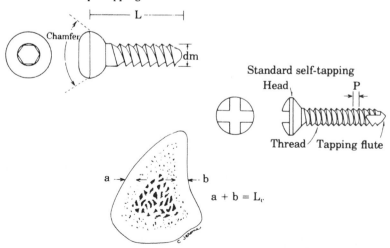

FIG. 10-4. Comparison between Association for the Study of Internal Fixation (ASIF) and standard cortical bone screws.

the chamfered head to the distal point of the screw (Fig. 10-4) . If a screw is installed in a plate, then additional length must be allowed. Given the fact that bone screws hold principally in cortical bone, a screw that is short by 4 mm may lose 50% of its holding power.

(3) When a screw is inserted on a **subcutaneous border of bone,** the hole should be **countersunk** before the depth is measured and the screw inserted.

(4) **Tighten the screw snugly and no more,** so as not to strip the threads of the bone when inserting the screw. Retighten cortical screws three times to allow for the obligate loss of strain between screw and bone resulting from loss of fluid in the bone and stress relaxation.

G. **General principles of plating** are described in the following paragraphs and generally follow the concepts and techniques advocated by the Association for the Study of Internal Fixation (AO/ASIF) group, which supplies the most widely used fracture fixation implants in use. The plates are listed by their general biomechanical functions (11).

1. Protection or **neutralization plates** are used in combination with lag or other screws and protect the screw fixation in diaphyseal fractures. Without the plates, the screw fixation by itself does not withstand much loading and does not allow for early range of motion. The lag screws provide for most of the interfragmental compression and the plate protects the screws from torsion, bending, and shearing forces (Fig. 10-5).

2. The dynamic compression plate (DCP) brings compression to the fracture site by its design. Recently, low-contact dynamic compression plates (LCDCPs) have been developed that allow greater freedom in screw insertion through the plate and also limit the pressure necrosis effect of the plate on the cortical bone surface (11) (Figs. 10-6, 10-7, 10-8).

3. By their nature, many epiphyseal and metaphyseal fractures are subject to compression and shearing forces. Lag screws are used to reconstruct the normal anatomy, but they cannot overcome the forces of shear and bending because of the thin cortical shells in these areas, especially in comminuted fractures. The fixation is supplemented with supporting or buttress plates to prevent subsequent fracture displacement from shear or bending stresses. Specially designed buttress plates include the T plate, the T **buttress plate,** the L buttress plate, the lateral tibial head plate, the spoon plate, the cloverleaf plate, and the condylar buttress plate. Additional plates for special locations (e.g., proximal and distal tibia, calcaneous) have recently been marketed.

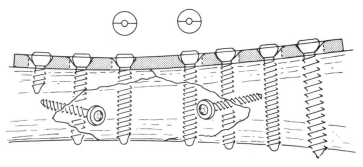

FIG. 10-5. Application of a conventional or neutralization internal fixation plate. The neutral drill guide is used. Neutralization plate allows for more loading of the fracture than simple lag screw fixation.

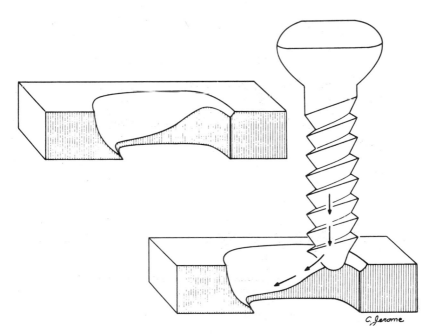

FIG. 10-6. A longitudinal section of the dynamic compression plate (DCP) screw hole. Insertion of the Association for the Study of Internal Fixation (AO/ASIF) screw causes self-compression of the fracture site by the plate by sliding down an inclined cylinder to a horizontal one. (Modified from Mueller ME, et al. *Manual of internal fixation*, 2nd ed. Berlin: Springer-Verlag, 1979:71, with permission.)

4. To restore the load-bearing capacity of an eccentrically loaded fractured bone and minimize the forces borne by the fixation device, it is necessary to absorb the tensile forces (the result of a bending movement) and convert them into compressive forces. This requires **tension band fixation,** which exerts a force equal in magnitude but opposite in direction to the bending force (assuming the bone is able to withstand compression) (11) . Therefore, comminuted fractures should be treated with other fixation devices or protected longer from bending moments.
   a. Ideally, **tension band plating** techniques are used on the femur, humerus, radius, and ulna (11).
   b. **Tension band wire internal fixation**
      (1) The **purpose** of tension band wire internal fixation is to secure the fragments of fractures in such a way that the application of normal forces (muscle forces, loads generated by walking) produces a compression of the fragments at the fracture site instead of pulling the fragments apart. The advantage of this technique is that the fixation is secure enough to allow early (if not immediate) use of the limb. Indications for tension band wiring are generally in the treatment of avulsion fractures at the insertion of muscles, tendons, or ligaments. If one has to deal with a rotational component or when accurate reduction of the fragments is vital, then introduce two parallel Kirschner wires before the insertion of the tension band. The tension band then is passed around the wire ends.

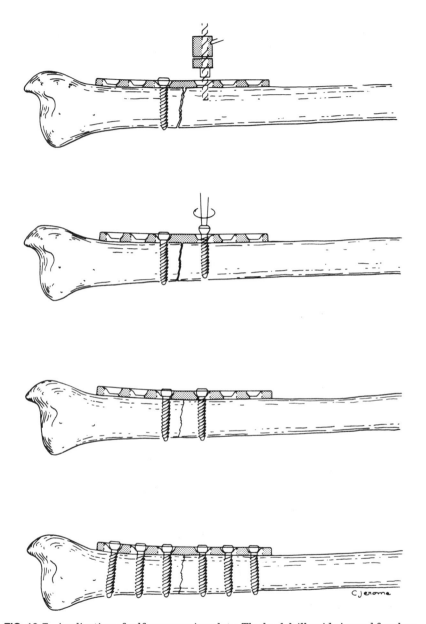

FIG. 10-7. Application of self-compression plate. The load drill guide is used for placement of the second drill as shown in the top illustration. The other holes are drilled with the neutral drill guide. (Modified from Mueller ME, et al. *Manual of internal fixation,* 2nd ed. Berlin: Springer-Verlag, 1979:67, 75.)

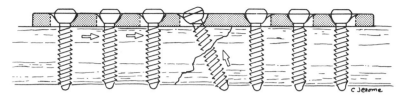

FIG. 10-8. Dynamic compression plate with lag screw. The compression through the plate is applied first; then the lag screw is added to prevent a shear force on the lag screw.

(2) The tension band **principle** works only when there are applied natural forces that tend to bend the bone at the fracture site. The olecranon, patella, and tip of the fibula are examples of such sites. Fig. 10-9 describes the principles of tension band wire internal fixation for the treatment of a transverse fracture of the olecranon.

(3) As shown on Fig. 10-9, **a single-screw fixation without a tension wire loop is not adequate,** because the screw bends with triceps activity and only half the fracture site is placed in compression.

(4) It is evident that the wire is pulled in tension by the bending effect of the muscle force. Therefore, whatever force is exerted across the bony interface must be **compressive and equal** in magnitude to the force carried by the wire.

(5) Note that the tension band wiring **does not provide the desired rigidity for loading from all directions.** It is intended to resist only the strong tension forces applied through the action of specific muscles or through loading.

(6) The **application** of tension band wire fixation is discussed in the treatment of olecranon fractures in Chap. 18 **(II.B.)** and of patellar fractures in Chap. 24 **(III.A.3.).**

5. **Numerous other plates and screws** serve the aforementioned functions with various shapes and sizes to adapt to the local anatomy. They include straight and offset condylar blade plates, reconstruction plates (more easily contoured in all three planes, which make them optimum for use in the pelvis and distal humerus), dynamic hip screws, and dynamic condylar screws.

6. **Contouring internal fixation plates.** Internal fixation plates may be contoured to fit the bone before application. Such contouring increases the bone-plate interface area so that the loads normally carried by the bone can be transferred to the plate by friction rather than pure shearing on the bone screws. To contour a plate template, press the aluminum template of the proper length against the bone, then bend the plate to match. Plate benders may be hand-held singular, hand-held pliers, and table-mounted bending presses.

a. The **bending press** gets the most use, because most contouring is two-dimensional. The anvil is adjustable so that the handle can be used in the position with the best control (near the end of its travel). The **hand press** is used mainly for small plates, for plates with a semitubular cross section, and reconstruction picks. There are three different anvils (straight, convex, and concave) to prevent squashing of the semitubular plates. The **bending irons** are for applying twists and are most conveniently used when the jaws are opened upward to prevent the plate from falling out and when the handles are on the same side of the plate. Theoretically, uniform twist occurs

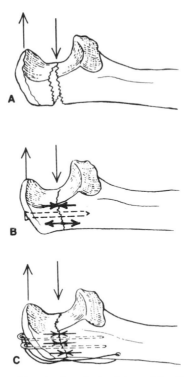

FIG. 10-9. The principles of tension band wire internal fixation as applied to a transverse fracture of the olecranon. Forces on an intact olecranon cause a bending moment. **A:** Same forces on a transverse fracture of the olecranon cause the fracture to open. **B:** Screw fixation provides only partial compression of fracture. **C:** Fixation of the cortex under tension creates equal compressive forces across the fracture site.

between the irons, so start with them at the ends of the desired twist length. Once the twist is started, move the irons closer together to get localized contours. DCPs are weakest through the holes, where most of the twist occurs, so try to position the irons to prevent excessive bends at any one hole. Use the press first because the plate does not fit the anvil if the bending irons are used to twist beforehand. LCDCPs have more uniform characteristics and do not bend at the holes. Fig. 10-10 illustrates the three types of instruments.
b. **Important guidelines in usage**
   (1) Bend the plate to form a **smooth, continuous contour.** Because the press causes a single, rather abrupt bend directly beneath the plunger, a long continuous curve is best formed by several small bends rather than a few sharp bends.
   (2) **Avoid bends through screw holes,** because they alter the shape of the countersunk surface of the hole so that the screw does not seat properly. If a bend must be made through a screw hole, go easy on the press handle, because the plate is weaker at a hole and less force is required to bend it.
   (3) If the required contour contains a series of **shallow and sharp bends,** do the shallow ones (greatest radius of curvature) first

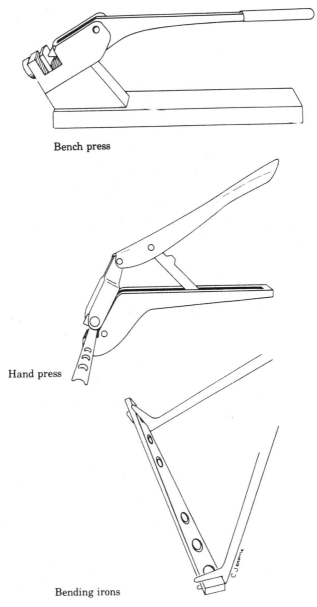

Bench press

Hand press

Bending irons

FIG. 10-10. Plate benders.

and progressively work toward the sharper bends, as shown in Fig. 10-11. This procedure tends to produce smooth contours and allows easier template matching. Contouring to fit a bump or knoll on the bone surface requires three bends: two convex and one concave.

(4) **Do not overbend but ease into a** contour (see Fig. 10-11). Overbending requires straightening, which, besides being time-consuming work, hardens the plate in that area and thus reduces the strength of the plate.

(5) When contouring the plate, do not match the template exactly, but rather alter (underbend or overbend) the shape so that

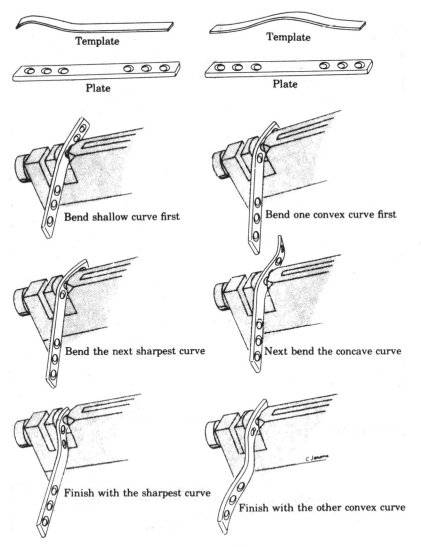

FIG. 10-11. Steps in plate contouring.

there is a **1- to 2-mm clearance between the plate and the bone at the site of a transverse fracture.** This technique causes compression of the cortex opposite the plate when the screws are tightened.

(6) **Minimize scratching or marking of the plate surface.** If the surface is scratched, then a potential corrosion site is created. Therefore, use the proper bending irons with smooth jaws rather than vise grips.

H. **Cerclage** is a technique of encircling a fractured bone with Parham-Martin band, stainless steel or titanium wire, Dahl-Miles cable, or other non-absorbable material to hold the fracture in reduction in conjunction with stronger, more permanent fixation. Cerclage is not recommended as a primary method of internal fixation of fractures. There are many techniques for applying cerclage wire.

1. **General rules of wire cerclage**
   a. **Avoid putting kinks in the wire.** Kinking is easy, particularly if the wire is coiled. Kinks result in stress concentrations that drastically reduce the fatigue strength of the wire.
   b. **Be sure the loop around the bone is perpendicular to the long axis of the bone.** Otherwise, the loop may appear tight, but any slight movement causes it to shift and loosen.
   c. Use the cerclage wire only to hold the fracture site in reduction, not to apply compression. The wire is not strong enough to apply useful compression. Tighten the wire only until it is snug; be careful not to overtighten while making the knot.
   d. Use the **proper-sized wire;** 18-gauge is common and has sufficient strength. The area of the wire is a measure of its load-carrying capacity, which depends on the square of the diameter. Thus, the load-carrying capacity decreases considerably with even moderate decreases in radius.

2. **Wire tighteners**
   a. The **Bowen wire tightener is an excellent tightener** (Fig. 10-12). Both wires are passed into the nose of the appliance and out the side. The outer wheel is turned to secure the wire against the inside cylinder. By turning the inside wheel, the inside cylinder is pulled up the handle of the device, effectively tightening the wire to the desired tension. The whole instrument is rotated to twist the wire, and the wires are then easily cut just distal to the last twist.
   b. The **Kirschner wire traction bows** (see Fig. 9-1) have a mechanical advantage that varies with the jaw opening. The lowest mechanical advantage is in the fully closed position; this increases gradually with increasing jaw width. The average mechanical advantage for both the large and small bows is 30:1. The last one-fourth inch of jaw opening coincides with a sudden increase in mechanical advantage of greater than 400:1, but this last one-fourth inch rarely is used.
   c. **Comparison of knot strength.** The types of knots described here were tied in 20-gauge steel wire and pulled apart in a tension test machine:
      (1) Type of knot/Maximum force before failure
         (a) ASIF loop/15.8 lb
         (b) Twist (one turn)/23.2 lb
         (c) Twist (three turns)/24.2 lb
         (d) Square knot/59.0 lb (wire broke)
      (2) These results are preliminary, but they do afford some conclusions. An ASIF loop is the weakest and is heavily dependent on careful knot formation for its strength. The twist is 47% stronger, but additional turns beyond the first 360-degree turn do not significantly increase the strength of the knot. The

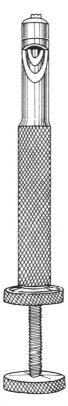

FIG. 10-12. The Bowen wire tightener.

reason for using several twists is to provide some residual resistance after untwisting begins, although whether this resistance actually occurs has not been determined. The square knot is the strongest of all. Failure occurs by wire fracture just below the knot.

I. Principles of intramedullary nailing

1. An intramedullary nail allows for internal splinting with a fixation device in the medullary canal. The **possibility of gliding along the dynamically locked nail promotes compression forces at the fracture site, and the stability from the long working length of the nail provides stiffness.**

2. This necessary reaming of the canal and resulting disruption of the endosteal blood supply in a severely open fracture that already has disruption of the periosteal blood supply may increase the chance for a non-union or infection. In these situations, the use of a smaller **unreamed nail** seems to give good results. Because these smaller unreamed nails have less mechanical stability, they generally require interlocking (placing one or two screws across the cortex and nail superiorly and inferiorly) (11). The incidence of implant failure by fatigue fracture is much greater than the larger diameter implants inserted with reaming.

3. In addition to the aforementioned indications, the treatment of complex fractures requires an **interlocking nail** to prevent excessive shortening and rotation. It is recommended to always statically lock the nail to avoid malrotation and shortening, which can occur related to unrecognized minimally displaced cracks.

J. External skeletal fixation

1. The **use** of external fixation, particularly in the treatment of comminuted or open fractures, **has regained popularity.**. Lambotte (1902) is generally given credit for the first use of external pin fixation. Anderson (1934), Stader (1937), and Hoffman (1938) all popularized a technique of external skeletal fixation. Vidal and Adrey, using the Hoffman approach, further refined the technique. Most recently, Ilizarov developed and popularized the ring fixator with small wire transfixion for use in limb lengthening, bone transport, and fracture fixation.

2. Multiple external fixators are currently on the market. Regardless of which technique is used, certain **basic principles** must be followed.

   a. The insertion of the pins and the attachment of the external skeletal fixation is a major procedure performed in the operating room **following all normal operating room procedures.**

   b. The skin and fascia must be incised so that there is **no pull on these structures** that could result in necrosis.

   c. The **pins** must be **inserted slowly** with a hand chuck after predrilling with a saline-cooled drill bit to avoid heat necrosis of bone.

   d. There must be a **minimum of two pins above and two pins below the fracture.** Three pins add a small amount of stability in some systems. Maximal fracture stability is achieved by using half pins separately within each bone segment and by placing the connecting bar as close to the skin as possible. Additional stability is attained by stacking a second bar (this must be done by planning ahead because parallel pins are required in some systems) or using a second row of pins and connecting bar.

   e. **Terminally threaded half pins** are used to prevent loosening and sliding of the unit in the bone.

   f. Avoid motion of skin and fascia against the pins.

   g. Use **strict aseptic techniques** when dressing the pin sites.

   h. **Avoid distraction.** Make adjustments to ensure coaptation or impaction of the fracture fragments during the course of healing.

   i. Studies have clearly shown that **external fixation devices can be used to treat fractures to union.** It was previously thought that the devices should be removed as soon as fractures are stabilized and be replaced by casts or cast-braces if necessary, to allow weight bearing across the fracture to stimulate healing.

   j. External pin fixation is a complex procedure that **requires skill and attention to detail.**

3. Possible **indications** for external skeletal fixation include the comminuted Colles' fracture and comminuted or open fractures of the tibia, particularly in the proximal and distal ends where intramedullary nailing is not feasible and the risk of infection from the more extensive soft-tissue stripping required for plating is significant. The apparatus should be used with caution for fractures in the humerus, femur, and pelvis because of the higher incidence of pin tract infection and pin loosening. Patient acceptance is also higher with other devices. The thin wire fixator technique developed by Ilizarov has made application in the metaphyseal region more secure, but because of the use of these "through" pins, the anatomic knowledge required in inserting them is greater. The Ilizarov frames are useful for fracture management, bone transport, and limb lengthening.

K. Obtaining bone graft material is a common procedure in orthopaedics. On most occasions, the iliac crest is used for the graft, although various bone grafts are available. After closure of the wound, installation of 0.5% bupivacaine without epinephrine reduces the postoperative pain. The following is the recommended surgical technique:

1. **For removal of a small amount of bone,** tension the skin over the iliac bone and cut to the ilium without entering muscle or fascial planes. A small periosteal flap is excised with sharp dissection from the superior aspect of the crest. A window then is cut through the cortical bone between the inner and outer tables. The periosteum is not stripped from the bone so pain is less.

2. **For removal of sizable grafts,** the surgeon must decide whether to use the anterior or posterior part of the iliac crest. Often, the choice is dictated by the position of the patient during operation. Anticipating the possible need for iliac bone grafting for proper positioning, prepping, and draping is required for the smooth flow of the operation. Whenever possible, the patient should be positioned so that the area of the posterior superior iliac spine can be used.

   a. **Removal of bone from the anterior part of the iliac crest.** The skin incision must be long enough to allow a comfortable exposure of the anterior 4–5 inches of the iliac crest. Sharp dissection is used to expose the crest. A periosteal elevator is used to expose the inner or outer surface of the ilium. The bone may then be removed by an osteotome or gouge. Care should be taken not to involve both tables of the ilium to minimize hematoma formation and postoperative pain. One should also be careful to avoid the anterior superior spine for reasons of cosmesis as well as to prevent injury to the lateral femoral cutaneous nerve. Absorbable gelatin sponges (Gelfoam) may be used to help control bleeding. The wound may be closed over suction drainage.

   b. **Removal of bone from the posterior iliac crest.** An oblique incision is made over the iliac crest approximately 1–2 inches lateral to the midline. The incision is not extended far enough over the crest to involve the superior cluneal nerves. The periosteum from the outer table is lifted with the periosteal elevator, and the detached muscles are protected with warm, moist lap sponges. Cancellous strips are then removed, and care should be taken not to enter the sacroiliac joint. Excessive bleeding is helped by absorbable gelatin sponges. The wound may be closed over suction drainage.

   c. **Removal of bicortical grafts.** These are wafers of bone taken from the iliac crest with the bone removed as a single block with both cortices. Generally, bicortical grafts are used in vertebral body fusions and in situations in which a structural graft is required. The same surgical techniques described in the preceding sections (**J.2.a** and **b**) are used, except that the incision and the donor site is between the anterior (or posterior) superior iliac spine and the most cephalad portion of the iliac crest. Bicortical graft donor sites are nearly always symptomatic for a significant postoperative period and often are deforming cosmetically.

L. **Basic skin suture techniques**

1. **General principles**

   a. Do not close the wound **if it may possibly be contaminated** (as in all open fractures). Delayed closure 3–5 days later is always preferable in doubtful cases.

   b. If skin edges are battered and ragged, then debride them so that healthy tissues are brought together.

   c. Good **closure of subcutaneous tissues** is the key to good skin closure.

   d. **Approximate,** do not strangulate.

   e. **Cutting needles with monofilament suture or thin wire** are used for skin. Skin staples are also used frequently. Cotton and silk sutures are not recommended for skin closure because of the increased inflammatory response to these materials and because of the wick effect that can draw organisms into the wound.

f. Before making a long incision, **mark it out with a surgical marking pen and make a crosshatch every 2 cm.** Then, when closing, make sure the crosshatches match up. Never make skin marks with a knife or needle because scarring results.

g. **Steri-Strips** are useful adjuncts for skin closure, but they should never be applied when the skin is under significant tension. They also can impede drainage because they provide a fairly watertight closure.

h. Consider placing a film of Polysporin ointment or a Betadine nonadherent dressing over the closed incision before applying outer dressings.

i. Use **pickups,** rather than pincers, **as skin hooks.**

2. **Types of skin suture.** All types of skin closure rely on good subcutaneous suturing to provide strength and to relieve some of the tension from the skin edges.

a. The needle path with a **box** or simple suture is perpendicular to the dermis. The depth of each half of the suture is equal. When tying the knot, have the edges just touch, as shown in Fig. 10-13. Never tie the knot so tightly that the skin bunches up.

b. Start the **everting** suture as for a large box-type closure, then reverse the direction, thus making a minibox suture of just the dermis. Match the depth in the opposite side, as shown in Fig. 10-14. Tie the knot so that the slightest skin pucker results.

c. An **intradermal** (or subcuticular) suture is entirely in the dermis and does not hold together with appreciable skin tension. Begin the closure several centimeters from the end of the wound and pass the needle from the starting point to the dermis at the apex of the wound. Obtain a secure amount of dermis on one side and then the other. Match the exit point on one side of the dermis with the entrance point on the other side, that is, directly opposite and of equal depth, as shown in Fig. 10-15. Occasionally pull the ends of the suture back and forth so that it slides well. End the suture as it was begun. The ends of the suture may be knotted or taped to the skin to prevent them from pulling out. The suture line is then splinted with Steri-Strips.

d. The **"near-far/far-near"** suture may be used when the skin must be closed under some tension. Begin with a deep box-type suture

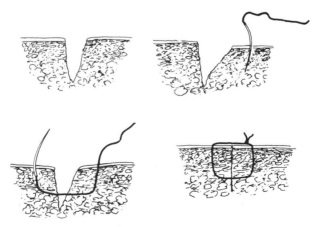

FIG. 10-13. Technique for a box suture.

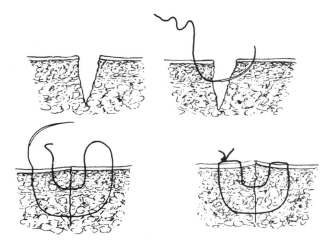

FIG. 10-14. Technique for an everting suture.

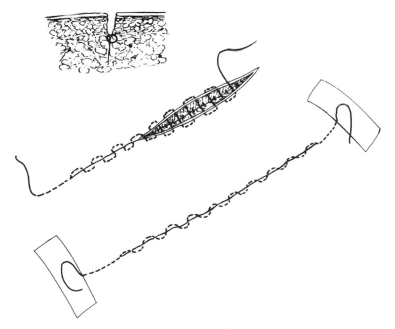

FIG. 10-15. Technique for an intradermal (subcuticular) suture.

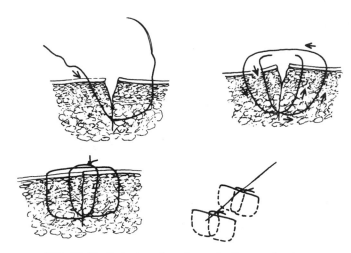

FIG. 10-16. Technique for a "near-far/far-near" suture.

that is near the wound edge on one side and far from it on the other. Complete the technique with a box-type suture with the near and far sides reversed. Tie the suture so the skin edges are approximated (Fig. 10-16).

e. The **Donati skin suture** technique, which was popularized by the ASIF group, is another modified mattress suture technique. It is useful when closing skin under tension. The suture courses deeply across the wound and then goes through the subdermal area without exiting the skin on the second side. Begin with a deep box-type suture on the first side of the wound. Pass back into the original side and exit between the wound and the original entrance site (Fig. 10-17).

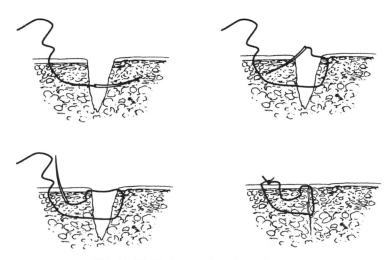

FIG. 10-17. Technique for a Donati suture.

References
1. Abramowicz M. *Med Lett Drugs Ther* 1992;34:5.
2. Arnold WD, Hilgartner MW. Hemophiliac arthropathy. *J Bone Joint Surg (Am)* 1977;59:287.
3. Benjamin JB, Volz RG. Efficacy of a topical antibiotic irrigant in decreasing or eliminating bacterial contamination in surgical wounds. *Clin Orthop* 1984;184:114.
4. Brod JJ. The concepts and terms of mechanics. *Clin Orthop* 1980;146:9.
5. Castles JJ. Clinical pharmacology of glucocorticoids. In: McCarty DJ, ed. *Arthritis and allied conditions,* 9th ed. Philadelphia: Lea & Febiger, 1979:399.
6. Lidwell OM. Clean air at operation and subsequent sepsis in the joint. *Clin Orthop* 1986;211:91.
7. Martin JT. Complications associated with patient positioning. *Anesth Analg,* 1988;67[Suppl 4S]:1.
8. McKenzie PJ, Loach AB. Local anaesthesia for orthopaedic surgery. *Br J Anaesth* 1986;58:779.
9. McLaren AC, Rorabeck CH. The pressure distribution under tourniquets. *J Bone Joint Surg (Am)* 1985;67:433.
10. Moore MR, Garfin SR, Hargens AR. Wide tourniquets eliminate blood flow at low inflation pressures. *J Hand Surg (Am)* 1987;12:1006.
11. Mueller ME, Allgower M, Schneider R, et al. *Manual of internal fixation,* 3rd ed. New York: Springer-Verlag, 1990.
12. Neimkin RJ, Smith RJ. Double tourniquet with linked mercury manometers for hand surgery. *J Hand Surg (Am)* 1983;8:938.
13. Nelson JP, et al. The effect of previous surgery, operating room environment, and preventive antibiotics on postoperative infection following total hip arthroplasty. *Clin Orthop* 1980;147:167.
14. Neu HC. Cephalosporin antibiotics as applied in surgery of bones and joints. *Clin Orthop* 1984;190:50.
15. Pencer G. What you should know about surgical instruments. *Surg Team* 1974;3:39.
16. Peterson AF, Rosenberg A, Alatary SD. Comparative evaluations of surgical scrub preparations. *Surg Gynecol Obstet* 1978;146:63.
17. Post M, Telfer MC. Surgery in hemophilia patients. *J Bone Joint Surg (Am)* 1975; 57:1136.
18. Raj PR, Cacodney A, Cannella J. Useful nerve blocks for pain relief and surgery. In: Browner B, ed. *Skeletal trauma.* Philadelphia: WB Saunders, 1992.
19. Reid HS, Camp RA, Jacob WH. Tourniquet hemostasis: a clinical study. *Clin Orthop* 1983;177:230.
20. Sapega AA, et al. Optimizing tourniquet application and release times in extremity surgery: a biochemical and ultrastructural study. *J Bone Joint Surg (Am)* 1985; 67:303.
21. Scherr DD, Dodd TA, Buckingham WW Jr. Prophylactic use of topical antibiotic irrigation in uninfected surgical wounds. *J Bone Joint Surg (Am)* 1972;54:634.
22. Shaw JA, Murray DG. The relationship between tourniquet pressure and underlying soft-tissue pressure in the thigh. *J Bone Joint Surg (Am)* 1982;64:1148.
23. Van Roekel HE, Thurston AJ. Tourniquet pressure: the effect of limb circumference and systolic pressure. *J Hand Surg (Br)* 1985;10:142.
24. Williams DN, Gustilo RB. The use of preventive antibiotics in orthopaedic surgery. *Clin Orthop* 1984;190:83.

Selected Historical Readings
Anderson R. An ambulatory method of treatment of the tibia and fibula. *Surg Gynecol Obstet*1934;58:639.
Bagby GW. Compression bone-plating. *J Bone Joint Burg (Am)* 1977;59:625.
Bechtol CO, Ferguson AB, Laign PG. *Metals and engineering in bone and joint surgery.* Baltimore: Williams & Wilkins, 1959.
Bowers WH, Wilson F C, Green WB. Antibiotic prophylaxis in experimental bone infections. *J Bone Joint Surg (Am)* 1973;55:795.
Boyd KS, Burke JF, Colton T. A double-blind clinical trial of prophylactic antibiotics in hip fractures. *J Bone Joint Surg (Am)* 1973;55:1251.

Burke JF. Sources of wound contamination. *Ann Surg* 1963;158:898.

Cooney WP, Linscheid RL, Dobyns JH. External pin fixation for unstable Colles' fractures. *J Bone Joint Surg (Am)* 1979;61:840.

Dineen P. Clinical research in skin disinfection. *AORNJ* 1971;14:73.

Dineen P. Microbial filtration by surgical masks. *Surg Gynecol Obstet* 1971;133:812.

Ha'eri GB, Wiley AM. The efficacy of standard surgical face masks: an investigation using tracer particles. *Clin Orthop* 1980;148:160.

Ha'eri GB, et al. Wound contamination through drapes and gowns: a study using tracer particles. *Clin Orthop* 1981;154:181.

Hamilton HW, et al. Penetration of gown material by organisms from the surgical team. *Clin Orthop* 1979;141:237.

Hargens AR, et al. Local compression patterns beneath pneumatic tourniquets applied to arms and thighs of human cadaver. *J Orthop Res* 1987;2:247.

Heppenstall RB, et al. A comparative study of the tolerance of skeletal muscle in ischemia: tourniquet application compared with acute compartment syndrome. *J Bone Joint Surg (Am)* 1986;68:820.

Jardon OM, et al. Malignant hyperthermia. *J Bone Joint Surg (Am)* 1979:61:1064.

Katz JF, Siffert RS. Tissue antibiotic levels with tourniquet use in orthopedic surgery. *Clin Orthop* 1982;165:261.

Hoffmann R. Rotules á os pour la reduction dirigé, non sanglante, des fractures (ostéotaxis) *Congrés Buisse de Chirurgie et Helvetica Medica Acta* 1938.

Jacobs JR, et al. Evaluation of draping techniques in prevention of surgical wound contamination. *JAMA* 1963;184:293.

Matthews LS, Hirsch C. Temperatures measured in human cortical bone drilling. *J Bone Joint Surg (Am)* 1972;54:297.

Whiteside LA, Lesker PA. The effects of extraperiosteal and subperiosteal dissection. *J Bone Joint Surg (Am)* 1978;60:26.

11. ACUTE SPINAL INJURY

I. **Fractures, dislocations, and fracture-dislocations**
   A. **Fracture of the C1 vertebra (Jefferson fracture)**
      1. **Mechanism of injury.** The superior articular processes of the atlas face upward, inward, and slightly backward. A vertical compression form can thrust the articular facets of the occipital condyles of the skull downward, push the lateral masses outward, and disrupt the ring of the atlas producing a C1 ring fracture, as shown in Fig. 11-1 (18). Less commonly, this same mechanism can produce an occipital condylar fracture, which can be isolated or associated with a basilar skull fracture (3).
      2. **Anatomic considerations.** The anteroposterior diameter of the ring of the atlas is approximately 3 cm. The spinal cord and the odontoid process each are approximately 1 cm in diameter, approximately one third the diameter of the ring. According to **Steel's rule of thirds,** the remaining centimeter of free space allows for some degree of pathologic displacement. Therefore, anterior displacement of the atlas exceeding 1 cm (the thickness of the odontoid process) threatens the adjacent segment of cord. This usually occurs with disruption of the transverse ligament of C1. This ligament maintains the proper relationship of the dens to C1 and is often ruptured as a pure ligamentous disruption from a flexion injury. Because the cardiac and respiratory centers lie at this level, displacement of the atlas threatens the life of the patient. If the ring of the atlas is capacious (greater than 3 cm in diameter either as an anatomic feature or as a result of a C1 ring fracture), there is less danger, whereas if it is narrow and unfractured, there is more (18).
      3. **History.** If consciousness is not lost as a result of a concurrent head injury, the history should suggest a mechanism for a vertical compression injury. The injury often results from a diving accident or any mechanism that applies axial force to the head.
      4. **Examination.** Clinical symptoms and signs vary from minimal complaints to severe pain and gross limitation of movement. Extension usually produces some pain, but rotation may be relatively pain-free. Because the suboccipital nerve crosses the ring posterior to each lateral mass and the greater occipital nerve emerges just below the posterior ring of the atlas to supply the skin over the occiput, testing of sensation can show involvement of the suboccipital or, more commonly, the greater occipital nerve. Damage to the spinal cord is uncommon, because a significant cord injury at this level causes immediate death.
      5. **Roentgenograms.** Anteroposterior films, including an open-mouth view and a lateral view, are routine. Tomograms or computed tomography (CT) scans are helpful. The common fracture sites are the anterior arch, either midline or just lateral to the midline, and the posterior arch at its narrowest portion just posterior to each lateral mass. Displacement of the fracture can be minimal. In an open-mouth roentgenogram of the odontoid process, when a comminuted fracture of C1 shows bilateral overhang of the lateral masses totaling 7 mm or more, a rupture of the transverse ligament may have occurred, rendering the spine unstable (Fig. 11-2).
      6. **Treatment.** Treat by immobilization in a cervicothoracic orthosis or halo vest until healing occurs, usually in 2–3 months. Initially, use 5–8 lb of tong traction in bed while the extent of the injury is assessed. Reduction of the fracture is best accomplished by adjusting the relative position of the head to the thorax. Head extension is required when the transverse ligament is ruptured (1,3).
   B. **Fracture of the odontoid process** (1,10)
      1. **Mechanism of injury.** The C1 vertebra and the odontoid process of C2 are a single functional unit. The apical/alar and transverse ligaments

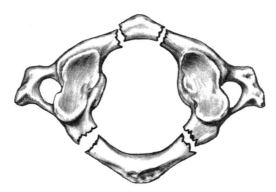

FIG. 11-1. Jefferson fracture.

on the posterior aspect of the odontoid process can remain intact following an injury, producing a fracture of the base of the process. The skull, the C1 vertebra, and the odontoid process of the C2 vertebra then move relatively independently of the body of the C2 vertebra.

2. **History.** Symptoms can be minimal, but severe pain behind the ears and stiffness following a flexion or extension injury are frequent. The patients often report a feeling of instability at the base of the skull and present themselves by holding their head with both hands. There is seldom any suggestion of weakness or numbness of the limbs following an acute injury.

3. **Examination.** Tenderness in the suboccipital region may be present.

4. **Roentgenograms.** A lateral roentgenogram demonstrates that the C1 vertebra has moved in relation to C2, and it is also usually seen that the anterior arch of the C1 vertebra and the odontoid process are in their normal relationship; that is, the odontoid process has been carried with the arch of the C1 vertebra (10). Translation of C1 or C2 of 3.0–4.5 mm, with neurologic symptoms or signs, can indicate clinical instability. When the translation is caused by traumatic disruption of the transverse ligament, then a C1-C2 fusion is indicated. Note the position of the posterior part of the C1 ring. It is normally equidistant between the

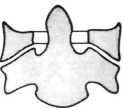

Stable   Unstable

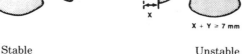

FIG. 11-2. Jefferson fractures. When a comminuted fracture of C1 shows bilateral overhang of the lateral masses that total 7 mm or more, rupture of the transverse ligament has probably occurred, rendering the spine unstable. (From White AA III, Panjabi MM. *Clinical biomechanics of the spine.* Philadelphia: JB Lippincott, 1978:203.)

base of the skull and the spinous process of C2. An open-mouth anteroposterior roentgenogram usually shows a fracture line at the base of the
odontoid process, and this fracture line may run inferiorly, possibly involving the upper part of the vertebral body. The fracture must be differentiated from congenital etiologies such as a secondary ossification
center with an open apophyseal plate, which may be seen in younger patients, or from a failure of segments of the odontoid process to fuse to
the body of C2, which may be seen in older patients. With a congenital
etiology, the radiolucency usually is situated more cephalad and is less
irregular than that seen with an acute fracture. In addition, an increased
incidence of anomalies of the anterior arch of C1 and of the atlanto-
occipital articulation is seen with congenital abnormalities of the odontoid process (1,10,24). Tomograms or CT scans are helpful.

5. **Treatment** (1,10)
   a. **Type I** is a fracture through the upper portion of the odontoid
      process. Treatment with a cervical orthosis is satisfactory. Non-
      union usually presents few problems, because the fracture is too far
      above the level of the transverse ligament to cause any loss of sta-
      bility. These fractures are rare.
   b. **Type II** is a fracture at the junction of the dens with the vertebral
      body of C2. Reduction of an anteriorly displaced C1 with a fractured
      odontoid process can often be achieved by allowing the head to sink
      into extension with the patient in a supine position in traction. This
      reduction is more easily done by sedating the patient adequately
      and inserting a pillow behind the shoulder to allow extension of the
      head and neck. Light traction in Gardner-Wells tongs should be ap-
      plied. Lateral roentgenograms should be obtained at frequent in-
      tervals until the reduction has been confirmed. Then the head and
      neck should be immobilized with the fracture reduced and held in a
      halo vest without distraction of the fracture. Apply the orthosis as
      soon as is feasible so the patient can sit up and become ambulatory.
      Immobilization of the fracture should be continued until the fracture
      is healed, usually 3–4 months; then progressive mobilization of the
      neck should be initiated. A soft collar is used until muscle strength
      has returned. This fracture is associated with a 15%–85% incidence
      of non-union (1,10,24).
   c. **Type III** is really a fracture through the body of the atlas at the
      base of the dens. Treat with very light traction for 2–3 days to pro-
      vide reduction of the fracture. Follow this with a halo vest that con-
      trols the spine effectively for an additional 12–14 weeks.
   d. Increasingly displaced type II fractures are treated with anterior
      screw fixation (1). Although technically demanding, the results are
      predictable in terms of fracture union, with rates in the range of
      90%. **An acceptable surgical technique** is a posterior fusion
      using an iliac graft, notched so as to fit over the spinous process of
      C2. The graft is firmly fixed in place by a wire carefully routed under
      and over the arch of C1, over the graft, and through a hole in the
      spinous process of C2. Fuse in situ, if the patient is neurologically
      intact. Rarely, a fusion of occiput to C2 is indicated by a modifica-
      tion of this technique. A larger "hot-pants" graft is used with two
      wires. The upper wire passes through a hole in the outer table of the
      occiput and around the upper graft. The lower wire loops about the
      upper wire and through a hole in the transverse process of C2. This
      may be indicated if the fracture is associated with a C1 ring frac-
      ture. When fixing grafts in the lower cervical spine, the wire can be
      placed through holes in the spinous processes above and below.

6. **Complications.** As revealed by roentgenography, union of the fracture
   may not be achieved in all cases. In a review of 60 odontoid fractures, it
   was found that fractures at the junction of the odontoid process with the

body of C2 had a non-union rate of 36%, which is the usual rate given to type II fractures (historical review, Anderson and D'Alonzo). With type III fractures, only 10% went on to non-union. It was theorized that the vertebral body consisted of more cancellous bone, which is associated with a higher union rate. The use of traction beyond the first few days is contraindicated, because it may produce distraction and it does not immobilize the fracture. This common practice may account for the high incidence of non-union. At 4 months after injury, flexion and extension films should be obtained. If there is instability, a posterior C1-C2 fusion should be recommended, although 10%–15% of neck rotation will be lost (1,10,24).

C. Fracture of C2 vertebra (hangman's fracture)

1. **Mechanism of injury.** Although the hangman causes this injury by distraction and extension, the other mechanisms of injury that produce the same fracture seem to be confusing and indefinite. Patients have remembered "hanging" their chins on the steering wheel or dashboard or striking their foreheads on the sun visor of cars involved in accidents. The classic injury is a bilateral fracture passing through the posterior part of the lateral masses or pars interarticularis of the axis and into the intervertebral notch (18). The body of the axis is then subluxated or dislocated in relation to the body of C3. The skull and C1 move as a unit with the body of C2, while the posterior elements of C2 remain as a unit with the posterior elements of C3, as shown in Fig. 11-3.

2. **Examination.** Involvement of the spinal cord in patients who survive the initial trauma is relatively uncommon, so the patient may complain of little more than local pain and stiffness. There is tenderness over the spinous process of C2, however.

3. **Roentgenograms.** Anteroposterior and lateral roentgenograms and tomograms or CT scans are essential. The retropharyngeal space may be widened on the lateral view (normal is 4–6 mm at C3). The injury is occasionally accompanied by other injuries in the lower part of the cervical spine, and these must be carefully excluded.

4. **Treatment.** The fracture tends to be reduced with the neck in a neutral position, but the most appropriate position should be adopted. Halo vest immobilization should follow a brief 1- to 2-day period of tong traction

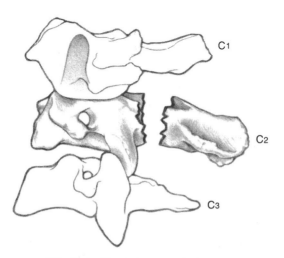

FIG. 11-3. Classic hangman's fracture.

and must often continue for 3 months. Traction can produce distraction and subsequent non-union or ligamentous instability. If minimally displaced, a cervical brace (such as a Philadelphia collar) may be used. The fracture usually heals solidly. Therefore, primary operative treatment is unwarranted.

5. **Complications.** Patients rarely require intubation or tracheostomy because of initial severe retropharyngeal swelling.

D. **Fractures and dislocations of the lower cervical spine** (5,6). In this region of the spine, dislocations without fractures are common, but fractures and fracture-dislocations do occur. The spinal cord and nerve roots frequently are involved; in addition to displaced bony elements, the intravertebral disc can become displaced and function as the leading "impact force" against the spinal cord (6,23). Injury to the vertebral arteries is not uncommon, particularly with injuries that produce quadriparesis (26).

1. **Mechanisms of injury**

a. Although the effects of a **vertical compression** or bursting injury are seen in C1, vertical compression can also produce injuries lower in the cervical spine. C5 is most commonly involved with this mechanism.

b. An **extension injury** produces tearing of the anterior longitudinal ligament with or without an avulsion fracture of the anterior aspect of one of the vertebral bodies. Fractures of the pedicles or facets and posterior subluxation can occur. This injury commonly is associated with a rear-end automobile accident. Subsequent symptoms may last for a prolonged period of time without objective documentation of any osseous or soft-tissue abnormalities (25) (see **I.E**).

c. **Flexion injuries**

(1) A **unilateral dislocation** or **fracture-dislocation** occurs with a dislocation of the facets on one side, with the facets on the other side remaining intact and in normal relationship to one another (5). This phenomenon generally occurs in the lower cervical spine, C5-C7.

(2) **Bilateral dislocations** or **fracture-dislocations** involve the facet joint on both sides. This diagnosis is easier to make on the lateral cervical roentgenogram because it is associated with more marked posterior displacement of the upper segment relative to the lower segment; displacement of disc material is common (23).

2. **Examination.** Carefully search for bruising or abrasions in the region of the face, forehead, and occiput (22). Presence and distribution of such lesions often gives an indication of the mechanism of injury. Assume that any patient with facial or forehead lacerations who has been involved in a high-speed impact has a cervical spine fracture until proven otherwise. Local examination of the neck reveals tenderness over one or more spinous processes, and there is limitation of movement and muscle spasm. The examination must include a careful neurologic assessment. It is not enough to decide whether there is evidence of cord damage. The level of a neurologic lesion must be accurately defined by both motor and sensory examinations as well as pathologic reflexes and must be recorded with the time and date, preferably in a flow-sheet format. Patients must be reexamined frequently in the first 24 hours after injury, especially those with incomplete spinal cord injury (6,20,22).

3. **Roentgenograms.** Good radiologic assessment (to include the first thoracic vertebra) is essential and frequently requires tomograms or CT scans. In patients with bilateral facet joints neurologically intact or with mild paresis, an emergent magnetic resonance imaging (MRI) scan is indicated to determine whether there is herniated disc material anteriorly that would place additional pressure on the spinal cord with close reduction. Some important points to look for in the plain radiographs are as follows (Fig. 11-4):

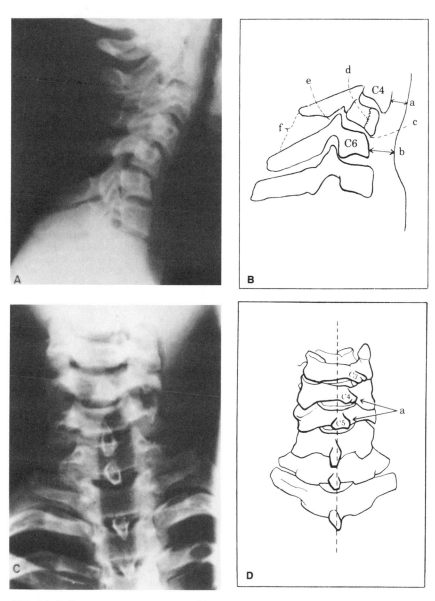

FIG. 11-4. Important roentgenographic signs of a cervical spine injury. **A and B:** (a) Normal width of the retropharyngeal space at C4 is 4–6 mm. (b) Normal width of the retropharyngeal space at C6 is 8–10 mm. (c) An alteration in the alignment of the bodies. (d) Look for fracture lines in the bodies or in the posterior elements. (e) A step-off in the line of the posterior intervertebral facet joint. (f) An increased distance between two spinous processes. **C and D:** The C4 spinous process is displaced laterally in relation to C5, demonstrating facet disruption.

a. Any alteration in the **alignment** of the bodies. Straightening of the cervical spine can result from muscle spasms or from positioning the patient's head in slight flexion.

b. Any **step-off** in the line of the posterior intervertebral **facet joints.**

c. Any increase in the **width of the retropharyngeal space** in front of the vertebral bodies (normal is 4–6 mm at C3 or above). This rule does not apply in a crying child.

d. Any **fracture lines** in the bodies or in the posterior elements.

e. Any **increase of distance between two spinous processes.**

f. Any **displacement of the spinous process** on the cephalad side, which is toward the side of any unilateral dislocation on the anteroposterior film.

g. Any **indication that the body of one vertebra has moved forward in relation to another on the lateral roentgenogram, because such movement usually indicates a dislocation or fracture-dislocation of one or both joint facets at that level.** If the amount of displacement is more than half the width of the vertebral body, the dislocation is bilateral and the spine is extremely unstable.

h. Pediatric patients can have severe neurologic deficits and normal radiographs; MRI scan identifies the soft tissue or hematoma associated with the injury (13).

4. **Initial treatment.** Once the association between neurologic deficit and spinal injury has been confirmed, parenteral steroids should be started. The efficacy of such treatment started within 8 hours of injury has recently been confirmed (8,9,14). An initial loading dose of 30 mg/kg of methylprednisolone IV is followed by 23 hours of 5.4 mg/kg of the same drug. Newer pharmacologic regimens are being studies to clarify their role in improving outcomes (9,14). Whether or not neurologic damage is present, reduction of any displacement should be undertaken. To reduce and treat the fracture properly, however, the fracture pattern must be understood. This usually is best assessed by attempting to understand the mechanism of injury as well as through high-quality roentgenograms. The suggested method for reduction of dislocations or fracture-dislocations, whether unilateral or bilateral, is with skull tongs inserted as described in Chap. 9, **V.B.** It is prudent to be sure that disc material has not been displaced into the spinal canal, especially with bilateral facet dislocations in a neurologically intact individual. If the dislocation is reduced before confirming the absence of herniated soft tissue by MRI scan, spinal cord injury may result. The patient is placed in skull tong traction, usually with 15 lb of weight. **Use traction in the direction of the deformity,** not in line with the patient's body. The weight may be gradually increased by 5 lb every hour. Obtain lateral roentgenograms every 30–60 minutes. Record a neurologic examination at 30-minute intervals. With a unilateral facet dislocation, after 60 lb (or one third of body weight) of traction force has been applied, then consider bending the head away while rotating the upper neck toward the side of the dislocation. Reduction should be achieved rapidly by this method, then the weight may be decreased to 5 lb. If reduction is not achieved rapidly or if the dislocation is old, then consultation with an experienced spinal surgeon is important because it may be necessary to proceed with an operation to achieve reduction. Reduction of the fracture or fracture-dislocation is the best and safest method of achieving decompression of the spinal cord or roots (6). Laminectomy is contraindicated because it may produce increased instability while adding surgical trauma.

5. **Management after reduction** is through immobilization by light tong traction for several days with the neck in the optimum position as demonstrated by lateral roentgenograms. In the absence of significant neurologic deficit, the patient may then be placed in a halo vest. If extensive

neurologic deficit is present, then immobilization in bed may be necessary. To avoid the complications of bed rest (e.g., pneumonia, urinary stasis, bed sores), operative stabilization is frequently indicated. Deep venous thrombosis prophylaxis must be used because of the very high rates of this complication in spinal cord–injured patients (17). In unstable injuries, it is wise to use a halo apparatus. Other types of cervical orthoses occasionally are used but are not as effective as the halo apparatus and are reserved for stable injuries. For unstable injuries, surgical stabilization and early mobilization of the patient is almost always indicated (6). The instability criteria of White and Panjabi may be used as guidelines. Posterior cervical fusion is recommended for all patients with bilateral facet dislocations. If reduction has been achieved by tong traction, then surgery is usually delayed 5–7 days to avoid the neurologic deterioration that can occasionally occur in quadriplegic patients. As noted earlier, before reduction and before surgery, the location of the intervertebral disc must be determined by CT scanning, myelography, or MRI. If the disc is retropulsed into the canal, then it must be removed before reduction and posterior fusion. The treatment of a unilateral facet dislocation is controversial (24). Many consultants recommend treatment in a halo vest following reduction in tong traction. The authors recommend posterior cervical fusion for this condition because anatomic alignment can then be maintained.

6. Spinal cord injuries are **classified** as complete or incomplete neurologic injuries (22). Patients with complete injuries have no motor or sensory function distal to the level of cord injury, and patients with incomplete injuries have some function, whether motor or sensory, distal to the lesion.

   a. The **anterior cord syndrome** involves loss of neural function in the anterior two thirds of the spinal cord. Patients with these injuries experience complete loss of motor function and of pain and temperature sensation but retain sensations of vibration, proprioception, and light touch. These preserved functions result in an improved prognosis.

   b. A penetrating injury or unilateral facet dislocation can result in hemiinjury to the spinal cord: the **Brown-Séquard syndrome.** Patients experience loss of ipsilateral motor and dorsal column function and contralateral pain and temperature sensation.

   c. The **central cord syndrome** is often associated with a cervical hyperextension injury, often in older patients. This syndrome consists of a disproportionately greater weakness in the upper extremities compared with lower extremities, various sensory changes at or below the site of the lesion, and urinary bladder dysfunction. Proposed causes include hematomyelia, contusion, cord swelling, and ischemia of the cervical spinal cord. The anterior horn cells at the level of injury may also be involved. Treatment is directed to reduction of cord edema and immobilization of the neck (8,9). The prognosis depends on the amount of initial neurologic involvement and the rapidity of subsequent recovery. The signs of neurologic damage tend to disappear in reverse order of their appearance.

E. The **hyperextension whiplash injury**

   1. The **mechanism of injury** is similar to that for the cervical spine extension injuries described in **D.1.b.** (26).

   2. Likewise, the **history** is similar; for example, the patient was an occupant in a car that was suddenly struck in the rear by another automobile.

   3. The **examination** shows tenderness along the scalene muscles and within the body of the trapezius muscle.

   4. In a pure soft-tissue injury without tearing of the anterior longitudinal ligament, the **roentgenograms are normal.**

   5. **Recommended treatment** for the first 10–14 days includes a properly sized soft collar to immobilize the neck, sufficient analgesics for

pain relief, and rest. Soft collars are preferable to rigid collars for comfort. Collars should be high posteriorly and low under the chin to keep the cervical spine in a neutral or slightly flexed position. Avoid hyperextension in whiplash injuries and cervical radiculopathy. Cold packs may be used for the first 24 hours, followed by warm packs. A folded towel can be used as a neck collar. Ice may be placed within the towel initially; then a damp warm towel may be used. Corticosteroid injection of the facet joints has not been proven to be effective in a randomized controlled trial (4).

6. The long-term **prognosis** for these injuries was reported as follows: 43% of the patients had residual symptoms 5 years after injury (historical readings, Hohl M). There were degenerative changes in 39% of the patients. A poorer prognosis was predicted if shortly after injury the following findings were present:

   a. **Pain or numbness in an upper extremity**
   b. Sharp **reversal of the cervical lordosis** as seen on the roentgenograms. This is not a completely reliable sign.
   c. **Restricted motion** at one interspace as seen in flexion-extension roentgenograms; these should not be obtained until 3 weeks after injury to improve their sensitivity in detecting instability.
   d. **Need for a cervical collar for more than 12 weeks or for home traction**
   e. **Need to resume physical therapy** more than once because of recurrence of symptoms

F. **Fractures and fracture-dislocations of the thoracic, thoracolumbar, and lumbar spine.** Denis improved upon Holdsworth's concepts to develop the three-column theory for thoracolumbar fractures (12). Recently, McAfee has shown the utility of using CT to classify fractures to aid in treatment decisions (21).

   1. **Types of injury** (21)

      a. **Compression fracture** (Fig. 11-5). A wedge compression fracture of the vertebral body is produced by a flexion force, but the posterior ligament complex (i.e., supraspinous ligaments, interspinous ligaments, ligamenta flava, and capsules of the intervertebral joint) remains intact. There is no fracture of the posterior elements. Kyphotic angulation (as measured by the angle between lines drawn from the end plates of the injured vertebrae to those of the adjacent uninjured vertebra) is usually less than 10 degrees and loss of anterior vertebral height is no greater than 40%. Therefore, this injury is classified as relatively stable but requires close observation for progressive kyphotic deformity.

      b. **Stable burst fracture** (Fig. 11-6). Burst fractures of the thoracolumbar spine are generally stable. By reviewing the plain roentgenograms and CT scan, the anterior and middle columns are parted with bone retropulsed into the spinal cord, but the posterior column is uninjured (the facet joints and ligaments are intact). Kyphosis is limited to 15 degrees and loss of vertebral height is less than 50%. These patients are neurologically intact.

      c. **Unstable burst fracture** (Fig. 11-7). In these injuries, the posterior column is disrupted as well. The hallmark is pedicle widening on the anteroposterior roentgenogram. The amount of neurologic injury varies based more on the level of the injury than the degree of canal compromise by bone fragments. One must remember that the spinal cord ends at L2 and fractures above this level have greater neurologic involvement. Stenosis of 80% is tolerated well below this level whereas stenosis of 30% in the thoracic spine may be associated with paraplegia.

      d. **Flexion-distraction injury** (Fig. 11-8). These injuries result from failure of the posterior elements in tension while the anterior and

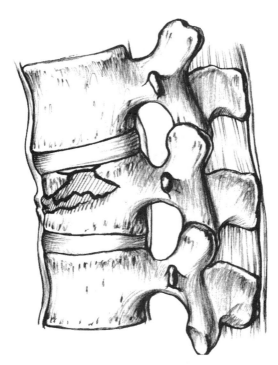

FIG. 11-5. Compression fracture of the thoracolumbar spine. (From Hansen ST, Swiontkowski MF. *Orthopaedic trauma protocols.* New York: Raven, 1993:216.)

middle columns are compressed. The most common mechanism is a lap belt in a motor vehicle accident. On the lateral roentgenogram, widening of the spinous processes is seen. The vertebral body is wedged anteriorly and occasionally a small fragment of bone is retropulsed into the canal. The neurologic injury is variable.

e. **Chance fracture** (Fig. 11-9). Generally, these fractures result from tension failure of all spinal bony elements as a result of hyperflexion over a secured lap belt. These injuries, which commonly occur in back seat passengers, are seen frequently in children (2). Bowel injuries occur in up to 65% of these patients because the lap belt provides the fulcrum against the abdominal wall. The injury can be ligamentous, bony, or both, but there is no compromise of the anterior elements if the injury is primarily ligamentous. Most often surgery is indicated.

f. **Translational injuries** (Fig. 11-10) are caused by shear forces that fracture or dislocate the facets. Paraplegia is generally the result. Anteroposterior translation of the vertebral bodies is present on the roentgenograms. Surgical stabilization is generally advisable.

2. **Diagnosis.** The diagnosis is suspected from the mechanism of injury or, in the elderly patient, following a sudden jolt or fall. Tenderness to palpation or percussion over the involved segment is common. Hematomas and gaps between spinous processes may be palpable.

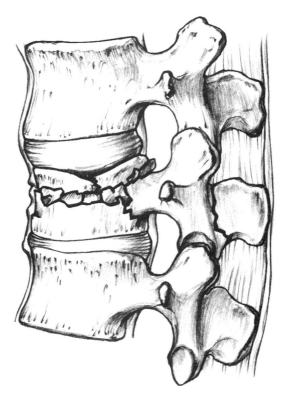

FIG. 11-6. Stable burst fracture. (From Hansen ST, Swiontkowski MF. *Orthopaedic trauma protocols.* New York: Raven, 1993:217.)

3. **Examination.** On initial examination, a neurologic assessment must be completed. If a sensory level is detected, mark it on the chart and on the trunk with the time and date of examination. If there is any motor deficit, then record it on a simple muscle chart. It is sufficient to record function of muscle groups rather than of individual muscles. A drawing of the patient can be helpful to illustrate pertinent neurologic findings. A flow sheet is another useful device to document changes in the neurologic status over time.
4. **Roentgenograms.** Excellent quality anteroposterior and lateral films are required, and CT scans often are indicated to evaluate the posterior elements and to assess stability (21). The pattern of injury must be accurately determined. If there is neurologic involvement and the roentgenograms and CT scans do not reveal a fracture, MRI is indicated. This study identifies herniated disc material or hematoma as the cause of the deteriorating neurologic examination (11,15).
5. **Treatment.** Logroll the patient on a firm mattress until stability of the fracture is assessed.
   a. **Minor fractures**
      (1) **Bed rest** on a firm bed for a few days with light analgesia is usually all that is required. Patients may be turned in a log-rolling fashion every 2–4 hours. An off-the-shelf Jewett brace or Risser cast is generally used for 12–16 weeks.

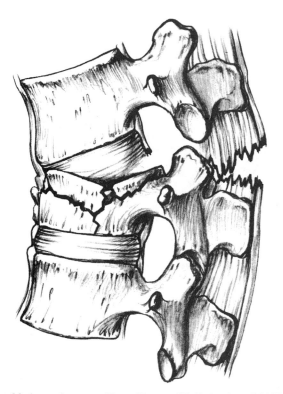

FIG. 11-7. Unstable burst fracture. (From Hansen ST, Swiontkowski MF. *Orthopaedic trauma protocols.* New York: Raven, 1993:218.)

   (2) Paralytic **ileus** tends to develop, particularly in patients with lumbar compression fractures. This development should be anticipated and the patient should take nothing by mouth until normal bowel activity is ensured; IV fluid maintenance is required.

   (3) As soon as the patient is comfortable in a cast or brace, start **extension exercises** to strengthen the thoracic and lumbar spinal extensor muscles. As soon as good muscle control is obtained, the patient may be allowed to ambulate.

   (4) **Lifting or flexion activities should be avoided** for 3 months.

 b. **Major fractures or fracture-dislocations.** Spinal fractures can be missed in unconscious obtunded patients; complete spine films must be obtained and carefully scrutinized (7). **Stable fractures** rarely require operative intervention. The exception is found in severe anterior compression fracture with a marked kyphosis, for which reduction with some type of posterior instrumentation such as a rod/hook or rod/pedicle screw construct may be indicated. Unstable fractures should be evaluated for stabilization with appropriate instrumentation by an orthopaedic surgeon trained in the use of these devices (12,15,16).

   (1) **Stable fractures without neurologic deficit** include most compression injuries and burst fractures resulting from verti-

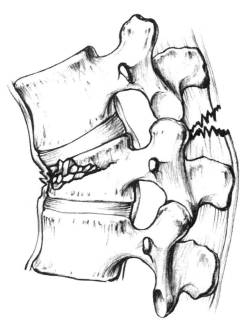

FIG. 11-8. Flexion-distraction injury. (From Hansen ST, Swiontkowski MF. *Orthopaedic trauma protocols*. New York: Raven, 1993:219.)

cal compression forces. Place the patient on strict bed rest until the pain is reduced sufficiently to allow an active exercise program. When good muscle function has been restored, the patient can be mobilized in a plaster or plastic body jacket or a suitable brace. Minor degrees of compression should be treated as are compression fractures elsewhere (see **F.5.a**).

(2) **Unstable injuries without neurologic involvement.** The most common of these injuries is the unstable burst type. If nonoperative treatment is selected, then provide external immobilization for 12–16 weeks, depending on the fracture pattern and physical build of the patient (19). Mild paresthesias or dysesthesias can be seen in this type of injury without other neurologic symptoms or signs; these do not constitute an indication for immediate operation. Consider operative intervention if motor, reflex, or sensory deficits develop. If significant deformity is likely, then surgery is generally recommended.

(3) **Unstable injuries with progressive neurologic damage.** This is one condition for which surgeons agree that reduction and internal stabilization with or without an immediate fusion is required (15). Methylprednisolone therapy is recommended (8,9).

(4) **Unstable injuries with incomplete neurologic deficit.** Treat these cases with a logrolling frame while the neurologic lesion is assessed. If it worsens or remains the same, then consider treatment as noted in the preceding paragraph. If it is improving, then no operative intervention for the lesion is needed, but the fracture instability should be evaluated to determine whether operative stabilization or early mobilization in a cast

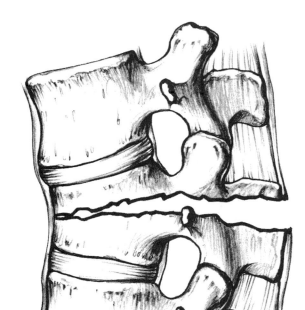

FIG. 11-9. Chance fracture. (From Hansen ST, Swiontkowski MF. *Orthopaedic trauma protocols.* New York: Raven, 1993:221.)

or custom plastic body jacket is the method of choice. Steroid therapy is also recommended.

  (5) **Unstable fractures with complete neurologic deficit.** If paraplegia is immediate and complete and there is no evidence of return of function within 48 hours, then early operative stabilization should be considered to allow earlier rehabilitation.

  c. **Indications for immediate operation**

   (1) **An advancing or progressive neurologic deficit**

   (2) **Paraplegia in the absence of bony injury and in the presence of a complete block as revealed by MRI or myelography,** which may indicate an acute traumatic disc prolapse or hematoma

   (3) **Severe root pain** from root compression at the level of the injury—another indication for exploration but seldom requiring immediate operation

G. **Fractures of the transverse process in the lumbar spine.** These fractures can result from different mechanisms of injury, and should be treated symptomatically. Patients tend to have significant pain and require heavier analgesia. Consider and rule out associated renal injury.

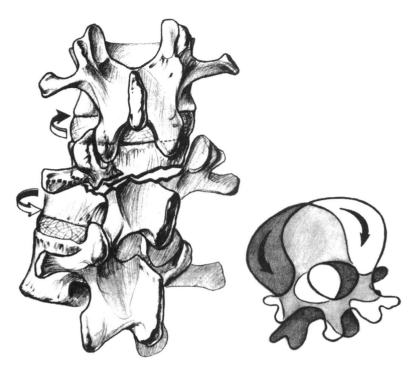

FIG. 11-10. Translational injuries. (From Hansen ST, Swiontkowski MF. *Orthopaedic trauma protocols.* New York: Raven, 1993:222.)

References
1. Aebi M, Etter C, Coscia M. Fractures of the odontoid process: treatment with anterior screw fixation. *Spine* 1989;14:1065–1070.
2. Anderson PA, Henley MB, Rivara FP, et al. Flexion distraction and chance injuries to the thoracolumbar spine. *J Orthop Trauma* 1991;5:153–160.
3. Anderson PA, Montesano PX. Morphology and treatment of occipital condyle fractures. *Spine* 1988;13:731–736.
4. Barnsley L, Lord SM, Wallis BJ, et al. Lack of effect of intraarticular corticosteroids for chronic pain in the cervical zygapophyseal joints. *N Engl J Med* 1994; 330:1047–1050.
5. Beyer CA, Cabarela ME, Berquist TH. Unilateral facet dislocations and fracture-dislocations of the cervical spine. *Orthop Trans* 1990;14:681.
6. Bohlmann HH, Anderson PA. Anterior decompression and arthrodesis of the cervical spine: long-term motor improvement. Part I—Improvement in incomplete traumatic quadriparesis. *J Bone Joint Surg (Am)* 1992;74:671–682.
7. Born CT, Ross SE, Iannacone WM, et al. Delayed identification of skeletal injury in multisystem trauma: the 'missed' fracture. *J Trauma* 1989;29:1643–1646.
8. Bracken MB, et al. A randomized controlled trial of methylprednisolone or naloxone in the treatment of spinal cord injury. *N Engl J Med* 1990;322:1405.
9. Bracken MB, et al. Administration of methylprednisolone for 24 or 48 hours or tirilazad mesylate for 48 hours in the treatment of acute spinal cord injury; results of the third national acute spinal cord injury randomized controlled trial. *JAMA* 1997;227:1597–1604.
10. Clark CR, White AA III. Fractures of the dens: a multicenter study. *J Bone Joint Surg (Am)* 1985;67:1340–1348.

11. Delamarter RB, Sherman JE, Carr JB. 1991 Volvo Award in experimental studies. Cauda equina syndrome: neurologic recovery following immediate, early, or late decompression. *Spine* 1991;16:1022–1029.
12. Denis F. The three-column spine and its significance in the classification of acute thoracolumbar spine injuries. *Spine* 1983;8:817.
13. Dickman CA, Zabramski JM, Hadley MN, et al. Pediatric spinal cord injury without radiographic abnormalities: report of 26 cases and review of the literature. *J Spinal Disord* 1991;4:296–305.
14. Geisler FH, Dorscy FC, Coleman WP. Recovery of motor function after spinal cord injury—a randomized, placebo-controlled trial with G-M-I ganglioside. *N Engl J Med* 1991;324:1829.
15. Gertzbein SD. Neurologic deterioration in patients with thoracic and lumbar fractures after admission to the hospital. *Spine* 1994;19:1723–1725.
16. Gumley G, Taylor TKF, Ryan MD. Distraction fractures of the lumbar spine. *J Bone Joint Surg (Br)* 1982;64:520.
17. Gunduz S, Ogur E, Mohur H, et al. Deep vein thrombosis in spinal cord injured patients. *Paraplegia* 1993;31:606–610.
18. Levine AM, Edwards CC. The management of traumatic spondylolisthesis of the axis. *J Bone Joint Surg (Am)* 1985;67:217.
19. Limb D, Shaw DL, Dickson RA. Neurological injury in thoracolumbar burst fractures. *J Bone Joint Surg (Br)* 1995;77:774–777.
20. Marshal LF, et al. Deterioration following spinal cord injury: a multicenter study. *J Neurosurg,* 1987;66:400.
21. McAfee PC, et al. The value of computed tomography in thoracolumbar fractures. *J Bone Joint Surg (Am)* 1983;65:461.
22. Mermelstein LE, Keenen TL, Benson DR. Initial evaluation and emergency treatment of the spine-injured patient. In: Browner BD, Jupiter JB, Levine AM, et al, eds. *Skeletal trauma,* 2nd ed. Philadelphia: WB Saunders, 1992:745–768.
23. Rizzolo SJ, Piazza MR, Cotler JM, et al. Intervertebral disc injury complicating cervical spine trauma. *Spine* 1991;16[Suppl 6]:S187–S189.
24. Ryan MD, Taylor TKF. Odontoid fractures. *J Bone Joint Surg (Br)* 1982;64:416.
25. Spence KF Jr, Decker S, Sell KW. Bursting atlantal fracture associated with rupture of the transverse ligament. *J Bone Joint Surg (Am)* 1970;52:543–549.
26. Williams N, Ratliff DA. Gastrointestinal disruption and vertebral fracture associated with the use of seat belts. *Ann R Coll Surg Engl* 1993;75:129–132.

Selected Historical Readings

Anderson LD, D'Alonzo RT. Fracture of the odontoid process of the axis. *J Bone Joint Surg (Am)* 1974;56:1663.
Bohler L. Fracture and dislocation of the spine. In: Bohler L, Bohler J, eds. *The treatment of fractures,* 5th ed. New York: Grune & Stratton, 1956.
Bohlman HH. Acute fractures and dislocations of the cervical spine. *J Bone Joint Surg (Am)* 1979;61:1119.
Braakman R, Vinken PJ. Unilateral facet interlocking in the lower cervical spine. *J Bone Joint Surg (Br)* 1967;49:249.
Chance GQ. Note on a type of flexion fracture of the spine. *Br J Radiol* 1948;452.
Clawson DK. Low back pain. *Northwest Med* 1970;69:686.
Dawson EG, Smith L. Atlanto-axial subluxation in children due to vertebral anomalies. *J Bone Joint Surg (Am)* 1979;61:582.
Dickson JH, Harrington PR, Erwin WD. Results of reduction and stabilization of the severely fractured thoracic and lumbar spine. *J Bone Joint Surg (Am)* 1978;60:799.
Fielding JW, et al. Tears of the transverse ligament of the atlas. *J Bone Joint Surg (Am)* 1974;56:1683.
Fielding JW, Hensinger RN, Hawkins RJ. Os odontoideum. *J Bone Joint Surg (Am)* 1980;62:376.
Griswold DM, et al. Atlanto-axial fusion for instability. *J Bone Joint Surg (Am)* 1978; 60:285.

Holdsworth F. Fractures, dislocations, and fracture-dislocations of the spine. *J Bone Joint Surg (Am)* 1970;52:1534.

Hohl M. Soft-tissue injuries of the neck in automobile accidents. Factors influencing prognosis. *J Bone Joint Surg (Am)* 1974;56:1675.

Johnson RM, et al. Cervical orthoses. *J Bone Joint Surg (Am)* 1977;59:322.

Rand RW, Crandall PH. Central spinal cord syndrome in hyperextension injuries of the cervical spine. *J Bone Joint Surg (Am)* 1962;44:1415.

Schatzker JE, Cecil H, Waddell JP. Fractures of the dens (odontoid process), an analysis of thirty-seven cases. *J Bone Joint Surg (Br)* 1971;53:392.

Schneider RC, et al. "Hangman's fracture" of the cervical spine. *J Neurosurg* 1965; 22:141.

Stauffer ES. Current concepts review: internal fixation of fractures of the thoracolumbar spine. *J Bone Joint Surg (Am)* 1984;76A:1136.

White AA III, Panjabi MM. *Clinical biomechanics of the spine.* Philadelphia: JB Lippincott, 1978.

12. DISORDERS AND DISEASES OF THE SPINE

I. **Low back pain and sciatica.** The lifetime incidence of low back pain is 50% to 70% and of sciatica is 30% to 40%. The cause of the low back pain in approximately 90% of the patients is related to disc degeneration.
   A. **Causes of low back pain.** Low back pain is a symptom, not a disease, and the pathologic basis of the pain frequently lies outside the spine. There are many causes, which are classified in Table 12-1.
      1. **Vascular back pain.** Aneurysms or peripheral vascular disease may give rise to backache or symptoms resembling sciatica.
      2. **Neurogenic back pain.** Tension, irritation, and compression of lumbar nerves and roots may cause pain down both legs. Lesions anywhere along the central nervous system, particularly of the spine, may present with back and leg pain.
      3. **Viscerogenic back pain** may be derived from disorders of the organs in the lesser sac, the pelvis, or the retroperitoneal structures such as the pancreas and kidneys.
      4. **Psychogenic back pain.** Clouding and confusion of the clinical picture by emotional overtones may be seen. A pure psychogenic component is rare.
      5. **Spondylogenic back pain.** Common conditions causing spondylogenic back pain are outlined in Table 12-2.
         a. **Disc degeneration** is by far the most common cause of back pain. Disc degeneration may occur anywhere along the spine and produce neck pain, thoracic spine pain, or lumbar or low back pain. Disc degeneration may be associated with nerve root irritation, which would then result in radicular leg pain. The nerve root irritation or compression may be due to an acute disc herniation or impingement by bony stenosis or a combination of soft-tissue and bony impingement.
            (1) **Anatomy.** The spine provides stability and a central axis for the limbs that are attached. The spine has to move, to transmit weight, and to protect the spinal cord. When the spine is viewed from the side, the thoracic spine is concave forward (kyphosis), the cervical and lumbar regions are concave backward (lordosis).
            (2) **Vertebral components**
               (a) Each segment of the vertebral column transmits weight through the vertebral body anteriorly and the facet joints posteriorly. Between adjacent bodies are the intervertebral discs, which are firmly attached to the vertebrae. The disc consists of an outer annulus fibrosis, which is made up of concentric layers of fibrous tissue. It surrounds and contains a central avascular nucleus pulposus, which consists of a hydrophilic gel made of protein, polysaccharide, collagen fibrils, sparsely chondroid cells, and water (88%). The spinal cord and caudal equina are found within the spinal canal. At each intervertebral level, nerve roots leave the canal through the intervertebral foramina.
               (b) A functional spinal unit or motion segment consists of two adjacent vertebrae and the intervertebral disc. It forms a three-joint complex with the disc in front and two facet joints posteriorly. The facet joints, like other joints in the body, have capsules, ligaments, muscles, nerves, and vessels. Changes in one joint affect the other two. Narrowing of the disc space, therefore, may result in malalignment of the facet joints and, with time, lead to wear-and-tear degenerative arthritic changes in those joints.

Table 12-1. Classification of low back pain causes

Spondylogenic
Vascular
Neurogenic
Viscerogenic
Psychogenic

(3) **Pathology.** Normal aging is associated with a gradual dehydration of the disc. The nucleus pulposus becomes desiccated and the annulus fibrosus develops fissures parallel to the vertebral end plates running mainly posteriorly. Small herniations of nuclear material may squeeze through the annular fissures and may also penetrate the vertebral end plates to produce Schmorl's nodes. If the nuclear material squeezes against the nerve, it may produce nerve root irritation. The flattening and collapse of the disc results in osteophytes along the vertebral bodies. Malalignment and displacement of the facet joints is an inevitable consequence of disc space collapse, leading to osteophytes that may narrow the lateral or subarticular recess of the spinal canal or the intervertebral foramina. This narrowing of the spinal canal or of the intervertebral neural foramina is called spinal stenosis.

(4) **Disc degeneration without nerve root irritation.** There are three patterns of low back pain associated with disc degeneration: **acute incapacitating backache,** which may occur a few times in a person's life and not be a regular problem; **recurrent aggravating backache,** which is the most common type and is associated with regular periods of recurrence and remission of back pain; and **chronic persisting backache,** which is the most difficult to treat and the patients have constant disabling back pain.

(b) The back pain associated with disc degeneration is mechanical in nature. It is aggravated or brought on by activity and relieved by rest. There may be a referred component of back pain into the legs, but this is usually down the back of the legs and rarely goes beyond the knee. The low back pain may be due to periods of hard work, prolonged

Table 12-2. Common conditions causing spondylogenic back pain

1. Disc degeneration
2. Spondylolisthesis
3. Trauma
    Myofascial sprains/strains
    Fractures
4. Infection (bacterial tuberculosis)
5. Tumor (benign, malignant, metastatic)
6. Rheumatologic
    Ankylosing spondylitis/spondyloarthropathy
    Fibrositis/fibromyalgia
7. Metabolic
    Osteoporosis
    Osteomalacia
    Paget's disease

standing or walking, or prolonged sitting in one position. The peak incidence of back pain in the general population is in the 40s and 50s. This is the time when the discs have collapsed and there is relative instability at the motion segment. The natural history, however, is for the spine to stiffen up with increased fibrosus around the facet joints and the discs. As the patient gets older, the physical demands become less and the spine becomes stiffer; the incidence of back pain, therefore, declines beyond the 60s.

(c) Patients who give a history of fever, weight loss, malaise, night and rest pain, morning stiffness, and colicky pain should be carefully evaluated for the possibilities of infection, tumor, spondyloarthropathy, or viscerogenic back pain.

(5) **Disc degeneration with root irritation**

(a) Nerve root irritation and compression may be due to an **acute disc herniation** or may be associated with **spinal stenosis.** Acute disc herniation results in "sciatica." Essentially, this involves severe, incapacitating pain that radiates from the back down the leg. It may be associated with paresthesia, neurologic symptoms, or motor sensory or reflex changes. The pain may be constant and is frequently aggravated by coughing, sneezing, and straining. Intradiscal pressure is increased in a bending and sitting position, especially if lifting is performed, therefore increasing the amount of pain. The pain may be lessened by lying down.

(b) The **most frequent sites of disc herniation** are in the spinal canal, resulting in impingement of the traversing nerve root. Less common disc herniation may be laterally in the foramen, resulting in impingement of the exiting nerve root. The leg pain or sciatica is accompanied by signs of nerve root tension, which can be diagnosed by a straight-leg raising test, bowstring sign, or Lasegue's test.

(c) In **spinal stenosis,** the leg pain or radicular pain is brought on by prolonged walking or standing (neurogenic claudication). The pain may be associated with paresthesia and is relieved by sitting or stooping. There are few physical findings or neurologic deficits unless the condition has been present for a long time and is advanced. Neurogenic claudication associated with spinal stenosis should be distinguished from vascular claudication caused by peripheral vascular disease.

(6) **Neurology of the lower extremities.** The nerve roots leaving the spine at each segmental level may be affected by acute disc herniations, bony foraminal stenosis, or a stenosis associated with both soft-tissue and bony compression. The nerve root may be affected within the central spinal canal, in the subarticular recess, or in the intervertebral foramen. The nerve root traversing the motion segment or the exiting nerve root may be affected. It is important to correlate the patient's symptoms and physical findings with the abnormalities seen on radiographs, magnetic resonance imaging (MRI) scans, and computed tomography (CT) studies. It is important, therefore, to have knowledge of the nerve roots and their enervation. The main nerve roots are listed in Table 12-3.

(7) **Imaging studies**

(a) **Radiographs** may appear normal or demonstrate disc space narrowing, osteophyte formation, or instability on

Table 12-3. Neurology of the lower extremity

Root	Muscles	Sensation	Reflex
L2	Hip flexion	Anterior thigh (proximal)	None
L3	Knee extension (quadriceps)	Anterior thigh (distal)	Patellar
L4	Anterior tibialis	Medial leg	Patellar
L5	Extensor hallucis longus	Lateral leg and dorsum of foot	None
S1	Gastrocsoleus Peroneus longus and brevis	Lateral foot	Achilles

lateral flexion and extension views. There is no clear-cut correlation between low back pain and the presence of disc degeneration.

(b) **Myleograms** are invasive and are less commonly used. They may be used in combination with CT scans in patients who have complex problems or who have had multiple surgeries.

(c) **CT scans** are generally helpful when MRI scans cannot be obtained. They give better detail of the bone.

(d) **MRI scans** of the lumbar spine are noninvasive and an excellent way to evaluate the compromise of neural structures.

(e) **Bone scans** of the spine and pelvis are useful if tumor and infection are suspected, although these abnormalities can also be picked up easily on an MRI scan.

b. **Spondylolisthesis.** Spondylolisthesis is the forward slippage of one vertebra on another. Spondylolysis is the presence of a bony defect of the pars interarticularis, which may result in spondylolisthesis.

(1) **Classification**
   (a) **Congenital**
   (b) **Isthmic**
   (c) **Traumatic**
   (d) **Pathologic**
   (e) **Degenerative**

(2) **Congenital spondylolisthesis** is a congenital deficiency of the facets. Isthmic spondylolisthesis is the typical defect in the pars interarticularis allowing forward slippage of the vertebrae. It may be related to an acute fracture, a fatigue fracture, or an elongation or attenuation of an intact pars interarticularis. Traumatic spondylolisthesis is an acute fracture of the pedicle, lamina, or facet. Pathologic spondylolisthesis is an attenuation of the pedicle caused by weakness of bone (e.g., osteogenesis imperfecta). The most common type of spondylolisthesis is **degenerative spondylolisthesis**.

(3) The **Meyerding grading system** is used to indicate the percentage of displacement of the superior vertebral body on the inferior vertebral body as follows: grade I, 0%–25%; grade II, 25%–50%; grade III, 50%–75%; grade IV, 75%–100%; grade V, greater than 100% spondyloloptosis.

(4) **Etiology.** The initial onset of a lesion occurs at approximately 8 years of age. History of minor trauma may exist. The onset of symptoms coincides closely with either the adolescent growth spurt or repetitive athletic activity. It is thought to originate in a stress or fatigue fracture. The shear stresses are greater on the pars interarticularis when the spine is extended. Such

stresses are seen with certain activities (e.g., back walkovers in gymnastics, carrying heavy backpacks, heavy lifting).

(5) **Clinical findings in isthmic spondylolisthesis.** Patients may be asymptomatic, but most patients have low back pain during the adolescent growth spurt. A few patients do have nerve root or radicular pain in the lower extremities. Hamstring tightness or spasm is commonly found in symptomatic patients. A palpable step-off may be felt at the level of the slip.

(6) Anteroposterior and lateral radiographs are helpful in making the diagnosis to demonstrate the slip of spondylolisthesis. An undisplaced spondylolysis is best seen on the oblique views of the lumbar spine. The "Scottie dog" sign describes the appearance of the facet joints and pars interarticularis on the oblique radiographs. The "Scottie dog's" neck representing the pars is broken in isthmic spondylolysis. There is no urgency about surgical treatment of spondylolisthesis unless serial radiographs have demonstrated progression of the slip or if there is significant neurologic impairment. The incidence of spondylolysis/ spondylolisthesis in the asymptomatic population is 3%–5%.

II. **Deformities of the spine.** There are three basic types of spinal deformity; **scoliosis**, **kyphosis**, and **lordosis**.

A. **A. Scoliosis**

1. Scoliosis is a side to side curvature when the spine is viewed in the coronal plane. This deformity may be flexible and reactive or fixed and structural. In the former, there is no structural change and the deformity is correctable. There are three causes: **postural, compensatory** (to another curve, pelvic tilt, or short leg), and **sciatic.** In structural scoliosis, there is a three-dimensional deformity. The vertebrae are deformed and are rotated toward each other. The resulting rotation of all the attachments and appendages of the vertebrae, such as ribs and processes, results in asymmetry of the body, waistline, and paravertebral prominences, as well as shoulder elevation.

2. The broad **categories of structural scoliosis** are as follows:
   a. Idiopathic (infantile, juvenile and adolescent)
   b. Osteopathic (congenital)
   c. Neuropathic (cerebral palsy, poliomyelitis)
   d. Myopathic (muscular dystrophies)
   e. Connective tissue (Marfan's, Ehlers Danlos)
   f. Neurofibromatosis

3. Scoliosis is also seen in the other disease processes such as spinal cord injuries, infections, metabolic disorders, and tumors.

4. **Curve types**
   a. A **structural curve** is a segment of the spine with lateral curvature lacking normal flexibility.
   b. A **primary curve** is the first or earliest of several curves to appear. A compensatory curve is a curve above or below a major curve. It may progress to be a fixed or secondary curve.

5. **Adolescent idiopathic scoliosis**. This is the most common type and has no known cause. It presents around puberty and may progress until skeletal maturity has been reached. There may be one, two, or three curves occurring most frequently in the thoracic and lumbar spine.
   a. **Risk factors for progression of adolescent idiopathic scoliosis.** Progression is related to the size of the curve, the area of the spine involved, and the physiologic age of a patient. Large thoracic curves progress to a greater degree than single lumbar or thoracolumbar curves. The younger the skeletal age, the more likely the curve progression. Progression is less likely to progress in boys than in girls.

6. **Clinical findings.** Presentation of a painless deformity occurs between 10 and 15 years of age. If severe and persistent pain is present, the pos-

sibility of a tumor (most commonly osteoid osteoma) sciatic scoliosis, or spondylolysis should be considered. The rotational deformity is more noticeable on forward flexion, creating a paravertebral prominence. Other clinical features include shoulder elevation, neckline prominence on side asymmetric waistline, or prominent hip. The term **spinal imbalance** refers to the head or the trunk being off center with respect to the pelvis. Clinically, this can best be measured by dropping a plumb line from the base of the skull. Any deviation of the line from the gluteal cleft measures the amount of spinal imbalance to the left or right. A complete history and physical examination is performed to exclude other causes of scoliosis.

   a. The **history** of a patient with spinal deformity should include age when the deformity was first noted, the perinatal history, the family history of scoliosis. In children and adolescents, scoliosis is generally not painful. If persistent pain is present, appropriate diagnostic tests should be performed to exclude bony or spinal tumor, herniated discs, or other abnormalities. The patient is examined, undraped, except for undershorts, and asymmetries in the shoulder, scapular, waistline, and pelvic region are identified. The balance of the thoracic area over the pelvis is assessed. The C7 plumb line test is used to evaluate the balance of the head over the pelvis and the range of motion of the spine in flexion and extension. Side bending is also noted. The patient should also be observed from the side for evaluation of kyphosis or lordosis. The forward bend test is useful to identify areas of asymmetry in the paravertebral areas. Prominence of the scapula or rib on one side is called a "rib hump." A complete neurologic examination should be performed. Pubertal stages in girls and boys are assessed. Leg length from the anterior-superior iliac spine to the medial malleoli is measured. The lower extremities are evaluated for deformities or contractures.

7. **Radiographic evaluation** includes full length views of the entire spine in a standing position. The angle of curvature is measured. The size of the curve is measured by the **COBB method**. The upper and lower end vertebrae are identified and perpendicular lines are erected to their transverse axis. The intersection of the perpendicular lines is the COBB angle. Radiographs are also used to evaluate the degree of skeletal maturity. The **Risser classification** evaluates the degree of ossification of the iliac epiphysis. This measures the degree of skeletal maturity. There are five grades.

8. **Treatment.** The natural history of these curves varies. Some curves remain the same, others progress, and yet others progress relentlessly. The goal of treatment is to prevent curve progression. Serial radiographs are obtained every 4 months until skeletal maturity. Risk of curve progression is greatest in younger patients with larger curves.

   a. Braces are indicated in the growing patient with curves of 20–40 degrees. Braces have distinct limitations. They brace the body and torso and indirectly exert forces on the spine (e.g., pressure pads on ribs attached to convex vertebrae) and are used to prevent further curve progression rather than straighten the curvature.

   b. Surgery is indicated for curves greater than 40 degrees in the skeletally immature patient who has failed conservative treatment. Anterior or posterior instrumentation is performed to correct the curvature and stabilize the spine. Bone grafting is added to achieve spinal fusion.

B. Kyphosis

1. The gentle posterior curvature of the normal thoracic spine when viewed from the side (sagittal plane) is kyphosis. The normal range is 20–40 degrees. Excessive posterior curvature beyond normal is also referred to as kyphosis.

2. **Adolescent round back** (postural kyphosis) is a flexible deformity evenly distributed throughout the thoracic spine and without any structural changes. It may be due to lax ligaments or poor muscle tone, and is associated with other postural defects such as flat feet. Treatment is the same as for Scheuermann's kyphosis.
3. **Structural kyphosis** refers to stiff curves with vertebral wedging. It is seen in Scheuermann disease and osteoporosis (round back of old age). Congenital kyphosis has underlying structural change and usually has a local sharp posterior angulation, also termed kyphus, which may also be seen in fracture or infection.
4. **Classification**
   a. Postural kyphosis
   b. Scheuermann's disease
   c. Myelomeningocele
   d. Traumatic kyphosis
   e. Post surgical kyphosis
   f. Post radiation kyphosis
   g. Metabolic disorders
   h. Skeletal dysplasia
   i. Tumors
5. **Scheuermann's disease** (adolescent kyphosis). This is a growth disorder of uncertain etiology involving the vertebral growth plates.
   a. **Clinical findings**
      (1) There are two types based on location. The **classic form** of Scheuermann's disease occurs in the thoracic spine. Criteria for diagnosis include wedging of at least 5 degrees of three adjacent vertebrae. End plates are irregular. This type is twice as common in girls as boys. The painless deformity is usually first noticed by parents. Pain may occur but is a rare symptom. Onset is usually around 10 years of age. A distinct hump at the apex of the kyphosis is frequently noted. The deformity is accentuated on forward flexion and its rigidity prevents correction on extension.
      (2) The **lumbar form** of Scheuermann's disease occurs more commonly in teenaged males. They present with chronic mechanical lumbar pain, which may improve with maturation.
      (3) Kyphosis is a change in the alignment of a segment of the spine in the sagittal (side view) plane that increases the normal posterior convex angulation. The COBB method of measuring kyphosis is used to measure angulation greater than 45–50 degrees in the thoracic spine.
6. **Treatment.** A progressive kyphosis of the thoracic spine in a skeletally immature patient is treated in a **Milwaukee brace** until maturity. Surgery is reserved for select cases with curves greater than 75 degrees that have pain or are unresponsive to bracing. Lumbar Scheuermann's disease is not responsive to bracing. It is treated by exercises and anti-inflammatories if painful.

13. FRACTURES OF THE CLAVICLE

  I. **Anatomy.** The clavicle is located superficially, providing the only bony articulation of the upper limb to the thorax. Medially, the clavicle is joined to the thorax via the sternoclavicular joint and the costoclavicular ligaments. Laterally, the clavicle attaches to the scapula by the acromioclavicular joint and the coracoclavicular ligaments.
 II. **Mechanism of injury.** Clavicular injuries may be caused by indirect force through a fall on the lateral shoulder or on an outstretched hand. A direct blow to the subcutaneous clavicle is also a common mechanism for a clavicle fracture (8). The incidence of the fracture is highest in the second decade, related to motor vehicle accidents and sports activity (7). The most common location of a clavicle fracture is its middle third (3).
III. **Diagnosis.** The diagnosis is confirmed by a history of injury with pain localizing to the clavicle. Often, an obvious deformity is evident.
 IV. **Roentgenographic findings.** A standard anteroposterior view of the clavicle usually confirms the diagnosis of a fracture. The amount of comminution and overriding of the fracture fragments should be noted.
  V. **Treatment.**
   A. Most fractures **medial** to the coracoclavicular ligaments are treated by nonoperative methods. Nondisplaced or minimally displaced fractures are easily treated with a sling-and-swathe bandage for comfort. Displaced fractures, or those with significant cosmetic disruption, may be treated with a commercially available figure-of-8 strap to maintain the shoulder in a retracted position in order to improve the alignment of the fracture. The strap should not be worn too tightly, because it will interfere with circulatory or nerve function in either arm. A pad (or longitudinally folded sheet) between the scapulae while sleeping also helps maintain reduction and comfort. If a commercial strap is not available, then a splint may be made of tubular stockinet (see Chapter 6, **II.B,** Fig. 6-2); this is most useful in children younger than 10 years of age. This splint is not effective in adults because the force necessary to keep the shoulder retracted stretches the stockinet. The commercial strap does not stretch because it is made of webbed material. In either case, a sling should be used for 1–2 weeks. A **well-applied** strap involves the following:
     1. **Pulling back both shoulders** against pressure in the center of the interscapular region during reduction of the fracture
     2. **Powdering** the axillae for comfort and hygiene
     3. **Using good padding**
     4. **Checking for interference with circulatory or nerve function** in either arm after reduction of the fracture and application of the splint. Because maintenance of fracture reduction is difficult, many surgeons recommend using a sling for comfort and foregoing the figure-of-8 splint.
   B. Fractures **lateral** to the coracoclavicular ligament that are not displaced may be treated with a sling. Fractures that involve the acromioclavicular joint often lead to symptomatic posttraumatic arthritis of the acromioclavicular joint. Displaced fractures have a tendency to go on to develop a non-union. The options of nonoperative treatment with a sling-and-swathe versus an open reduction and internal fixation should be discussed with the patient. If the fracture is lateral to the coracoclavicular ligament but is displaced more than half the diameter of the clavicle, then it should be reduced and internally fixed, as described for a complete acromioclavicular dislocation in Chap. 14 **II.** This is recommended because of the high incidence of non-union.
 VI. **Follow-up.** Close follow-up of individuals in a figure-of-8 strap is required to ensure that it is being worn tightly enough to achieve a reduction, but not so tightly as to cause neurovascular compromise or excessive pain. The figure-of-8 strap must be tightened by a family member **frequently**. The parents of young patients may be instructed in how to tighten the strap if it becomes loosened at home. Children (younger than 10 years old) wear the strap or splint for 3–4 weeks until they

are pain-free. Adults typically need to wear a sling for 4–6 weeks. Patients are allowed to return to all activities as their symptoms abate. Often, it is not possible to produce or maintain a reduction that is optimum for cosmetic reasons, and, rarely, open reduction and internal fixation are necessary. Patients should be advised that a "bump" in the region of the fracture is a likely outcome, but that this rarely affects function. Some authors have recommended open reduction with internal fixation when fracture overlap is more than 2 cm because there is a high incidence of non-union and poor function (4). Other authors have not found any relationship between fracture shortening and shoulder function (6).

VII. **The indications for surgery** include an open fracture, fractures associated with vascular injury requiring repair, fractures associated with a scapulothoracic dissociation (floating shoulder), or those associated with displaced glenoid neck fractures. The author's preferred method of treating established non-unions and those acute fractures that require repair is to use a contoured plate and screws, adding iliac crest graft for atrophic non-union (5). Other authors prefer intramedullary pin fixation (1).

VIII. **Complications.** Complications with this injury are rare when it is managed nonoperatively. Fractures with greater than 2.5 cm of override, or those associated with a gap of greater than 1 cm between fragments, have a higher incidence of going on to a delayed union or non-union. In adults, roentgenographic evidence of a union may not be present for several months, and asymptomatic fibrous nonunions are not uncommon. Complications may occur following internal fixation; primarily they are infection and non-union (2).

HCMC Recommendations and Protocols
Clavicle Fractures
    Diagnosis: Anteroposterior shoulder radiograph, 15-degree cephalad oblique view, clinical examination
    Treatment: Sling and/or figure-of-8 bandage for comfort: 2–4 weeks, institute range-of-motion exercises at 2 weeks
    Indications for Surgery: Open fractures, vascular injuries, non-unions, or initial displacement of greater than 2 cm
    Recommended Technique: 3.5-mm reconstruction plate or low contact dynamic compression plate (LCDCP), applied to anteroinferior surface of the clavicle

---

References
1. Boehme D, Curtis RJ, DeHaan JT, et al. Non-union of fractures of the mid shaft of the clavicle; treatment with a modified Hagie intramedullary pin and autogenous bone grafting. *J Bone Surg (Am)* 1991;73:1219–1226.
2. Bostman O, Manninen M, Pihlajamaki H. Complications of plate fixation in fresh displaced midclavicular fractures. *J Trauma* 1997;43:778–783.
3. Craig EV. Fractures of the clavicle. In: Rockwood CA Jr, Matsen FA III, eds. The shoulder. Philadelphia: WB Saunders, 1990:367–412.
4. Hill JM, McGuire MH, Crosby LA. Closed treatment of displaced middle-third fractures of the clavicle gives poor results. *J Bone Joint Surg (Br)* 1997;79:537–539.
5. Jupiter JB, Leffert RD. Nonunion of the clavicle: associated complication and surgical management. *J Bone Joint Surg (Am)* 1987;69:753.
6. Oroko PK, Buchan M, Winler A, et al. Does shortening matter after clavicular fractures? *Bull Hosp Joint Dis* 1999;58:6–8.
7. Robinson CM. Fractures of the clavicle in the adult; epidemiology and classification. *J Bone Joint Surg (Br)* 1988;70:461.
8. Stanley D, Trowbridge EA, Norris SH. The mechanism of clavicular fracture. *J Bone Joint Surg* 1988;70B:461.

Selected Historical Readings
Allman FL. Fractures and ligamentous injuries of the clavicle and its articulation. *J Bone Joint Surg* 1967;49A:774–784.

14. STERNOCLAVICULAR AND ACROMIOCLAVICULAR JOINT INJURIES

I. **Sternoclavicular joint injuries** (see Chap. 13, I)
  A. **Injury classification** (9)
    1. **A first-degree sternoclavicular sprain** results from an incomplete rupture of the sternoclavicular and costoclavicular ligaments.
    2. **A second-degree sternoclavicular sprain** (subluxation) consists of a complete tear of the sternoclavicular ligaments and a partial tear of the costoclavicular ligaments.
    3. **A third-degree sprain** (dislocation) results from a complete disruption of the sternoclavicular and costoclavicular ligaments.
    4. The medial clavicle can **dislocate anteriorly** to lie over the first rib and is indicated by an enlarged sternoclavicular joint. Less commonly, the medial clavicle may **dislocate posteriorly** (retrosternal dislocation) and result in a clinically less prominent sternoclavicular joint as compared with the normal side.
  B. **Roentgenographic findings.** Oblique views of the sternoclavicular joint may help demonstrate the direction and degree of dislocation as well as whether a fracture of the medial clavicle is present. The author prefers to obtain a **computed tomography (CT) scan** of the normal and injured sternoclavicular joints to more clearly define the pathology present.
  C. **Treatment**
    1. **Anterior dislocations** are generally treated nonoperatively. A prominence of the sternoclavicular joint often remains but is rarely symptomatic.
    2. **Posterior dislocations** can be an emergency if the medial end of the clavicle compromises the vital structures of the mediastinum (great vessels, trachea, esophagus, and thoracic duct).
      a. **Nonoperative treatment** consists of a gentle attempt at reduction by placing a sandbag between the scapulae and applying a posteriorly directed force over the lateral clavicle and shoulder. If this is not successful, the patient is taken to the operative suite. Under a general anesthetic with good muscular relaxation, a more forceful reduction is attempted. If necessary, a towel clip may be used to grasp the medial end of the clavicle to help elevate it into position. Meticulous control of the patient's airway as well as the capacity to handle significant mediastinal hemorrhage should be available. After reduction, the patient is maintained in a snug-fitting figure-of-8 splint.
      b. **Operative treatment** is indicated in symptomatic individuals with a posterior, irreducible dislocation. In patients with chronic instability and pain, a resection of the medial 1 cm of the clavicle with or without an associated ligament augmentation is indicated. Metal pins or wires should not be used because of the risk of migration into the mediastinum.
    3. **Medial physeal injuries.** The medial ephysis does not fuse with the shaft of the clavicle until around 24 years of age. Many sternoclavicular dislocations in this young age group are actually fractures of the physis. Most heal and remodel with time. If posterior displacement is present, a reduction is indicated.
II. **Acromioclavicular joint injuries**
  A. **Anatomy.** The acromioclavicular (AC) joint is a true synovial joint that contains a small, round meniscus composed of a fibrocartilage similar to the menisci of the knee. The AC joint capsule is strongest superiorly and

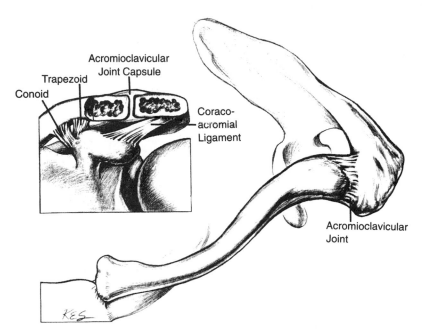

FIG. 14-1. Acromioclavicular joint anatomy. The relatively thick joint capsule and conoid and trapezoid portions of the coracoclavicular ligament stabilize this articulation. (From Hansen ST, Swiontkowski MF. *Orthopaedic trauma protocols.* New York: Raven Press, 1993:80.)

posteriorly (2). The scapula is also suspended from the clavicle by the strong coracoclavicular ligaments, which are located medial to the AC joint (Fig. 14-1).

B. Mechanism and grading of injury

    1. The most common **mechanism of injury** is a force applied directly over the superior or lateral aspect of the acromion and shoulder. Depending on the amount of force and the speed at which it is applied, a capsular disruption of the AC joint occurs and may be associated with disruption of the coracoclavicular ligaments in more severe cases (7).

    2. The **grading of injuries** (9) is based on the classification of Tossy (10). A *first-degree AC sprain* is an incomplete tear of the AC capsule without subluxation of the joint. A *second-degree AC sprain* is a more severe injury to the AC capsule that allows subluxation of the AC joint, but the CC joints are at least partially intact. A *third-degree AC sprain* is a complete AC joint dislocation with the joint capsule disrupted and the CC ligaments torn. The classification system has been expanded (5,12), adding a grade IV (posterior instability), a grade V (marked superior displacement), and a grade VI (inferior dislocation under coracoid process), each of which represents a more severe soft-tissue injury to the suspensory mechanism of the clavicle to the scapula (Fig. 14-2).

C. First- and second-degree injuries

    1. Diagnosis. The patient has point tenderness over the AC joint with a mild amount of swelling present in this region. If the AC joint is partially subluxed by palpation, then a second-degree sprain is present.

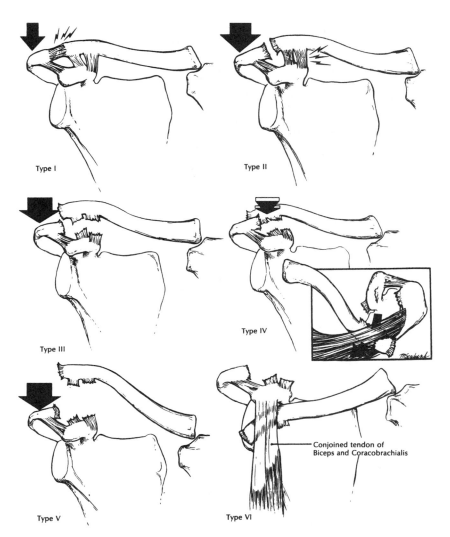

FIG. 14-2. Schematic drawings of the classification of ligamentous injuries that can occur to the acromioclavicular ligament. Type I: A mild force applied to the point of the shoulder does not disrupt either the acromioclavicular or the coracoclavicular ligaments. Type II: A moderate to heavy force applied to the point of the shoulder will disrupt the acromioclavicular ligaments, but the coracoclavicular ligaments remain intact. Type III: When a severe force is applied to the point of the shoulder, both the acromioclavicular and coracoclavicular ligaments are disrupted. Type IV: In this major injury, not only are the acromioclavicular and coracoclavicular ligaments disrupted but also the distal end of the clavicle is displaced posteriorly into or through the trapezius muscle. Type V: A violent force has been applied to the point of the shoulder, not only rupturing the acromioclavicular and coracoclavicular ligaments but also disrupting the deltoid and trapezius muscle attachments and creating a major separation between the clavicle and the acromion. Type VI: Another major injury is an interior dislocation of the distal end of the clavicle to the subarachnoid position. The acromioclavicular and coracoclavicular ligaments are disrupted. (From Rockwood CA, Williams GR, Young DC. Injuries to the acromioclavicular joint. In: Rockwood CR, Green DP, Bucholz RW, et al, eds. *Fractures in adults,* 4th ed. Philadelphia: Lippincott-Raven, 1996:1354.)

2. **Roentgenographic findings.** Visualization of the AC joint is best obtained on a single 7- × 14-inch roentgenograph positioned to include both AC joints. A concurrent view obtained with a 10-lb weight tied to each wrist may increase the deformity seen but is **rarely** necessary to confirm the diagnosis. A spot view with a 10-degree cephalic tilt (Zanca view) of the affected joint is necessary to rule out any interarticular fractures.

3. **Treatment.** Nonoperative therapy for first- and second-degree AC sprains is advocated. The degree of disability is small, and the final deformity is usually minor. The author recommends the use of a sling until symptoms have subsided. An active exercise program is initiated early to maintain the range of motion and strength in the shoulder girdle. Patients are allowed back to all activities as their symptoms abate. Often, discomfort in the shoulder when sleeping at night may exist for several months.

4. **Complications.** Rarely, symptomatic posttraumatic osteolysis or arthritis of the AC joint develops. In these individuals, an arthroscopic or open resection of the distal clavicle is indicated.

D. **Third-degree injuries**
1. **Diagnosis.** The patient typically holds the arm tightly against the side in a supported adducted position. There is an obvious clinical deformity, with the lateral clavicle tenting the skin over the superior shoulder. The deformity can be reduced by supporting the arm in a cephalad direction.

2. **Roentgenograms.** The radiographic workup is similar to that for first- and second-degree injuries. The distal clavicle is seen to be completely displaced above the level of the acromion, and the distance between the coracoid process and clavicle is widened.

3. **Treatment.** Clinical studies (1,3,8,11) comparing operative versus nonoperative treatment for grade III sprains have generally indicated that operative management is **not superior** to nonoperative treatment. Controversy still exists on how to best treat the overhead laborer.

   a. **Nonoperative treatment** is the author's preferred method. A sling for general support of the upper extremity is indicated for pain control. A physical therapy program is initiated as pain allows and early return of use of the extremity is encouraged. A specialized sling to aid in reduction of the deformity (Kenny Howard sling) has been used, but complications with skin breakdown and neurovascular compression limit its usefulness.

   b. **Operative treatment.** Multiple surgical procedures (4,6) have been described to repair an AC joint separation. They fit broadly into two categories: fixation of the distal clavicle directly to the acromion and repair or augmentation of the CC ligament to maintain the AC joint reduced. The indications for an acute repair are mainly cosmetic to correct the prominent distal clavicle. Rarely, patients remain chronically symptomatic with weakness in the shoulder and vague brachial plexus tension type symptoms. These cases can be successfully managed by a CC ligament reconstruction combined with a limited distal clavicle resection.

E. **Type IV, V, and VI injuries**
1. **Diagnosis.** These injuries are rare and are easily detected by clinical evaluation.

2. **Treatment.** These three types of injury represent severe soft-tissue injuries to the shoulder girdle. Operative repair is generally indicated. Type VI (subcoracoid) injuries are often associated with neurovascular symptoms.

HCMC Treatment Recommendations
AC Injuries

- *Diagnosis*: Anteroposterior shoulder radiograph, 15-degree cephalad oblique radiograph, clinical examination
- *Treatment*: Grade I-III, sling for comfort for 7–10 days, then range-of-motion exercises
- *Indications for surgery*: Grade IV, V, or VI injuries.
- *Recommended technique*: Subcoracoid suture loop with CC ligament and deltotrapezial fascial repair

---

References
 1. Bannister GC, Wallace WA, Stablforth PG, et al. The management of acute acromioclavicular dislocation: a randomized prospective controlled trial. *J Bone Joint Surg* 1989;71B:848–850.
 2. Fukuda K, Craig EV, An KN, et al. Biomechanical study of the ligamentous system of the acromioclavicular joint. *J Bone Joint Surg* 1986;68A:434–439.
 3. Galpin RD, Hawkins RJ, Grainger RW. A comparative analysis of operative versus non-operative treatment of grade III acromioclavicular separations. *Clin Orthop* 1985;193:150–155.
 4. Kawabe N, Watanabe R, Sato M. Treatment of complete acromioclavicular separation of coracoacromial ligament transfer. *Clin Orthop* 1984;185:222.
 5. Post M: Current concepts in the diagnosis and management of acromioclavicular dislocation. *Clin Orthop* 1985;200:234.
 6. Roper BA, Levack B. The surgical treatment of acromioclavicular dislocations. *J Bone Joint Surg* 1982;64B:597.
 7. Rosenorn N, Pedersen EB. The significance of the coracoclavicular ligaments in experimental dislocation of the acromioclavicular joint. *Acta Orthop Scand* 1974; 45:346.
 8. Smith MJ, Stewart MJ. Acute acromioclavicular separations: a 20-year study. *Am J Sports Med* 1979;7:62.
 9. Subcommittee on Classification of Sports Injuries. *Standard nomenclature of athletic injuries*. Chicago: American Medical Association, 1976.
10. Tossy JD, Mead NC, Sigmond HM. Acromioclavicular separations: useful and practical classification for treatment. *Clin Orthop* 1963;28:111–119.
11. Urist MR. Complete dislocation of the acromioclavicular joint: the nature of the traumatic lesion and effective methods of treatment with an analysis of 41 cases. *J Bone Joint Surg* 1946;28:813–837.
12. Williams GR, Nguyen VD, Rockwood CA. Classification and radiographic analysis of acromioclavicular dislocations. *Appl Radiol* 1989;18:29–34.

Selected Historical Readings
Allman FL. Fractures and ligamentous injuries of the clavicle and its articulations. *J Bone Joint Surg* 1967;49:774.

15. ACUTE SHOULDER INJURIES

I. General principles

A. **Anatomy.** The glenohumeral joint is one of the most unconstrained joints in the human body. This allows for our ability to perform work both in an outstretched (reaching) position and to do overhead activity. This degree of flexibility comes from a very small glenoid surface articulating with a large humeral head. The depth of the glenoid cavity is augmented by the labrum, which also serves as the anchor point for the capsular ligaments to the glenoid. The ligaments serve as static restraints at the extremes of range of motion. The rotator cuff muscles (subscapularis, long head of the biceps, supraspinatus, infraspinatus, teres minor) are very important dynamic stabilizers of the joint (3). The scapulothoracic articulation provides approximately one third of the total active motion of the shoulder girdle. The periscapular muscles are extremely important in positioning the glenoid correctly as well as providing a stable platform for the glenohumeral joint to function from. The neurovascular bundle lies directly anterior and inferior to the glenohumeral joint, which accounts for the frequency of neurovascular injuries, especially with anterior dislocations, that are associated with shoulder trauma.

B. **Differential diagnosis**
1. Cervical disc disease, particularly C5 root irritation
2. Diaphragmatic irritation
3. Pleural irritation
4. Superior sulcus tumors (Pancoast's)
5. Thoracic outlet
6. Brachial neuritis
7. Cholecystitis

C. The shoulder is prone to stiffness. Therefore, early treatment is directed at maintaining motion. An appropriate exercise program is prescribed initially and should be closely monitored by the treating physician.

II. Shoulder dislocations

A. **Classification.** The glenohumeral joint is involved in almost 50% of all major joint dislocations. Dislocations are commonly classified as anterior, inferior, posterior, or multidirectional (more than one direction). Anterior dislocations are the most common. Dislocations that occur in patients younger than 20 years typically involve an avulsion of the labrum and ligaments from the glenoid. Dislocations that occur in patients older than 30 years of age tend to involve interligamentous tears. Dislocations in patients older than 50 years are frequently associated with rotator cuff tears and greater tuberosity fractures. These older patients have a low rate of recurrence of dislocations and have a high rate of posttraumatic shoulder stiffness (10).

B. **Anterior dislocations**
1. **Mechanism of injury.** The injury usually results from a traumatic event in which the position of the arm is in an externally rotated and forward flexed or abducted position.
   a. In patients younger than 20 years of age, the anterior capsule and labrum are avulsed from the glenoid, often with a small fragment of bone (Bankart lesion). The humeral head dislocates anterior to the glenoid fossa and under the coracoid process. A compression fracture occurs on the posterolateral humeral head (Hill-Sachs lesion) from impaction of the head on the anterior edge of the glenoid (2).
   b. In patients older than 40 years of age, intrasubstance failure of the anterior capsule occurs. This injury is frequently associated with acute tears of the rotator cuff.

    c. Recent basic science studies have shown that sectioning of the anterior capsule alone does not cause gross anterior instability. Damage to the posterior or superior capsule must also occur to allow for a complete dislocation.

2. **Examination.** Individuals with an acute dislocation hold their arm in an adducted position. There is a loss of symmetry of their shoulders and the humeral head can be palpated anterior and inferior to the coracoid process. Any attempt at range of motion of the shoulder is extremely painful. A thorough neurovascular check of the upper extremity is necessary before any attempt is made to reduce the dislocation. Attention to checking the sensory function of the axillary nerve over the lateral aspect of the shoulder is important.

3. **Roentgenograms.** In all patients with a suspected initial dislocation of the shoulder, a standard trauma series should be obtained (7). This series includes an anterior posterior and a transscapular lateral ("Y") view. If the presence and direction of the dislocation is not clearly evident, an axillary view is obtained. This view is difficult to obtain and painful for the patient; it may require physician assistance to position the patient's shoulder. Any associated tuberosity fractures or epiphyseal injuries should be clearly visualized.

4. **Treatment of the first dislocation**

    a. Reduction without general anesthesia. Prompt reduction of the dislocation provides a great deal of pain relief. To achieve a gentle and pain-free reduction, muscle relaxation and pain relief are required. Several methods of reduction have been described, but the authors prefers one of the following methods:

        (1) Prone reduction under lidocaine block (11). The patient is allowed to remain sitting on the examination table and the posterior aspect of the shoulder is sterilely prepped. Ten to 20 mL of 1% lidocaine is injected into the glenohumeral joint from posteriorly. The patient is then placed prone on the examination table with the involved arm and shoulder hanging in a dependent position over the edge of the table. A 10-lb weight is suspended from the patient's wrist. After 10–15 minutes, good analgesia and relaxation are present and the shoulder can be reduced by elevation and forward rotation of the medial border of the scapula.

        (2) Reduction by traction. If the first method fails, the patient is repositioned supine and additional IV sedation is administered. A sheet is placed around the patient centered in the axillary region. An assistant holds the two ends of the sheet above the patient and provides countertraction while the physician grasps the forearm of the involved shoulder and gently pulls in a line of 30 degrees of abduction and 20–30 degrees of forward flexion. Sustained traction for 5 minutes may be necessary. Vigorous and forceful attempts at reduction may result in a fracture, especially in older patients.

    b. Reduction under anesthesia. If the aforementioned methods fail or if a significant fracture is present, a reduction under general anesthetic with complete muscle relaxation is indicated. The shoulder typically reduces easily with little risk of further damage to the glenohumeral joint or its surrounding structures.

5. **Postreduction treatment.** The length of immobilization has no effect on the incidence of redislocations (9). The shoulder should be immobilized for a brief period to allow for pain control after a dislocation or subluxation episode. A range of motion and rotator cuff strengthening program is initiated early, but the extremes of range of motion for forward flexion or external rotation are avoided. Patients are allowed to return to sports and other activities when the shoulder has good

strength and minimal apprehension in an abducted, externally rotated position (1).

6. **Recurrent dislocations of subluxations.** If necessary, the shoulder is reduced as in section four (above), and a physical therapy program is prescribed as in section five (above). Recurrent instability episodes tend to be painful and disabling. Many different types of surgical repairs have been described (9,12,16). The author prefers either an open or arthroscopic Bankart repair or capsular shift reconstruction (12,14). The open type of repair has been associated with success rates of 97% with few significant complications. Arthroscopically assisted repairs are technically possible, but have not yet achieved success rates comparable to open capsular repairs.

7. **Complications**

   a. **Damage to the nerves** originating with the brachial plexus occurs in 5%–14% of shoulder dislocations. The axillary nerve and musculocutaneous nerve are most commonly injured. Most injuries are a neuropraxia, and a full recovery is typical. The same is true with postoperative neurologic injuries.

   b. **Rotator cuff tears** are common in patients older than 40 years with an anterior dislocation. If good range of motion and strength have not returned in 3–4 weeks after the injury, a workup of the rotator cuff with magnetic resonance imaging (MRI) is indicated.

C. **Posterior dislocations**

1. **Mechanism of injury.** Posterior instability results from a fall on an adducted and forward flexed arm, which drives the head of the humerus posterior to the glenoid fossa. A compression fracture of the anterior lateral aspect of the humeral head develops (reverse Hill-Sachs lesion). In younger individuals, an avulsion of the posterior labrum with a small fragment of the posterior glenoid rim (reverse Bankart lesion) occurs. Seizures or electrocution are other mechanisms that often produce posterior instability.

2. **Examination.** An obvious clinical deformity is typically not present and the patient may be complaining of only minimal symptoms. Many posterior dislocations are not diagnosed and reduced in the emergency department. External rotation of the shoulder is limited and painful, and is the hallmark of a posterior shoulder dislocation.

3. **Roentgenograms.** Anteroposterior views often are normal and misleading, except that the arm is positioned in a markedly internally rotated position, which produces a "light bulb sign" with the proximal humerus. A transscapular "Y" view and an axillary view show the posterior position of the humeral head.

4. **Treatments.** Muscle relaxation via IV sedation is recommended. Reductions can usually be obtained by gentle traction on the arm with an additional anterior and laterally directed force applied to the posterior aspect of the humeral head. After reduction, treatment is similar to the treatment for anterior dislocations **(B.5),** except internal rotation and adduction extremes are avoided. If the shoulder redislocates after being reduced, the arm should be braced in an externally rotated and abducted position for 4 weeks to maintain stability.

5. **Recurrent dislocations** that occur as a result of traumatic events and have evidence of ligament damage may be treated with a reverse capsular shift. Many patients with posterior instability do not have a history of a significant traumatic event that initiated the instability and may be able to **voluntarily dislocate** or sublux their shoulder. These patients have poor operative results and should undergo treatment with physical therapy and activity or lifestyle restrictions (5).

D. **Multidirectional instability (MDI)**

1. **Mechanism of injury.** MDI is diagnosed when there is clinical evidence that the shoulder is unstable in two or more directions. There

is often no history of significant trauma and the patient may be able to voluntarily dislocate the shoulder.

2. **Examination.** The typical patient is a "double jointed" adolescent female. A sulcus sign is present and the patient is apprehensive with the arm in positions that stress both the anterior and posterior capsule.
3. **Roentgenograms.** Often, radiographs are normal. The presence of a Hill-Sachs or a reverse Hill-Sachs lesion is detected on a Stryker notch view.
4. **Treatment.** Nonoperative treatment is strongly advised because operative management has a high failure rate (15). A new procedure using thermal energy to arthroscopically "shrink" the redundant anterior capsule may be successful, but clinical results are limited (6).

E. **Inferior dislocations.** Inferior dislocations are rare. The patient's arm is locked in an overhead position. Reduction is obtained by IV sedation and relaxation. The arm is then reduced with lateral distraction while the arm is brought out of an abducted position.

III. **Acute tears of the rotator cuff**
A. **Mechanism of injury.** Acute tears of the rotator cuff are rare and occur mainly in individuals younger than 40 years old who have a history of significant trauma. Attritional tears of the rotator cuff are more common and occur in older individuals (see Chap. 16).
B. **Examination.** (see Chap. 16).
C. **Roentgenograms.** Damage to the glenohumeral joint, including the greater tuberosity, is best assessed on an anteroposterior view, obtained with the arm in 30 degrees of external rotation. An outlet view and an axillary view should also be obtained. Young individuals who are suspected of having a rotator cuff tear on history or examination should undergo an MRI scan to assess the status of their rotator cuff.
D. **Treatment.** In patients with a true acute rotator cuff tear, early (within 3 months) operative repair is indicated. Early repair is also indicated in those cases associated with a displaced avulsion fracture of the greater tuberosity (4).

IV. **Ruptures of the long head of the biceps brachii**
A. **Mechanism of injury.** Injuries of the long head of the biceps (LHB) tendon may occur with forceful elbow flexion or hand supination. Eighty percent of the cases are associated with ongoing rotator cuff problems and shoulder impingement syndrome. Steroid use for body conditioning is becoming another common etiology.
B. **Examination.** A visible asymmetry of the injured versus noninjured upper arm is evident when the patient is asked to "make a biceps" muscle. This deformity is called a "Popeye" sign.
C. **Treatment.** Ruptures of the LHB tendon are treated nonoperatively. The indications for repair are mainly cosmetic in nature, because little functional disability results. In patients with evidence of impingement syndrome, an appropriate workup of the rotator cuff is indicated.

V. **Rupture of the pectoralis major.** The pectoralis major muscle or tendon typically ruptures with a bench press lift or similar functional maneuver. The patient has pain and an ecchymosis in the anterior shoulder. On examination there is a loss or defect in the anterior axillary line. Treatment is usually symptomatic, except in the heavy laborer or athlete in whom early operative repair is indicated. Ruptures medially at the muscle tendon junction are difficult to repair. A preoperative MRI scan is indicated in those individuals for whom operative repair is being considered to determine at what level the defect occurred.

VI. **Scapular fractures.** These injuries are frequently treated **nonoperatively**, with early range of motion of the shoulder girdle. Displaced fractures involving greater than 25% percent of the articular surface of the glenoid or glenoid neck fractures with medially displacement are generally treated operatively (8).

HCMC Treatment Recommendations
Shoulder Dislocation

* *Diagnosis*: Anteroposterior, transscapular lateral, axillary lateral radiographs, clinical examination
* *Treatment*: Reduction in emergency department under analgesia or intra-articular lidocaine, sling for comfort followed by assisted range-of-motion exercises beginning at 2–3 weeks after injury
* *Indications for surgery*: Recurrent dislocation
* *Recommended technique*: Bankart repair, open or arthroscopic

---

References

1. Arciero RA, Wheeler JH, Ryan JB, et al. Arthroscopic Bankart repair vs non-operative treatment for acute, initial, anterior shoulder dislocations. *Am J Sports Med* 1994;22:589–594.
2. Baker CL, Uribe JW, Whitman C. Arthroscopic evaluation of acute initial anterior shoulder dislocations. *Am J Sports Med* 1990;28:25–28.
3. Bassett RW, Browne AO, Morrey BF, et al. Glenohumeral muscle force and moment mechanics in a position of shoulder instability. *J Biomech* 1990;23:405–415.
4. Bassett RW, Cofield RH. Acute tears of the rotator cuff: the timing of surgical repair. *Clin Orthop* 1983;175:18.
5. Bigliani LU, Pollock RG, McIlveen SJ, et al. Shift of the posteroinferior aspect of the capsule for recurrent posterior glenohumeral instability. *J Bone Joint Surg* 1995;77:1011–1020.
6. Burkhead WZ, Rockwood CA. Treatment of instability of the shoulder with an exercise program. *J Bone Joint Surg Am* 1992;74:890–896.
7. Engebretsen L, Craig EV. Radiologic features of shoulder instability. *Clin Orthop* 1993;291:29–44.
8. Hardegger FH, Simpson L. The operative treatment of scapular fractures. *J Bone Joint Surg* 1984;66B:315.
9. Hovelius L. Anterior dislocation of the shoulder in teenagers and young adults: five-year prognosis. *J Bone Joint Surg* 1987;69A:393.
10. Johnson JR, Bayley JIL. Early complications of acute anterior dislocation of the shoulder in the middle-aged and elderly patient. *Injury* 1982;13:431–434.
11. Lippitt SB, Kennedy JP, Thompson TR. Intraarticular lidocaine verses intravenous analgesia in the reduction of dislocated shoulders. *Orthop Trans* 1992; 16:230.
12. Morgan CD, Bodenstab AB. Arthroscopic Bankart suture repair: technique and early results. *Arthroscopy* 1987;3:111.
13. Morrey BF, James JM. Recurrent anterior dislocation of the shoulder: long-term follow up of the Putti-Platt and Bankart procedures. *J Bone Joint Surg* 1976;58A:252–256.
14. Rowe CR, Pierce DS, Clark JG. Voluntary dislocation of the shoulder. *J Bone Joint Surg* 1973;55A:445.
15. Rowe CR. Acute and recurrent dislocations of the shoulder. *J Bone Joint Surg* 1962;44A:998.
16. Torg JS, et al. A modified Bristow-Helfet-May procedure for recurrent dislocation and subluxation of the shoulder: report of two hundred and twelve cases. *J Bone Joint Surg* 1987;69A:904.

Selected Historical Readings

Bankart ASB. Recurrent or habitual dislocation of the shoulder joint. *BMJ* 1923;2:1132.
Mosley HF. The basic lesions of recurrent anterior dislocation of the shoulder. *Surg Clin North Am* 1963;43:631.

16. NONACUTE SHOULDER DISORDERS

I. Rotator cuff disorders

A. Anatomy. The rotator cuff is composed of the teres minor, infraspinatus, supraspinatus, long head of the biceps, and subscapularis muscle. Each has its own specific muscle body but they coalesce together as they come together through the subacromial space. The borders of the subacromial space are as follows: superiorly, the undersurface of the acromion and the acromioclavicular (AC) joint; anteriorly, the coracoacromial ligament and coracoid; inferiorly, the humeral head. The subacromial bursa also exists in the subacromial space above the rotator cuff.

B. Mechanism of injury. The rotator cuff goes through the confined opening of the subacromial (SA) space. Any anatomic influence that narrows this space has the potential to compromise the rotator cuff tendon and irritate the subacromial bursa. Thickening of the bursa, undersurface spurring of the AC joint, instability of the glenohumeral joint, or changes in the shape of the acromion (Fig. 16-1) are the most common reasons for rotator cuff compromise. This process of rotator cuff attrition is described as **impingement syndrome.** The process of cuff disease begins with bursitis and reversible tendinitis and gradually progresses to full-thickness cuff pathology over time.

C. History. The typical patient with impingement syndrome is older than age 40 years and complains of anterolateral shoulder pain, which is worse with overhead activities and worse at night.

D. Examination. Shoulder motion is usually nearly symmetric. Weakness and pain to supraspinatus strength testing is usually present. Tenderness is present over the anterior rotator cuff and SA bursa. Significant weakness to external strength testing often indicates that a large rotator cuff tear is present.

E. Roentgenograms. Plain roentgenograms should be obtained in patients with a history of acute trauma or those who do not improve with standard nonoperative treatment. Sclerosis of the greater tuberosity, narrowing of the acromiohumeral distance, or spur formation at the AC joint or the anterior acromion are all evidence of ongoing impingement syndrome. An acromion that has an inferiorly directed hook at its anterior edge is classified as a type III acromion (1) (Fig. 16-1). This hooked acromion predisposes some patients to developing rotator cuff pathology by narrowing the subacromial space. Usually the supraspinatus tendon is affected first. In patients in whom operative intervention is indicated, further imaging studies may be obtained. Arthrograms are widely available and easily used to detect the presence of a rotator cuff tear. However, they do not give good information regarding tear location, size, or other associated subacromial pathology. A magnetic resonance imaging (MRI) scan, if available, gives more detailed information regarding pathology in the subacromial space. However, it is more expensive and may be susceptible to technical problems and misinterpretation.

F. Treatment

1. Bursitis/tendinitis

a. Nonoperative treatment is successful in the majority of patients. The cornerstone of treatment is **physical therapy** to rehabilitate the rotator cuff muscles (especially the supraspinatus), to regain scapulothoracic stability, and to correct any contractures (typically loss of internal rotation). If physical therapy alone is not successful, an **injection** of corticosteroid and lidocaine into the subacromial space often brings the patient's symptoms under control. If the diagnosis of impingement syndrome is correct, the lidocaine should give excellent relief of pain for 2–3 hours. If no lidocaine effect is obtained, alternative diagnoses should be considered. The steroid typically

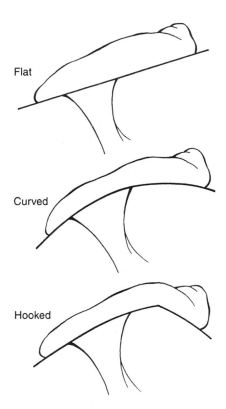

Flat

Curved

Hooked

FIG. 16-1. Bigliani classification of acromial morphology: type I, flat; type II, curved; type III, hooked. (Adapted from Bigliani LU, Morrison DS, April EW. The morphology of the acromion and rotator cuff impingement. *Orthop Trans* 1986;10:288.)

takes 2–4 days to take effect. The indications for a subacromial injection at the initial visit include significant night pain or symptoms severe enough to make progress in physical therapy difficult.

   b. **Operative treatment** is indicated in individuals who fail a minimum 6-month course of nonoperative treatment. The goal of the surgery is to open the subacromial space. This is typically accomplished by excision of the thickened and scarred bursa, recession of the coracoacromial ligament, and an anterior acromioplasty. Any other factors (AC joint hypertrophy or glenohumeral instability) that may predispose the patient to impingement syndrome should also be addressed. This opening of the subacromial space is termed a **decompression.** A decompression may be completed through either open or arthroscopic techniques.

2. **Rotator cuff tears**

   a. **Younger patients** (younger than 55 years) or those with true acute tears typically undergo surgical repair.

   b. **Older patients** often do well with physical therapy and nonoperative treatment. MRI studies of asymptomatic patients older than 60 years of age have shown that 50% have some form of rotator cuff pathology. A late subacromial decompression and rotator cuff repair are indicated only after nonoperative measures have failed. In older, low functional demand patients with large rotator cuff tears, a subacromial decompression alone often yields good pain relief, but only limited improvement in function. In those patients with a massive, unrepairable rotator cuff tear and glenohumeral arthritis, a hemiarthroplasty of the joint is indicated.

3. **Calcific bursitis** involves deposition of a calcium salt into the substance of the rotator cuff tendon. This paste-like material may escape into the subacromial bursa, causing an acute inflammatory bursitis. Severe symptoms of impingement syndrome result. A subacromial injection with corticosteroids with lidocaine and physical therapy are effective in controlling acute symptoms. If repetitive episodes of pain occur, an arthroscopic excision of the calcific deposit is indicated.

4. **Long head of biceps tendinitis** (see Chap. 15, IV) often occurs as part of impingement syndrome and is treated with the same program.

II. **Glenohumeral disorders**
   A. **Arthritis**
      1. **Etiology.** Arthritis of the glenohumeral joint may be idiopathic (osteoarthritis), secondary to inflammatory disease (rheumatoid arthritis), or posttraumatic. Symptomatic arthritis of the glenohumeral joint is not as common as arthritis of the knee and hip.
      2. **History.** Nonspecific lateral shoulder pain is present, which is made worse with increased activities. Stiffness is also a frequent presenting complaint. Polyarticular complaints should arouse the suspicion of an inflammatory disorder.
      3. **Examination** reveals loss of active and passive range of motion, crepitus on joint motion, and mild diffuse muscle atrophy. Strength is usually not significantly affected. Distal neurovascular changes are rare.
      4. **Roentgenographic** studies should include an anteroposterior view of the shoulder in 30 degrees of external rotation and an axillary view. Narrowing of the glenohumeral joint space is present. Inferior spur formation on the humeral head is an indication of osteoarthritis. Periarticular erosions are suspicious for inflammatory disease. A computed tomography scan to exactly determine glenoid version, or an MRI scan to assess rotator cuff status may be indicated preoperatively.
      5. **Treatment**
         a. **Nonoperative treatment** is directed toward controlling inflammation with nonsteroidal antiinflammatory agents, injections of the glenohumeral joint with corticosteroids, and improvement of joint mechanics (especially range of motion) with physical therapy and lifestyle modification.
         b. **Operative treatment.** In early cases of inflammatory arthritis, an arthroscopic synovectomy may yield improvement of symptoms. Once the articular surface is eroded to bone, either a hemiarthroplasty, a total shoulder replacement, or an arthrodesis is indicated. A total shoulder replacement results in the best function of the glenohumeral joint and pain relief (3), but may not be indicated in young patients or patients with heavy occupational demands.
   B. **Adhesive capsulitis** (frozen shoulder)
      1. **Etiology**
         a. **Idiopathic adhesive capsulitis results from capsular fibrosis. The pathologic mechanism for this fibrosis is not well understood (2).**
         b. Adhesive capsulitis may result from capsular fibrosis from a traumatic or surgical event, or may be associated with a systemic disease such as diabetes, thyroid disorders, cervical disc disease, or neoplastic disorders of the thorax.
      2. **History.** The patient complains of a deep, achy pain in the shoulder that is present at rest as well as with activities. Complaints of loss of

motion follow the onset of the pain by several weeks. A careful past medical history and review of systems is necessary to rule out any systemic causes. Distal neurovascular complaints are rare.

3. **Examination.** A global loss of active and passive range of motion is noted. Internal and external rotation are typically affected first. Nonspecific tenderness is usually present early in the disease process. Rotator cuff strength is often normal.

4. **Roentgenographs** are typically unremarkable.

5. **Treatment**

    a. **Nonoperative** management with a home-based stretching program as well as pain medication if necessary is successful in 90% of patients. Symptoms may take up to 18 months to resolve. Occasionally, an injection of the glenohumeral joint with corticosteroid is necessary to control pain (4).

    b. **Operative treatment** is directed at releasing the contracted capsule in a sequential fashion to improve range of motion. This may be accomplished arthroscopically. Any associated pathology (especially in the subacromial space) should also be addressed (8).

III. **Acromioclavicular joint disorders**

  A. **Arthritis**

    1. **Etiology.** Osteoarthritis of the AC joint is extremely common in individuals older than 50 years of age. Most are asymptomatic (7). Inflammatory processes such as rheumatoid arthritis or fractures of the distal clavicle can also cause AC joint symptoms.

    2. **History.** Pain is localized to the superior aspect of the AC joint. Symptoms are worse when sleeping on the affected side. Overlap symptoms with impingement syndrome are common.

    3. **Examination.** Tenderness over the subcutaneous aspect of the AC joint is present. The extremes of motion of forward flexion and cross body are limited and painful. Frequently coexisting rotator cuff findings are present.

    4. **Roentgenograms** are similar to those obtained for patients with impingement syndrome. A Zanca view is helpful.

    5. **Treatment** is directed at controlling local symptoms with physical therapy, a nonsteroidal antiinflammatory medication, and, if necessary, a corticosteroid and lidocaine injection to the AC joint. A typical AC joint will accept one to two cc's of volume. If nonoperative treatment fails, a distal clavicle resection is indicated. This may be completed either via arthroscopic or open techniques (9).

  B. **Osteolysis** of the clavicle may occur following a traumatic injury to the AC joint or in individuals who place repeated unusual stress on the AC joint, such as weight lifters. Radiographic changes consist of osteopenia and erosive changes in the articular surface. Treatment is similar to that described for arthritic conditions.

IV. **Scapulothoracic disorders**

  A. **Scapulothoracic bursitis** (snapping scapula)

    1. **Etiology.** The scapula has a significant excursion across the chest wall with range of motion of the shoulder girdle. This motion requires the presence of a large bursa between the scapula and the thorax. Inflammation of this bursa can be caused by overuse of the shoulder, serratus anterior contracture, or a bony deformity on the undersurface of the scapula (5).

    2. **History.** Patients complain of pain deep and medial to the scapula on the thorax posteriorly. The hallmark symptom of this disorder is catching with motion of the scapula.

    3. **Examination.** Scapulothoracic motion may be limited. The patient can usually reproduce a palpable sensation of crepitus under the scapula.

    4. **Imaging studies** are not typically useful unless there is a history of trauma or there is suspicion of an osteochondroma under the scapula.

5. **Treatment** is directed at increasing motion of the scapula away from the thorax and strengthening the periscapular muscles. Occasionally, a corticosteroid injection into the scapulothoracic bursa is necessary. If nonoperative methods fail, an arthroscopic or open excision of the bursa and the superior medial angle of the scapula is indicated (10).

B. **Winging of the scapula**
   1. **Etiology.** The scapula is held against the thorax by the serratus anterior muscle, which is innervated by the long thoracic nerve. Anything that disrupts either of these two structures results in winging of the scapula.
   2. **History.** Weakness and loss of active motion of the shoulder is noticed first. Secondary symptoms of rotator cuff inflammation may develop. A history of trauma to the chest wall in the location of the long thoracic nerve may be present. However, most patients do not have a readily identifiable cause for their serratus anterior dysfunction (6). Fascioscapulohumeral muscular dystrophy often initially presents with isolated winging of one or both scapulae.
   3. **Examination.** Winging of the scapula occurs when the medial border of the scapula is rotated outward and laterally, causing the scapula to give the appearance of "wings" on the patient's back. (Fig. 16-2)
   4. **Treatment** is directed at strengthening the periscapular muscles and waiting in observation to determine whether the long thoracic nerve will recover. If after 18 months no recovery is present, either a pectoralis major tendon transfer or a scapulothoracic fusion is indicated.

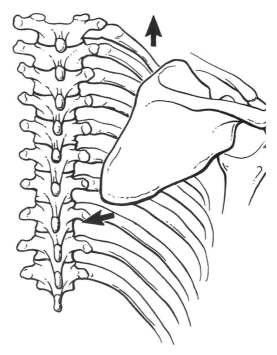

FIG. 16-2. Position of the scapula with primary scapular winging due to serratus anterior palsy. The scapula pulls away from the back and does not protract on arm elevation. (From Kuhn JE, Hawkins, RJ. Evaluation and treatment of scapular disorders. In: Warner JJP, Iannotti JP, Gerber C, eds. *Complex and revision problems in shoulder surgery.* Philadelphia: Lippincott-Raven, 1997: 357–375.)

References

1. Bigliani LU, Morrison DS, April EW. The morphology of the acromion and its relationship to rotator cuff tears. *Orthop Trans* 1983;175:18.
2. Bunker TD, Anthony PP. The pathology of frozen shoulder. A Dupuytren-like disease. *J Bone Joint Surg* 1995;77B:677–683.
3. Cofield RII. Uncemented total shoulder arthroplasty: a review. *Clin Orthop* 1994;66(A):899–906.
4. Dacre JE, Beeney N, Scott DL. Injections and physiotherapy for the painful stiff shoulder. *Ann Rheum Dis* 1989;48:322–325.
5. Edelson JG. Variations in the anatomy of the scapula with reference to the snapping scapula. *Clin Orthop* 1996;322:111–115.
6. Foo CL, Swann M. Isolated paralysis of the serratus anterior: a report of 20 cases. *J Bone Joint Surg* 1983;65B:552.
7. Grimes DW, Garner RW. The degeneration of the acromioclavicular joint. *Orthop Rev* 1980;9:41–44.
8. Harryman DT II, Sidles JA, Matsen FA III. Arthroscopic management of refractory shoulder stiffness. *Arthroscopy* 1997;13:133–147.
9. Peterson CJ. Resection of the lateral end of the clavicle: a 3 to 30-year follow-up. *Acta Orthop Scand* 1983;54:90–907.
10. Strizak AM, Cowen MH. The snapping scapula syndrome. *J Bone Joint Surg* 1982;64A:941–942.

Selected Historical Readings

Neer CS II: Anterior acromioplasty for the chronic impingement syndrome in the shoulder. *J Bone Joint Surg* 1972;54A:41.

17. FRACTURES OF THE HUMERUS

I. **Fractures of the proximal humerus**
   A. **General principles.** Epiphyseal fractures are considered separately. Fractures of the proximal humerus are seen in all age groups but are more common in older patients. In young adults, they are a result of high-energy trauma. In the older patients, treatment is designed to maintain glenohumeral motion. Considerable angulation at the fracture site may be accepted; motion is begun early to avoid shoulder stiffness.
   B. **Classification and treatment.** Neer divides proximal humeral fractures into six groups, as shown in Fig. 17-1, and this concept is useful in considering the management of the injury. There can be difficulty in interpreting radiographs to accurately classify proximal humerus fractures. Elderly patients who are too ill to be considered for surgery are treated as described for the first group.
      1. **All fractures with minimal displacement and displaced anatomic neck fractures.** Approximately 85% of all fractures of the proximal humerus are in this category. Any fracture pattern can be seen, but the displacement of all components must be less than 1 cm, except anatomic neck fractures, to be considered in this group according to Neer's concept. Angulatory or rotatory deformity should not exceed 45 degrees. Stability is usually afforded by some impaction and the preservation of soft-tissue attachments. A sling is the preferred treatment. Wrist and hand exercises are begun immediately. Circumduction exercises should be started as soon as they can be tolerated, generally within 5–7 days. The patient is instructed to bend to 90 degrees at the waist, allowing the arm to either hang or swing in a gentle circle and avoid active contraction of the shoulder muscles (12). Assisted forward elevation and assisted external rotation exercises in the supine position can generally be started approximately 10–14 days after injury. The fracture site is often completely pain-free after 2–3 weeks, and full range of motion is possible in 4–6 weeks. Some form of protection may be needed for 6–8 weeks; then more vigorous physical therapy may be prescribed, including wall climbing, overhead rope-and-pulley, passive range of motion, and rotator cuff strengthening exercises.
      2. **Displaced surgical neck fractures.** The fracture is produced with the arm in abduction. The rotator cuff is usually intact. Undisplaced linear fractures can occur that extend into the humeral head. The humeral shaft is often angulated more than 45 degrees or malrotated. Neurovascular injury can occur in this type of fracture because the shaft may be displaced into the axilla. This is more common in elderly patients with calcified arteries.
         a. **Treatment is by closed reduction** under general or supraclavicular regional anesthesia. Align the distal fragment to the proximal one. This alignment usually requires abduction and flexion. Reduction of the fracture depends on an intact posteromedial periosteal sleeve. The fracture may be stable enough to permit immobilization of the arm at the side in a sling-and-swathe, but may require a spica cast or abduction pillow splint to hold the arm in the reduced position. Fixation can be added percutaneously to maintain the reduction; this is advised in younger patients. As soon as the immobilization is concluded, generally in 2–3 weeks, a program to regain shoulder motion is started as for fractures with minimal displacement and anatomic neck fractures. Unstable reductions may necessitate percutaneous pin or screw fixation. In unreliable patients, the fixation may need to be protected with a shoulder spica cast for

Displaced fractures

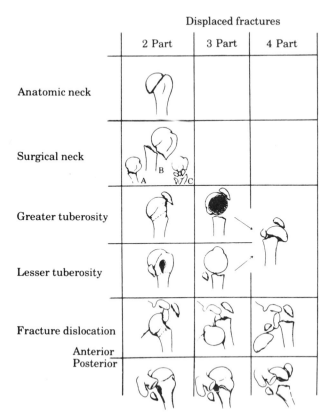

FIG. 17-1. Neer's anatomic concept for standardizing the terminology of fractures of the proximal humerus. (From Neer CS. Displaced proximal humeral fractures. Part I. *J Bone Joint Surg (Am)* 1970;52:1077.)

3 weeks. With reliable patients, circumduction exercises can be started immediately after pinning and the exercise program advanced as described at 4–6 weeks after surgery for pin removal.

  b. **If closed reduction is impossible,** then consideration is given to open reduction and plate fixation or tension band wiring. A low profile plate such as the AO/ASIF (Association for the Study of Internal Fixation) cloverleaf small fragment plate or Blade plate is preferred.

3. **Displaced greater or lesser tuberosity fracture, or both.** Rarely, a three-part fracture is encountered involving the lesser or greater tuberosity as well as the surgical neck. If the fracture is displaced, then the rotator cuff function is compromised and open reduction of the fracture is indicated. The fracture should be anatomically reduced and held firmly with tension band wiring or screw fixation. It is also possible to fix these fractures percutaneously, but this will not address a rotator cuff tear.

4. **A fracture-dislocation of the shoulder,** whether anterior or posterior, may be reduced by a closed method under general anesthesia. If closed reduction fails, then open reduction with internal fixation or prosthetic replacement in older patients is indicated.

5. Neer (see Selected Historical Readings) states that open reduction is indicated for any displaced **three-part fracture** and that prosthetic

replacement is preferable treatment for any displaced **four-part fracture.** This is because of the high rate of posttraumatic humeral head osteonecrosis in four-part fractures. We believe that, at best, these are difficult fractures to treat and that operative treatment should be undertaken only by surgeons with special expertise in managing shoulder trauma.

C. **Complications**
   1. The most common complication is **loss of some glenohumeral motion,** especially of internal rotation and abduction. This often occurs as a result of malposition of tuberosity. The best way to rehabilitate the glenohumeral joint is to start motion early and to achieve primary fracture union. Careful attention to starting an early physical therapy program can markedly improve the end result. Home programs where exercises are performed by a motivated patient two to three times per day with weekly physical therapy monitoring seems to produce the best results. Open treatment may be indicated to achieve adequate stability of displaced fractures to allow early motion.
   2. **Delayed union or non-union** is not uncommon with displaced fractures, especially surgical neck fractures. When it occurs, joint motion is probably incomplete, regardless of subsequent treatment. If the patient experiences pain in association with loss of motion, then the treatment is either replacement arthroplasty or internal fixation with bone grafting.
   3. **Associated nerve and vascular damage** is not rare with displaced fractures and should be identified early so that prompt, effective treatment can be instituted. Involvement of the axillary, median, radial, and ulnar nerves is reported with nearly equal frequency.

II. **Proximal humeral epiphyseal separation**
   A. **Examination.** The injury is most often seen in children 8–14 years of age. On examination, the shoulder usually is deformed. Roentgenograms reveal the correct diagnosis. The epiphyseal slip is usually a Salter class 2 or, less commonly, a class 1 fracture (see Chap. 1, **VII.B**).
   B. **Treatment.** The fracture may usually be reduced by closed methods after appropriate anesthesia. Reduction requires aligning the distal fragment to the proximal one, usually by abduction and external rotation of the distal fragment. Up to the age of 9 years in a girl and 10 years in a boy, remodeling produces a normal shoulder as long as the rotation is correct. Up to 11 years in a girl and 12 in a boy, 50% apposition is acceptable, but varus malalignment should not exceed 45 degrees and rotary deformity must be minimal. The younger child is placed in a shoulder spica cast with the arm in the reduced position. The cast is maintained for 4–6 weeks, at which time it may be removed and the arm brought to the side. Treatment is then carried out in a sling with circumduction exercises. Open reduction rarely is indicated, but closed manipulation and percutaneous pin fixation should be considered if closed reduction fails to achieve an acceptable degree of correction and stability. The mature adolescent should be treated as an adult.

III. **Diaphyseal fractures**
   A. The **diagnosis** is usually self-evident, and the exact fracture pattern is confirmed by anteroposterior and lateral roentgenographic examination. The incidence of this fracture is bimodal occurring at the highest rate in young adults and individuals 60 years of age and older (9). Although the fracture may occur in any part of the diaphyseal bone, the middle third is most commonly involved.
   B. **Physical examination** should be thorough to rule out any nerve or vascular damage. Radial nerve injury is common with this fracture. The time of onset of any nerve involvement must be accurately documented. There are three separate mechanisms by which the nerve may be involved.

1. **Damage at the time of injury** usually produces a neurapraxia, less commonly an axonotmesis or traction injury, and rarely a neurotmesis. Neurotmesis is most commonly associated with open fractures (4).
2. **During the process of manipulation and immobilization,** neurapraxia can occur, and if the pressure is not relieved, then it can become an axonotmesis. This usually is a result of the nerve's becoming trapped between the fracture fragments.
3. **During the process of internal fixation,** neurapraxia or axonotmesis can develop from manipulation of the nerve.

C. **Treatment** (1–5,10,11)

1. The **fracture** should be treated by placing the forearm in a collar and cuff by immobilizing the arm against the thorax with plaster coaptation splints, as shown in Fig. 17-2. The splint can be removed and the patient placed into a snug-fitting commercial or custom fracture orthoses at 2–3 weeks after injury (8,10,11). Shoulder and elbow motion is then initiated. Bayonet apposition is acceptable as long as alignment is good and is preferable to distraction. Open reduction is indicated for a vascular injury, for Holstein's fracture (an oblique distal third fracture with radial nerve injury where the nerve can be trapped in the fracture), for an open fracture (where the nerve should be explored), for bilateral fractures, for massive obesity (where closed reduction is not possible), and for polytrauma. Plates and screws, reamed intramedullary nails, and flexible intramedullary nails seem to be equally efficacious. Intramedullary nails can be placed without opening the fracture site, but they do result in a 20%–30% incidence of postoperative shoulder pain (1–5).
2. Treatment of an associated **radial nerve injury**
   a. **Nerve involvement at the time of injury** calls for passive range-of-motion exercises of the wrist and fingers and for use of a **radial**

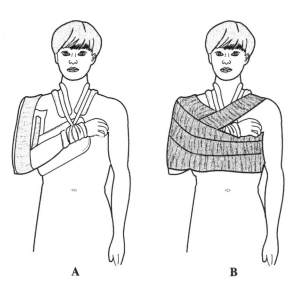

A   B

FIG. 17-2. Treatment of the humeral shaft fractures. **A:** The first step is to apply coaptation splints to the arm and then to apply a commercial collar and cuff or one made of muslin. Stockinet should not be used because it stretches. The neck and wrist are padded beneath the collar and cuff with felt. **B:** After adequate padding in the axilla and beneath the forearm, the arm and forearm can be immobilized against the thorax with a swathe.

nerve splint for the wrist and fingers. Follow up the patient for nerve recovery as outlined in Chap. 1 **(V.E.)** for nerve injuries. The prognosis for recovery is excellent, with 90% or more patients regaining full function.

    b. Nerve involvement at the time of closed reduction should be treated with nerve exploration and fixation as soon as possible.

    c. Late nerve involvement is also an indication for exploration and neurolysis.

  D. Complications. Delayed unions and non-unions do occur. They are best treated with compression plating and a cancellous bone graft. Longer plates and the use of methylmethacrylate in screw holes may be necessary in osteoporotic patients.

IV. Supracondylar fractures

  A. A supracondylar fracture is most common in children and elderly patients, but it may occur at any age (10). The **mechanism of injury** is extension or flexion, or a direct blow as a result of high-energy trauma. The extension type of injury is produced by a fall on the extended elbow and is stable only in significant flexion. Such a fracture may have an intracondylar or intracapsular component. The flexion type is produced by a fall on the flexed elbow and is relatively stable in extension.

  B. Examination. The elbow injury is obvious clinically, but the full extent of the damage must be demonstrated with good roentgenograms. Because of the potential for associated vascular and nerve injury, it is essential to conduct a careful assessment for such injuries. Vascular damage, nerve damage, or marked displacement constitutes a surgical emergency. At times, it is possible to bring about relief by reducing the fracture with sedation and applying a splint.

  C. Treatment

    1. Children

      a. Because of the seriousness of the potential complication of Volkmann's contracture with a **supracondylar fracture,** nearly all children with a displaced fracture are admitted to the hospital. As soon as the condition of the patient allows, a definitive reduction under general anesthesia is attempted. The technique of reduction is illustrated in Figs. 17-3 and 17-4. The authors prefer percutaneous or open cross Kirschner-wire fixation after reduction. If the patient is seen late and the swelling is massive, an alternative is the use of Dunlop's traction until the swelling resolves (see Fig. 9-5). In the younger child, there is some latitude in anteroposterior angulation or displacement. The direction of the initial displacement provides a clue for the proper forearm position after reduction. If the initial displacement is medial, then placing the forearm into pronation tightens the medial hinge, closes any lateral gap in the fracture line, and helps prevent subsequent cubitus varus. If the initial displacement is lateral, then placing the forearm in supination tightens the lateral soft-tissue hinge, closes the medial aspect of the fracture line, and helps prevent cubitus deformity. The use of **Baumann's angle** to guide treatment was described in the German literature in 1929. To use this technique, bilateral roentgenograms of the distal humerus are ordered. A line is drawn down the center of the diaphysis of the humerus, and another is drawn across the epiphyseal plate of the capitellum. If the angle is 5 degrees different from the unaffected side, the reduction is not complete and a significant abnormality in the carrying angle, such as cubitus varus, may result. The reduction is generally off in rotation. Open reduction may be necessary if repeated attempts at closed reduction fail. Internal fixation or percutaneous smooth pins are often required to maintain a satisfactory reduction. Because there is the serious possibility of causing nerve and vascular damage

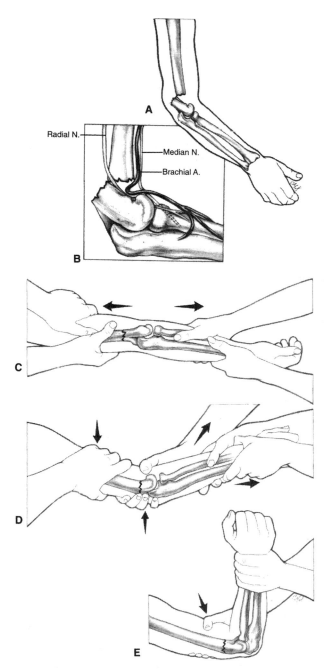

FIG. 17-3. Reduction technique for supracondylar humeral fractures that occur with the elbow in flexion. **A:** Distal fragment is displaced posteriorly. **B:** The brachial artery may become entrapped at the fracture site. **C:** Restore length by applying traction against countertraction. **D:** With pressure directed anteriorly on the distal fragment, provide reduction. **E:** The reduction is generally stable with the elbow in flexion with the forearm pronated.

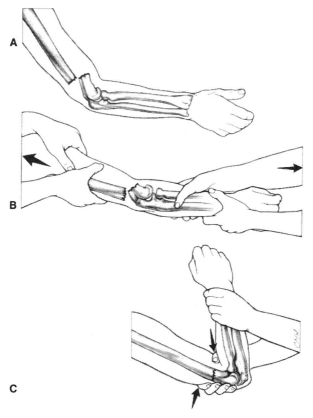

FIG. 17-4. Reduction technique for supracondylar fractures that occur with the elbow in extension. **A:** The distal fragment is displaced anteriorly relative to the proximal fragment. **B:** Restore length by applying traction against countertraction. **C:** With pressure directed posteriorly on the distal fragment, the fracture is reduced. The elbow is then extended to enhance stability of the reduction in most circumstances.

in this region, repeated manipulation should be infrequent and the rule "one doctor, one manipulation" applies. Splint the elbow in 20–30 degrees of flexion after pinning the fracture to allow for swelling. This is only possible when the fracture has been stabilized by pin fixation. The patient must be observed for at least 24 hours for the signs and symptoms of compartment syndrome. Frequent checks of the radial pulse by palpation and Doppler are recorded in the chart and the patient is closely observed for the signs of compartmental syndrome (see Chap. 2, **III**). The pins are removed after 3–4 weeks, and intermittent active motion is started out of splint. The splint is discarded 6 weeks after the injury. Stiffness may result from overzealous attempts of family, friends, and therapists to aid the child in regaining motion quickly. The child should be allowed to use the elbow, and the family should be reassured that he or she will gain extension of the joint with time and growth.

   b. **Distal humeral epiphyseal slips** are rare, but when they occur, they should be treated as supracondylar fractures.
2. **Adults.** These injuries occur rarely and generally in quite elderly individuals. Stiffness in the elbow develops rapidly in the older patient when the elbow is immobilized for any length of time. One of the requirements for any method of treatment is to allow early mobilization. Therefore, treatment should be as follows:
   a. If the fracture is **minimally displaced and stable,** then supination-pronation exercises are begun within 2–3 days without removal of the posterior splint. After 2 weeks, the splint may be removed during these sessions to allow some active flexion and extension.
   b. If the fracture is displaced, the **percutaneous pins** may be used for stability to allow early motion as outlined in **1.a** (above).
   c. **Open reduction and internal fixation** should be considered if steps **a** and **b** do not produce satisfactory alignment and stability (6,7).
   d. If the elbow is grossly swollen and difficult to treat by the aforementioned methods or if marked comminution precludes stable fixation, then **olecranon pin traction** with early movement is an option; it is rarely indicated.
D. **Complications**
   1. **Cubitus varus and valgus (varus is far more common)**
   2. **Loss of elbow motion**
   3. **Tardy ulnar nerve palsy**
V. **Intercondylar fractures**
A. **Type of injury.** "T" and "Y" fractures are typically supracondylar fractures of the lower end of the humerus with a vertical component running into the elbow joint, but any combination of fractures in this area (e.g., comminuted fractures, fractures of the capitulum) are included in this category. Some comminution usually is present.
B. **Roentgenograms.** Films must be of excellent quality to assess the fracture pattern adequately. Intraoperative traction films may be helpful in defining the fracture pattern.
C. **Treatment.** If the fracture is one in which reduction and firm fixation can be achieved by open reduction and internal fixation, then this is performed (6). Highly comminuted fractures are referred to experienced fracture surgeons to prevent the situation of open reduction and unstable fixation. Optimum exposure for anatomic reduction of the joint surface often requires an olecranon osteotomy; patients undergoing ORIF should be started on active range-of-motion exercises within 3–5 days of the procedure. If the degree of comminution is so great that the internal fixation cannot be satisfactorily achieved and referral is not an option, then the fracture may be treated by olecranon pin traction and early motion. Begin movement of the hand and fingers, and commence shoulder movements after 2 weeks. If traction is not used, active flexion from the position of immobilization is encouraged if it does not cause pain. Tenderness usually disappears in 4–6 weeks; the splint is then discarded, and further active elbow movement is encouraged. This injury commonly results in significant loss of elbow extension.
VI. **Lateral condyle fractures**
A. **Type of injury.** These are nearly always seen in children and are a serious injury type of the disruption of the joint surface.
B. **Roentgenograms.** Routine anteroposterior and lateral films are obtained, but oblique films and films of the uninjured elbow often are needed to define the injury accurately.
C. **Treatment.** If displacement is present, then open reduction and pin (two small Kirschner wires) fixation are essential. If no displacement is evident, then additional roentgenograms should be obtained in 5–7 days to check position. Open reduction is done through a lateral approach with minimal stripping of the bony fragment. Rotation of the fragment must be accurately assessed. The pins are removed at 3 weeks; gentle exercises are started at 6 weeks.

D. **Complications**
  1. **Failure to achieve accurate reduction of the fracture** results in cubitus valgus, late arthritic changes, non-union, or a tardy ulnar nerve palsy.
  2. When the epiphysis is open, **overgrowth of the lateral condyle** occasionally occurs, with a resulting cubitus varus.
VII. **Medial epicondyle fractures**
  A. **Mechanism of injury.** The center of ossification of the medial epicondyle of the humerus appears at 5–7 years of age. Displacement of the medial epicondyle as an isolated injury is uncommon. The common mechanism is the result of an elbow dislocation with avulsion of the fragment. This is most common in children but can occur in adults. The medial ligament of the elbow maintains its inferior attachment and pulls the medial epicondyle from the humerus.
  B. The **diagnosis** may be made clinically in a great majority of cases. When the medial epicondyle has been avulsed, there is a surprisingly large defect, which is easily palpated even in a swollen elbow.
  C. **Roentgenograms** are used to identify the position of the medial epicondyle. Roentgenograms of the normal elbow are helpful.
  D. **Treatment.** Reduce any elbow dislocation by linear traction with sedation and assess the position of the fragment roentgenographically. The medial epicondyle may be trapped within the joint, causing incomplete motion. If the epicondyle is in the joint, then open reduction is required. The medial epicondyle fracture can be reduced and held by pin fixation. In adults, consider small fragment screws. If open reduction is undertaken, the ulnar nerve must be protected but need **not** be transpositioned anteriorly.
  E. **Complications** are largely those of an elbow dislocation. If the medial epicondyle remains displaced, ulnar nerve problems are not uncommon. If the epicondyle is anatomically reduced and the elbow joint space is roentgenographically sound, then the injury can be treated by splinting for 7–10 days followed by early active motion exercises (earlier in adults).

HCMC Treatment Recommendations
Proximal Humerus Fractures
   Diagnosis: Anteroposterior shoulder radiograph with axillary view and transscapular lateral (shoulder trauma series). Consider computed tomography scan with reconstructions if a displaced three- or four-part fracture is noted on plain radiographs and the patient is a surgical candidate.
   Treatment: Be sure the humeral head is located. If the fracture is impacted or minimally displaced, apply sling for comfort and begin assisted range-of-motion exercises at 7–14 days.
   Indications for surgery: Marked (greater than 1 cm) displacement of tuberosity fragments, varus angulation of head, dislocated humeral head, head-splitting fracture, or open fractures.
   Technical options: Based on age of the patient, type of fracture, and bone quality:

   • Greater tuberosity fractures: open reduction and screw or tension band fixation
   • Two-part surgical neck fractures: closed reduction and percutaneous pinning. In pediatric fractures, plate or intramedullary nail fixation in adults
   • Three-part fractures: closed reduction and pinning versus open reduction with internal fixation with tension band technique.
   • Four-part fractures, head-splitting fractures: prosthetic replacement is advisable for elderly patients with markedly comminuted fractures or those associated with humeral head dislocation.

HCMC Treatment Recommendations

Humeral Shaft Fractures

   Diagnosis: Anteroposterior and lateral radiographs, physical examination. Be sure to check radial nerve function.

   Treatment: Closed reduction and application of coaptation splints—convert splints to functional brace and begin range-of-motion exercises for shoulder and elbow 2 weeks following injury.

   Indications for surgery: Multiply injured patient or extremity, open fractures, non-union.

   Recommended technique: 4.5-mm large fragment low contact dynamic compression plate (LCDCP), explore and protect radial nerve. Alternatively, use an antegrade interlocking humeral nail but expect shoulder pain in 20–30% of individuals.

HCMC Treatment Recommendations

Distal Humerus Fractures

   Diagnosis: Anteroposterior and lateral elbow radiographs and physical examinations.

   Treatment: Initial long arm splint after documenting neurocirculatory status.

   Indications for surgery: Any displacement of the joint surface greater than 2 mm, open fractures.

   Recommended technique: Posterior approach with olecranon osteotomy where articular displacement is severe. Fixation with two 3.5-mm reconstruction plates at right angles. Olecranon osteotomy fixed with 6.5-mm cancellous screw with tension band wire.

References

1. Bell MJ, et al. The results of plating humeral shaft fractures in patients with multiple injuries: the Sunnybrook experience. *J Bone Joint Surg (Br)* 1985;67:293.
2. Brumback RI, et al. Intramedullary stabilization of humeral shaft fractures in patients with multiple trauma. *J Bone Joint Surg (Am)* 1986;68:960.
3. Dabezies EL, Banta CJ, Murphy CP, et al. Plate fixation of the humeral shaft with and without nerve injuries. *J Orthop Trauma* 1992;6:10–13.
4. Foster RF, et al. Internal fixation of fractures and nonunions of the humeral shaft. *J Bone Joint Surg (Am)* 1985;67:857.
5. John H, Rosso R, Neff U, et al. Operative treatment of distal humerus fractures in the elderly. *J Bone Joint Surg (Br)* 1994;76:793–796.
6. Jupiter JB, et al. Intercondylar fractures of the humerus: an operative approach. *J Bone Joint Surg (Am)* 1985;67:226.
7. Pereles TR, Koval ICJ, Gallagher M, et al. Open reduction and internal fixation of the distal humerus. Functional outcome in the elderly. *J Trauma* 1997;43:578–584.
8. Sarimento A, et al. Functional bracing of fractures of the shaft of the humerus. *J Bone Joint Surg (Am)* 1977;59:596.
9. Tytherleigh-Strong G, Walls N, McQueen MM. The epidemiology of humeral shaft fractures. *J Bone Joint Surg (Br)* 1997;80:249–253.
10. Vandergriend R, Tomasin L, Ward EF. Open reduction and internal fixation of humeral shaft fractures. *J Bone Joint Surg (Am)* 1986;68:430–433.
11. Wallny T, Westermann K, Sagebiel C, et al. Functional treatment of humeral shaft fractures: indications and results. *J Orthop Trauma* 1997;11:283–287.
12. Young TB, Wallace WA. Conservative treatment of fractures and fracture-dislocations of the upper end of the humerus. *J Bone Joint Surg (Br)* 1985;68:373.

Selected Historical Readings

Baumann, E. Beiträge zur Kenntnis der Frakturen an Ellbogengellenk unter besonderer Berücksichtigung der Spätfolgen. I. Allgemeines und Fractura supra condylica. *Beitr f Klin Chir* 1929;146:1–50.

Brown RF, Morgan RG. Intercondylar T-shaped fractures of the humerus. *J Bone Joint Surg (Br)* 1971;53:425.

Hardacre JA, et al. Fractures of the lateral condyle of the humerus in children. *J Bone Joint Surg (Am)* 1971;53:1083.

Holstein A, Lewis GB. Fractures of the humerus with radial nerve paralysis. *J Bone Joint Surg (Am)* 1963;45:1382.

Nacht JL, et al. Supracondylar fractures of the humerus in children treated by closed reduction and percutaneous pinning. *Clin Orthop* 1983;177:203.

Neer CS II. Displaced proximal humeral fractures. Part I. *J Bone Joint Surg (Am)* 1970;52:1077.

Neer CS II. Displaced proximal humeral fractures. Part II. *J Bone Joint Surg (Am)* 1970;52:1090.

Risenborough EI, Radin EL. Intercondylar T fractures of the humerus in the adult. A comparison of operative and nonoperative treatment in twenty-nine cases. *J Bone Joint Surg (Am)* 1969;51:130.

Weiland AJ, et al. Surgical treatment of displaced supracondylar fractures of the humerus in children. *J Bone Joint Surg (Am)* 1978;60:657.

18. ELBOW AND FOREARM INJURIES

I. **Ruptures of the distal biceps brachii**
   A. **Location.** Rupture of the distal biceps may occur at the muscle tendon junction or more commonly at its tendinous insertion into the radial tuberosity.
   B. **Mechanism of injury.** Often a chronic case of distal biceps tendinitis has been present, making the tendon susceptible to failure with forceful supination of the hand or elbow flexion.
   C. **Examination.** A palpable defect is present at the elbow and the bulk of the biceps muscle is retracted proximally. Often, this shortened muscle is prone to spasm for several weeks after the injury occurs. The patient has minimal weakness to elbow flexion, but does have weakness to hand supination.
   D. **Treatment.** If the rupture occurs at the muscle tendon junction, nonoperative care with early range-of-motion (ROM) exercises is indicated. Treatment of distal tendon tears is controversial. The biceps functions as a weak elbow flexor, but is a strong supinator of the hand. Individuals who do not like the cosmetic deformity or are involved in activities that require supination strength should undergo operative repair. A single curvilinear incision is made that allows exposure to locate the retracted tendon proximally and the original biceps tunnel to the radial tuberosity is used. A repair of the tendon to the tuberosity with suture anchors is completed. A sling is used for 4 weeks postoperatively with an active assisted ROM program initiated immediately postoperatively.
II. **Dislocation of the elbow joint** accounts for 20% of all dislocations, second only to glenohumeral and interphalangeal joints.
   A. The **mechanism of injury** is usually a fall on a hyperextended arm.
   B. The **history** of an elbow injury must document, if possible, the mechanism of injury, type and location of pain, amount of immediate sensory, motor, and circulatory dysfunction, treatment before examination, time when swelling began, and any history of elbow injuries.
   C. The **examination** of an injured elbow must document, if possible, the degree of effusion, location of any ecchymosis, ROM, and stability of the joint when compared with that of the opposite side. In the examination of an injured elbow, there may be confusion about whether the deformity arises from a dislocation of the elbow or from a supracondylar fracture, but this can be resolved clinically by comparing the relative positions of the two epicondyles and the top of the olecranon by palpation. These **three bony points** form an isosceles triangle. The two sides remain equal in length in a supracondylar fracture. If the elbow is dislocated, however, the two sides become unequal (Fig. 18-1). The position of the proximal radius should also be palpated on the lateral surface of the elbow to rule out a radial head dislocation. The function of the peripheral nerves and the state of the circulation to the hand, including capillary refill and presence of radial pulse, should be carefully noted. The anterior interosseous branch of the median nerve and the radial nerve are most frequently involved.
   D. **Roentgenograms** demonstrate whether the displacement is directly posterior (most common), posterolateral, or posteromedial. Roentgenograms should include a lateral view of the elbow, an anteroposterior view of the humerus, and an anteroposterior view of the forearm. Fractures of the coranoid process have been identified in 10%–15% of elbow dislocations.
   E. **Treatment** consists of immediate reduction, which is essential, and usually requires anesthesia for proper muscle relaxation. Reduction can usually be achieved by gentle traction on the slightly flexed elbow, applying countertraction to the humeral shaft. After reduction, motion should be nearly full, and medial and lateral stability should be assessed. With a simple posterior elbow dislocation, a portion of the collateral ligaments are generally intact so the joint is fairly stable and early motion may be instituted after 3–5 days of

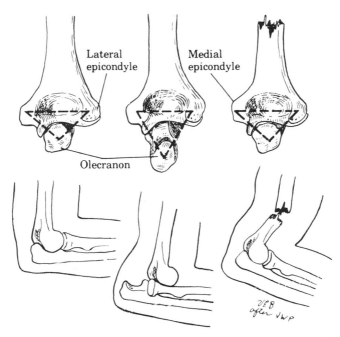

FIG. 18-1. The two epicondyles and the tip of the olecranon form an isosceles triangle. This triangle is maintained with a supracondylar humeral fracture, but with an elbow dislocation, the two sides of the triangle become unequal or distorted.

splinting. With other dislocations, the collateral ligaments may be completely disrupted, creating an unstable joint and necessitating longer immobilization before active exercises are started. Postreduction roentgenograms are mandatory, because they, too, help determine postreduction treatment. If the joint space is not congruent, generally cartilaginous, bony debris or ligament is in the joint, and open reduction and collateral ligament repair is indicated. If significant articular fragments are displaced, they should be internally fixed with a recessed small or "minifragment" implants at the same time. Coranoid fractures, unless involving more than 50% of the length, do not require external fixation. If the elbow is stable after collateral ligament repair, motion should be initiated as with stable reductions treated in a closed manner (17).

F. **Postreduction treatment**
   1. If the medial and lateral ligaments are intact and are providing a **stable elbow joint,** the elbow is placed in a padded posterior splint in 90 degrees of flexion that extends far enough to support the wrist. The elbow is kept elevated above the heart until the swelling recedes. Active flexion is begun in 3–5 days to achieve as much ROM as possible. Passive ROM is contraindicated. Repeat radiographs should be obtained within 3–5 days to make certain the joint remains congruent. The elbow is kept in the posterior splint when not being exercised. As soon as the patient can achieve near full extension, use of the splint may be discontinued.
   2. If the **elbow is unstable** and the joint is congruent on roentgenograms, it is splinted in 90 degrees of flexion for 2–3 weeks with initial elevation to help control swelling. Radiographs must be obtained in the splint initially and at 3–5 days to ensure that the elbow is congruous. An active exercise program is then begun to regain ROM. Open reduction is

generally not necessary; there is no documented advantage to open reduction over closed reduction (8,11,16).

G. **Complications**

1. **Up to 10 degrees limitation of full extension** as well as some limitation of flexion is common unless an intensive rehabilitation program is instituted.

2. Traumatic **peripheral nerve injuries** may occur: Ulnar, median, combined ulnar and median, and brachial plexus injury have all been reported.

3. **Compromise of circulation** can occur as a result of posttraumatic swelling or injury to the brachial artery. See Chap. 2, **III,** for a discussion of compartmental syndromes.

4. **Myositis ossificans** can develop, and its treatment should follow the guidelines in Chap. 2, **V.** Posttraumatic elbow stiffness can be successfully treated by open release (7). If associated with postresection instability, a hinged external fixator distractor can be used with good results in motivated patients (15).

5. **Chronic instability** can be difficult to diagnose; when recognized, surgical reconstruction is generally successful (16).

III. **Fractures of the olecranon**

A. **Fractures of the olecranon may be divided into four groups:**

1. **Transverse and undisplaced**

2. **Transverse and displaced**

3. **Comminuted and minimally displaced** with clinical findings suggesting an intact triceps aponeurosis.

4. **Comminuted and displaced,** indicating a disrupted extensor mechanism

B. **Treatment**

1. **Undisplaced fractures** should be treated in a posterior splint with the elbow flexed 90 degrees. Pronation and supination movements are started in 2–3 days, and flexion-extension movements are started at 2 weeks. Protective splinting or a sling is used until there is evidence of union (usually approximately 6 weeks). Closed clinical and roentgenographic follow-up is essential to ensure full ROM and to identify any displacement.

2. **Displaced fractures** should be reduced anatomically and fixed internally with tension band wiring technique or by tension band plating via a posterior approach. An olecranon lag screw should not be used without tension band wire. If used alone, the screw does not provide maximum stabilization when the elbow flexes, because half of the fracture is placed in compression and the other half is placed in tension, as shown in Fig. 10-9. Regardless of the type of internal fixation used, motion should be started within the first few days postoperatively.

a. The **tension band wiring technique for a transverse displaced fracture** of the olecranon begins with reduction without devitalization of the fragments. Stabilization of the fragments is accomplished by two Kirschner wires introduced parallel to each other and to the anterior cortex of the ulna. Place the drill hole just distal to the fracture, transversely through the posterior cortex of the ulna. Thread the 1.2-mm (or 16–18 gauge) wire through the drill hole, cross the ends in a figure-of-8 style, pass the wire around the protruding ends of the Kirschner wires, and tie the wire under tension, providing two twists, one on each side of the ulna. This makes the tension even across the fracture site. The result should be a figure-of-8 tension band wire with the crossover point lying over the fracture. Finally, shorten the projecting ends of the Kirschner wires and bend them to form U-shaped hooks that are then impacted gently into the bone over the tension wire (Fig. 18-2) and reconstruct the triceps incision over the bent wires. Similar results can be obtained by inserting a 6.5-mm cancellous screw across the fracture and using the same figure-of-8 technique.

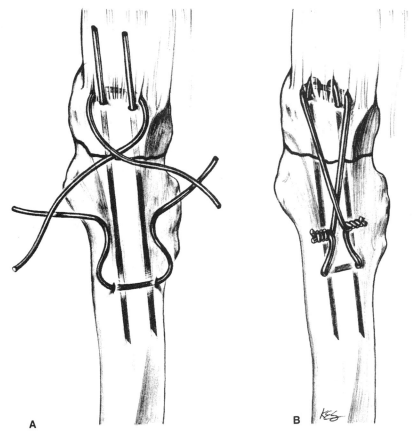

FIG. 18-2. The tension band wiring technique. Two parallel Kirschner wires cross an olecranon fracture at right angles. One strand of 18-gauge wire has been inserted within the triceps tendon anterior to the Kirschner wires. The second wire is inserted through the dorsal ulnar cortex of the ulna **(A)**. The fixation is secured **(B)**. (From Hansen ST, Swiontkowski MF. *Orthopaedic trauma protocols.* New York: Raven Press, 1993:112.)

      b. The tension-band wiring technique for comminuted displaced fractures of the olecranon is much the same except that an anatomic reduction is more difficult to achieve and small Kirschner wires may be required for stabilization of minor fracture fragments.
IV. Epiphyseal fractures of the proximal radius
    A. Mechanism of injury. These pediatric injuries occur from a fall on the outstretched hand.
    B. Examination. Pain, occasionally swelling, and tenderness are usually present over the upper end of the radius. There is also limitation of motion.
    C. Treatment
      1. Fractures with less than 15 degrees of angulation are immobilized in a long-arm splint for 2 weeks. Active exercise is then initiated while the arm is protected in a sling.
      2. Angulation of greater then 15 degrees calls for manipulation under anesthesia. If this fails, operative reduction is required. After reduction,

the fracture is usually stable. If not, internal fixation is used with a fine, smooth Kirschner wire introduced from distal to proximal, stopping short of the articular surface of the radial head. The pin can be removed at 3 weeks and active motion initiated. The radial head should never be removed in children.

V. Fractures of the head and neck of the radius

    A. Mechanism of injury. This injury should be suspected following a fall on the outstretched hand whenever there is swelling of the elbow joint, tenderness over the head of the radius, and limitation of elbow function (especially painful pronation and supination).

    B. Roentgenograms. If the fracture is not apparent on the anteroposterior and lateral roentgenograms, films obtained with the head of the radius in varying degrees of rotation are helpful. An anterior fat pad sign, indicative of an elbow effusion, should alert the treating physician to order these special roentgenograms.

    C. Treatment

        1. Minimally displaced (<1 mm) fractures of the head (mason 1) or impacted fractures of the radial neck are treated with a posterior splint with active motion exercises beginning in the first 3–5 days. This treatment is followed by the wearing of a sling and active movement of the elbow. Acutely, it is helpful to aspirate the elbow effusion and inject 5 mL of 1% lidocaine to be sure that elbow motion is full and unimpeded.

        2. Displaced fractures involving less than one third of the articular surface (Mason 2) are treated by early motion if the postaspiration and lidocaine injection examination reveals a full ROM. If motion is blocked or if there is an associated elbow fracture or dislocation, the fracture is treated by open reduction with minimal fragment screws and early motion (9). The radial head should not be excised.

        3. Comminuted or displaced fractures of the head that involve more than one third of the articular surface and displaced or unstable fractures of the neck are treated by early excision of the radial head with or without placement of a metal prosthesis if it is anticipated that after 4–5 days pain will restrict active exercises (8). If adequate movement can be achieved before the fifth day after injury, excision may be avoided. The end result of excision of the radial head is good, but a normal elbow mothion is generally not achieved. 50% of the patients have a late complication of subluxation and pain at the distal radioulnar joint (4,13). Insertion of a Silastic prosthesis to prevent late complication appears warranted, but complications from the prosthesis itself are not uncommon (synovitis, prosthesis fracture); therefore the authors recommend metal prosthesis when indicated.

VI. Monteggia's fracture-dislocation of the elbow

    A. This is a dislocation of the radial head and a fracture of the proximal ulna. There are **four types,** as described by Bado (see Selected Historical Readings), depending on the direction of radial head dislocation and associated radial fracture.

    B. The **mechanism of injury** may be a "failed" posterior dislocation of the elbow, that is, the ulna fractures instead of dislocating because of an axial loading force. Alternatively, the injury may occur as a result of an anteriorly or posteriorly directed blow.

    C. Treatment

        1. Children. Closed reduction of the ulna is carried out. If the radial head has not been indirectly reduced by realigning the ulna, reduction of the radial head is attempted by supination of the forearm and direct pressure on the head, which usually is successful. When the radial head cannot be anatomically reduced, removal of the interposing capsule with repair of the annular ligament is advisable.

        2. Adults. Operative treatment is recommended (12,21). Open reduction with compression plate fixation of the ulna is generally followed by indirect reduction of the radius. If reduction of the radius is not obtained, an open reduction must be done. If the radial head is unstable, cast for approximately 6 weeks in supination, then start active exercises. If the radial head is stable after closed reduction or open repair, start early active motion with a hinged elbow orthosis, maintaining the forearm in supination. Protect the arm until the fracture is healed. With anterior dislocation and an unstable closed reduction, the arm may be immobilized in 100 to 110 degrees of elbow flexion, which relaxes the biceps and helps maintain reduction of the radial head. If the radial head remains subluxed after ulnar fixation, the forearm should be supinated while applying pressure over the radial head.

VII. **Diaphyseal fractures of the radius and ulna** (5,20–24)
  A. **Roentgenograms.** Of all fractures, this type best exemplifies the need for visualizing the joint above and below fractures of long bones.
  B. **Treatment**
    1. **Children.** The fractures are usually of the greenstick type, and even with considerable displacement, a dense periosteal sleeve ordinarily remains. This sleeve is usually sufficient to make satisfactory closed reduction possible. Greenstick fractures tend to redisplace unless the fracture is overreduced, that is, unless the opposite cortex has been fractured with the reduction. For the closed reduction in which angulation is the only deformity to be corrected, sedation and hematoma block may be adequate. Where there is total displacement with shortening of either of both bones, a brief general anesthetic enhances atraumatic reduction. In the child, operative treatment is undesirable because remodeling with growth is excellent and there is an increased likelihood that cross-union will develop after operative treatment. In the mature adolescent, failure to obtain a satisfactory closed reduction is an indication for open reduction and treatment as for the adult. Bone grafting of operatively reduced fractures in the adolescent is not necessary.
    2. **Adults** (5,20–23)
       a. **Principles.** It is difficult to achieve a satisfactory closed reduction of displaced fractures of the forearm bones, and, if achieved, it is hard to maintain. Unsatisfactory results of closed treatment have been reported to range from 38% to 74% (18). For this reason, open reduction with internal fixation is routine except in cases of undisplaced fractures.
       b. **Undisplaced single bone fractures** should be treated in a long-arm cast until there is roentgenographic evidence of union or definitive evidence or delayed union.
       c. **Fractures of both bones or a displaced isolated fracture** of the radius or ulna should be treated by open reduction, plate fixation, and cancellous bone grafting whenever there is bone loss. Bone grafting should not be performed routinely (22,23). This treatment is carried out as a semielective procedure as soon as the patient's condition warrants; reduction is easiest when the fracture is treated within the first 48 hours. At a minimum, there must be screws engaging six cortices above and below the fracture site. Great care must be exercised to restore the length and curvature of the radius relative to the ulna to prevent loss of pronation and supination (18,20). The use of a 3.5-mm plate system has nearly eliminated the problem of refracture after plate removal (3,21). Previously, this problem was thought to be related to "stress-protection" of the underlying cortical bone but is now understood to be related to cortical bone ischemia (21). Plates should not be routinely removed from healed adult diaphyseal forearm fractures. Eight-hole plates are used most often. If bone grafting is indicated because of significant bone loss, the graft should be taken without disturbing either table of iliac bone or its muscle attachments, as described in Chap. 10, **II.K;** postoperatively, morbidity from the graft site is minimized. Reliable patients may be placed in a removable splint and early motion started as soon as wound healing is complete.

VIII. Galeazzi's fracture of the radius (14)

  A. Description. This fracture is at the junction of the middle and distal third of the radius and is combined with a subluxation of the distal radioulnar joint (said to represent approximately 5% of forearm fractures).

  B. Treatment. The treatment of choice is the same as for an isolated displaced fracture of the radius with forearm immobilization in supination for 6 weeks. The radius is fixed anatomically with a volar approach and plate fixation as for bone forearm fractures. If the distal radioulnar joint remains stable in supination as documented radiographically, a long-arm splint is applied to this position. In a reliable patient, elbow motion can be started with the forearm in supination using a hinged orthoses or Munster cast as soon as wound healing is confirmed. Occasionally, an open reduction of the distal radioulnar joint is necessary because of inability to reduce the joint. If the reduction is unstable, fixation with two Kirschner wires from the ulna to the radius is advisable; the wires are removed in 4 weeks. The Kirschner wire should be a minimum size of .062″or larger to avoid breaking. The distal radioulnar joint must be confirmed to be reduced by roentgenograms during the immobilization period.

IX. Isolated ulna fractures

  A. Mechanism. This fracture frequently occurs as the result of a blow across the subcutaneous surface of the bone, thus the term "nightstick fracture."

  B. Treatment. If the fracture is displaced and not associated with radial head subluxation, it can be well treated conservatively. Functional bracing or treatment with casting yields 95%–98% union rates with good fixation (2,6,19).

X. Colles' fracture (1)

  A. This extraarticular fracture of the distal radius was first described by Abraham Colles in 1814. In this important paper, he differentiated this injury from the rare dislocation of the wrist on clinical grounds without the aid of roentgenograms.

  B. Examination. The wrist and hand are displaced dorsally in relation to the shaft of the radius (Fig, 18-3) to form the classic silver-fork deformity. Tenderness is found over the distal radius and over the ulnar styloid.

  C. Roentgenograms. Anteroposterior and lateral films are essential and often show the following:

    1. Comminution of the dorsal cortex

    2. The following **displacements,** in varying degrees, of the distal fragments:

      a. Dorsal displacement
      b. Dorsal angulation
      c. Proximal displacement
      d. Radial displacement
      e. Articular extension. If the articular fractures are displaced, treatment is different.

  D. Treatment must be directed as vigorously toward maintaining hand, elbow, and shoulder function as toward obtaining an acceptable cosmetic result.

    1. The **radiocarpal joint normally faces palmarward** anywhere from 0 to 18 degrees, so any amount of dorsal angulation is usually unacceptable, and better alignment should be attempted. Reduction of extraarticular fractures that are angulated palmarward between 1 and 15 degrees depends on the age of the patient and the activity level desired; ordinarily, no reduction is necessary. If the palmar tilt is between 10 and 20 degrees, the fracture should be immobilized with no attempt at reduction. The normal radial deviation of the radiocarpal joint ranges from 16 to 28 degrees.

    2. Reduction of this fracture usually is easy to achieve but difficult to maintain. It may be performed under a hematoma block, a Bier block (intravenous regional anesthetic), or an axillary block. Reducing the deformities that have been described previously involves the following steps:

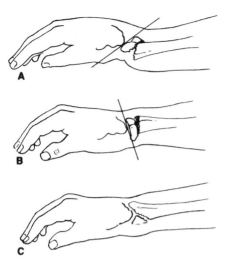

FIG. 18-3. A: Colles' fracture. **B:** Smith's fracture (reversed Colles' fracture). **C:** Barton's fracture (causes displacement of the anterior portion of the articular surface).

    a. Fingertrap traction with a 10-lb weight hung from a strap across the arm is used, and the elbow is flexed 90 degrees in the line of the forearm to **disimpact the fracture.**

    b. While traction is maintained, pressure is applied to the dorsal aspect of the distal fragment and to the palmar aspect of the proximal fragment to **correct dorsal displacement and rotation.**

    c. Pressure is applied on the radial aspect of the distal fragment to **correct radial deviation.**

  3. The following are useful clinical **tests of reduction:**

    a. Palpation of the normal wrist shows that the radial styloid lies 1 cm distal to the ulnar styloid, and this relationship should be restored on the injured side.

    b. There should be **no tendency toward recurrence of the deformity;** that is, when one holds the elbow with the forearm parallel to the ground, the wrist contour appears normal. This may be difficult to assess with severe swelling.

  4. Methods of immobilization

    a. The **wrist usually is immobilized** with the hand in ulnar deviation, the wrist neutral to no more than 15 degrees of flexion, and the anterior splints or single posterior splint extending over the first and second metacarpals to maintain the full ulnar deviation. Splints should be placed over a single layer of Webril applied with an adherent. Splints are wrapped in place by bias-cut stockinet or by an elastic bandage. Because of the potential for swelling, a circular cast is not advisable as initial treatment. The splints may be incorporated into a circular cast after all adjustments for swelling have been made. It is essential to allow full (90-degree) flexion of all metacarpophalangeal joints.

    b. Short-arm versus long-arm casting. If the surgeon wishes to maintain an accurate reduction, the elbow joint should be immobilized. A forearm splint-cast is appropriate, however, in the following situations:

      (1) When the individual is **debilitated or elderly**

      (2) When an **incomplete reduction is to be accepted**

(3) When **no reduction is attempted,** and the **impacted position of the fragments is accepted**

   c. In the younger individual with a severely comminuted and displaced extraarticular fracture, consider **external skeletal fixation** through the radius and the second metacarpal to maintain proper position and length (22). Immobilization in the fixator for at least 6 weeks is usually necessary, followed by mobilization of the wrist. In the older patient with badly comminuted fractures, early excision of the distal ulna and acceptance of radial shortening may also be considered (1). See Chap. 10, **II.J,** for a discussion of external skeletal fixation.

   d. The presence of **intraarticular extension** changes the treatment paradigm in all but the most debilitated patients. A displacement of more than 3–4 mm mandates an attempt at closed reduction. Displacement of more than 2 mm warrants reduction in an adult because of the association of residual displacement with degenerative joint disease of the radiocarpal joint (10). Closed reduction of articular displacement is rarely successful. Therefore, an open reduction through a dorsal approach, Kirschner wire fixation, bone graft for the dorsal defect, and pins, external fixation, or small fragment plates for neutralization is generally recommended.

E. Aftercare

   1. Frequent **active movements of the fingers and elevation of the hand** are both essential to reduce swelling and relieve pain. **Full movement of the shoulder joint also must be maintained.**

   2. Within 1 week of treatment, the following criteria should be met:

      a. There is **full, active movement of the fingers and the shoulder.**

      b. **Pain is minimal** and readily controlled with minimal analgesics.

      c. The **immobilization is satisfactory and comfortable.**

   3. **Follow-up roentgenograms** obtained through the splint should be obtained:

      a. **After reduction**

      b. On the **third day or when the swelling subsides**

      c. After **10–14 days**

      d. At **6 and 12 weeks after injury**

   4. **Duration of immobilization.** If the fracture is unreduced, it should be immobilized for 4–6 weeks. If the fracture is reduced, it should be immobilized for 6–8 weeks. Diminishing of tenderness over the site of fracture is evidence of progressive union. The wearing of a removable dorsal splint for several weeks after cast removal can improve patient comfort while allowing mobilization of the extremity.

F. Complications

   1. The most frequent complication is **stiffness of the finger joints and shoulder.**

   2. Pain with finger movement or numbness in the radial three digits often can signify a **carpal tunnel syndrome.** The pain usually is associated with complaints or abnormal neurologic findings in the median nerve distribution. If the abnormal findings persist for 3 days or increase in severity over 4–12 weeks, the carpal tunnel should be released. If the patient has severe median nerve deficit, carpal tunnel release should be part of the initial management, which generally involves percutaneous pinning, external fixation or open reduction.

   3. **Pain over the distal radioulnar joint** on supination of the forearm is a common complaint when immobilization is discontinued. The symptoms usually disappear within 6 months. Warn the patient of this problem in advance; if symptoms persist after full mobilization of the hand, excision of the distal ulna should be considered.

   4. **Some recurrence of deformity** is common. It is rare for the fractured wrist to have the same appearance as a normal wrist. Give the patient

advance warning about this discrepancy and stress the desirability of good function rather than cosmesis.

5. **If rupture by attrition of the extensor pollicis longus** is reported, early repair is indicated. This may occur even with nondisplaced fractures. This is thought to be due to damage to the blood supply to the paratenon.

XI. **Distal radial and ulnar fractures in children**

   A. **Description.** These fractures are often referred to incorrectly as Colles' fractures because the deformity of the wrist is similar.

   B. **Roentgenograms.** Roentgenographic examination is diagnostic. Be certain that the fracture is not one of the types of epiphyseal slips described in **XIII.**

   C. **Treatment.** When completely displaced, these fractures can be difficult to reduce. Manipulation should be done with the patient anesthetized, and the rule "one doctor, one manipulation" applies. Direct traction alone is rarely successful and should not be attempted, especially without complete patient relaxation under an anesthetic.

   1. **Manipulative reduction** consists of either

      a. **Traction in line with the deformity** until the bone ends can be "locked on," followed by correction of the deformity.

      b. **Increasing the angulation of the distal fragments by manipulation (re-creating the deformity) until the bone ends can be "locked on,"** followed by alignment of the distal fragment to the proximal fragment to correct the deformity.

   2. **If reduction can be achieved,** it is usually stable, and treatment then consists of immobilization as for a Colles' fracture in a long-arm splint with the elbow at 90 degrees.

   3. The fracture infrequently requires **open reduction.**

XII. **Smith's and Barton's fractures of the distal radius**

   A. **Smith's fracture** is a fracture of the distal radius with the distal fragment and accompanying carpal row displaced volarly (reversed Colles' fracture; Fig. 18-3**B**). The articular surface of the radius is not involved. This injury is usually secondary to a blow on the dorsum of the wrist or distal radius with the forearm in pronation.

   1. **Treatment** may initially consist of a closed reduction under anesthesia. Longitudinal treatment is applied in a line with the deformity (pronation and flexion) until the fragments are distracted. Supination and pushing dorsally on the distal fragment reduce the fracture. The fracture should be immobilized with the forearm positioned in supination and the wrist in extension. These fractures are highly unstable and the patient should be informed that this may occur and that open reduction with pins or small fragment plates is generally necessary.

   2. **Postmanipulative care is the same as for a Colles' fracture.**

   B. **Barton's fracture** is a fracture-dislocation in that the triangular fragment of the volar surface of the distal radius is sheared off (Fig. 18-3**C**). This fragment long with the carpus is displaced volarly and proximally.

   1. The **mechanism of injury** is usually forced pronation under the axial load.

   2. **Treatment** of this fracture by closed methods is difficult. Unless there is significant comminution, open reduction and fixation with a volar buttress plate is recommended.

XIII. **Distal radial epiphyseal separation**

   A. The usual **mechanism of injury** is a fall on the outstretched hand with a forced rotation of the wrist into dorsiflexion, resulting in dorsal displacement of the distal radius through the epiphyseal plate.

   B. This fracture follows the rule of epiphyseal injuries (see Chap, 1, **VIII.B**). It is usually a **Salter class 1 or 2 fracture of the epiphysis;** hence, growth arrests may occur. The parents of an injured child must be gently acquainted with this fact.

   C. **Good-quality roentgenograms** are essential in determining the type of epiphyseal separation.

D. Treatment. The younger the child, the more angulation and displacement can be accepted with assurance of normal subsequent function and cosmesis. In a child of any age, **angulation exceeding 25 degrees or displacement exceeding 25% of the radial height should be reduced.** A less-than-automatic reduction is preferable to repeated manipulations. The reduction is accomplished after adequate anesthesia to ensure complete muscle relaxation. Traction is applied in the line of deformity. The manipulation and postreduction treatment are the same as for a Colles' fracture. The patient should be immobilized in a long-arm cast for 3–4 weeks, followed by a short-arm cast for 2–4 weeks. Parents should be reassured that remodeling of the plate and joint motion will occur.

HCMC Treatment Recommendations
Elbow Dislocations
Diagnosis: Anteroposterior and lateral radiographs of the elbow, physical examination
Treatment: Reduction under sedation in the emergency department— longitudinal traction with the elbow slightly flexed—postreduction stability examination and radiographs are essential for planning. If the elbow has good stability, start ROM exercises at 7–10 days.
Indications for surgery: Unstable elbow after reduction, intraarticular fragments, associated fractures, especially of the coronoid process or radial head/neck.
Recommended technique: Repair of the collateral ligaments, joint irrigation, fixation of associated fractures, particularly coronoid fractures of any significant size. Splint for 7–10 days and then start Active Range of Motion (AROM) exercises.

HCMC Treatment Recommendations
Proximal Ulna Fractures
Diagnosis: Anteroposterior and lateral radiographs, physical examination
Treatment: Splint initially, then generally open reduction with internal fixation (ORIF)
Indications for surgery: Displacement of fracture of more than 2 mm or any persistent angulation, especially when associated with radial head dislocation
Recommended technique: Posterior approach, ORIF with tension band wire loop (figure-of-8) around K wires. ORIF with small fragment plates for more complicated fractures.

HCMC Treatment Recommendations
Radial Head Fractures
Diagnosis: Anteroposterior and lateral elbow radiographs, physical examination
Treatment: Aspiration of intraarticular hematoma, injection of lidocaine followed by ROM (especially pronation and supination) of the elbow
Indications for surgery: A markedly displaced (greater than 3–4 mm) Mason 2 fracture that inhibits pronation and supination or a displaced type 3 fracture
Recommended technique: ORIF wherever technically possible using minifragment screws (or plates for Mason 3). Excision of radial head where reduction is not possible using spacer where there is an ipsilateral wrist injury.

HCMC Treatment Recommendations

Forearm Shaft Fractures

Diagnosis: Anteroposterior and lateral radiographs of the forearm, physical examination

Treatment: ORIF with 3.5-mm plates and screws for any displaced forearm shaft fracture in an adult. The exception is the isolated ulna fracture with minimal shortening (<1–2 mm) and at least 50% apposition of bone fragments. Generally use eight-hole plate length or longer; plates should be left in wherever possible.

- Galeazzi variant—fixation of radius as described, with examination of distal radioulnar joint. If stable in supinated position, hold forearm in supinated position for 6 weeks; if joint is unstable, apply temporary K wire fixation
- Monteggia variant—fixation of ulna fracture as described, examination (radiographic and clinical) of radiocapitellar joint. If not reduced, check ulna reduction for anatomicity and, if perfect, undertake open reduction of radius.
- Isolated ulna—ORIF with technique described for fractures with significant displacement
- Isolated radius—ORIF with technique described for fractures with significant displacement (>2–3 mm of shortening) or loss of radial bow

---

HCMC Treatment Recommendations

Distal Radius Fractures

Diagnosis: Anteroposterior and lateral radiographs of the forearm, physical examination. Computed tomography scan can be helpful for intraarticular fractures.

Treatment:

- Extraarticular variant—closed reduction under intravenous regional or hematoma block. Follow-up radiographs in 3–7 days to be sure that reduction is maintained. Comminution at the fracture site makes redisplacement likely. The reduction must be neutral on the lateral with <4 mm loss of radial length on anteroposterior view—this is age dependent. External fixation is also an option.
- ORIF or closed reduction with percutaneous pinning for intraarticular fractures with greater than 2-mm displacement.

Recommended technique: ORIF with K wires or small fragment specialized plates. Volar approach with small t-plate for Barton's (volar, partial articular fractures).

References

1. Altissimi M, Antencci R, Fiacca Mancini GB. Long-term results of conservative treatment of fracture of the distal radius. *Clin Orthop* 1986;206:202.
2. Atkin DM, Bohay DR, Slabangh P, et al. Treatment of ulnar shaft fractures: a prospective, randomized study. *Orthopedics* 1995;18:543–547.
3. Beaupre GS, Csongrad LL. Refracture risk after plate removal in the forearm. *J Orthop Trauma* 1996;10:87–92.
4. Broberg MA, Morrey BF. Results of delayed excision of the radial head after fracture. *J Bone Joint Surg (Am)* 1986;68:669–674.
5. Chapman MW, Gordon JE, Zissimos AG. Compression plate fixation of acute fractures of the diaphysis of the radius and ulna. *J Bone Joint Surg (Am)* 1989;71:159.
6. Gebuhr P, Holmich P, Orsnes T, et al. Isolated ulnar shaft fractures: comparison of treatment by a functional brace and long-arm cast. *J Bone Joint Surg (Br)* 1992; 74:757–759.

7. Husband LB, Hastings H. The lateral approach for operative release of posttraumatic contracture of the elbow. *J Bone Joint Surg (Am)* 1990; 72:1353.
8. Josefsson PO, et al. Surgical versus nonsurgical treatment of ligamentous injuries following dislocations of the elbow. *J Bone Joint Surg (Am)* 1987;69:605.
9. King GJW, Evans DC, Kellom JF. Open reduction and internal fixation of radial head fractures. *J Orthop Trauma* 1991;5:21.
10. Knirk JL, Jupiter JB. Intraarticular fractures of the distal end of the radius in young adults. *J Bone Joint Surg (Am)* 1986;68:647.
11. Melhoff TL, Noble PC, Bennett LB, et al. Simple dislocation of the elbow in the adult. *J Bone Joint Surg (Am)* 1988;70:244–249.
12. Mih AD, Cooney WP, Idlers RS, et al. Long-term follow-up of forearm bone diaphyseal plating. *Clin Orthop* 1994,199:156–158.
13. Mikic ZD, Vukadinovic SM. Late results in fracture of the redial head treated by excision. *Clin Orthop* 1983;181:220.
14. Moore TM, et al. Results of compression plating of closed Galeazzi fractures. *J Bone Joint Surg (Am)* 1985;67:1015.
15. Morrey BF. Treatment of the contracted elbow: distraction arthroplasty. *J Bone Joint Surg (Am)* 1990;72:601–618.
16. O'Driscoll SW, Morrey BF, Korinek S, et al. Elbow subluxation and dislocation: a spectrum of instability. *Clin Orthop* 1992;280:17–28.
17. Regan W, Morrey BF. Fractures of the coronoid process of the ulna. *J Bone Joint Surg (Am)* 1989;71:1348.
18. Sarmiento A, Ebramzaden R, Brys D, et al. Angular deformities and forearm function. *J Orthop Res* 1992;10:121–133.
19. Sarmiento A, Lotta LL, Zych G, et al. Isolated ulnar shaft fractures treated with functional braces. *J Orthop Trauma* 1998;12:420–424.
20. Schmeitsch EH, Richards RR. The effect of malunion on functional outcome after plate fixation of both bones of the forearm in adults. *J Bone Joint Surg (Am)* 1992; 74:1068–1078.
21. Unthoff HK, Boiscert D, Finnegan M. Cortical porosis under plates, reaction to unloading of necrosis? *J Bone Joint Surg (Am)* 1994;76:1502–1512.
22. Vaughan PA, et al. Treatment of unstable fractures of the distal radius by external fixation. *J Bone Joint Surg (Br)* 1985;67:385.
23. Wei SY, Born CT, Abene A, et al. Diaphyseal forearm fractures treated with and without bone graft. *J Trauma* 1999;46:1045–1048.
24. Wright RR, Schmeling GL, Schwab JP. The necessity of acute bone grafting in diaphyseal forearm fractures: a retrospective review. *J Orthop Trauma* 1997; 11:288–294.

Selected Historical Readings

Bado JL. The Monteggia lesion. *Clin Orthop* 1967;50:71.
Burwell HN, Charnley AD. Treatment of forearm fractures in adults with reference to plate fixation. *J Bone Joint Surg (Br)* 1964;46:404.
Fowles JV, et al. The Monteggia lesion in children: fracture of the ulna and dislocation of the radial head. *J Bone Joint Surg (Am)* 1983;65:1276.
Fuller DJ, McCullough CJ. Malunited fractures of the forearm in children. *J Bone Joint Surg (Br)* 1982;64:364.
Linscheid RL, Wheeler DK. Elbow dislocations. *JAMA* 1965;194:1171.
Mason M. Some observations on fractures of the head of the radius with a review of 100 cases. *J Bone Joint Surg (Br)* 1954;42:123.
Monteggia GB. *Instituzione Chirugiche*, 2nd ed. Milan: G. Masdero, 1813–1815.
Morrey BF, Chao EY, Hui FC. Biomechanical study of the elbow following excision of the radial head. *J Bone Joint Surg (Am)* 1979;61:63.
Taylor TKF, O'Connor BT. The effect upon the inferior radioulnar joint of excision of the end of the radius in adults. *J Bone Joint Surg (Br)* 1964;46:83.

19. WRIST AND HAND INJURIES

I. Fractures and dislocations of the carpal bones (16)

A. Principles. Fractures and dislocations of the carpal bones can be difficult to diagnose and manage. Roentgenograms frequently do not reveal the full extent of the osteocartilaginous or ligamentous injury. Numerous classifications have been proposed, but none of them readily assist the treating physician in delineating fractures or suggesting appropriate treatment. When a patient complains of wrist pain, it is essential to have excellent quality roentgenograms obtained in several projections. Stress films often are helpful in determining the severity of the injury and the stability of the wrist. Tomograms, computed tomography (CT) scans, bone scans, magnetic resonance imaging (MRI), or arthrography may be necessary to define fractures or ligamentous injuries. Many nondisplaced fractures are not apparent on initial radiographic examination, but they usually are evident after 10 days; this is particularly true of undisplaced fractures of the scaphoid. Bone scans and MRI can be particularly helpful. If TcMDP uptake is not increased on a bone scan 7–10 days after injury, then no carpal fractures are present and persistent pain must be attributed to ligamentous injury, tendonitis, or soft-tissue contusion.

B. Fractures of the carpal scaphoid

1. **Examination.** Limitation of extremes of wrist motion is usually present because of pain on the radial side of the wrist and tenderness in the anatomist's snuffbox.

2. **Roentgenograms.** The roentgenographic evaluation includes anteroposterior and lateral wrist views as well as scaphoid views. Fractures of the carpal scaphoid cannot be ruled out following a wrist injury until roentgenograms made especially for viewing this bone are negative at 10–14 days. A suspected sprained wrist should be treated as a fractured scaphoid until this possibility has been ruled out.

3. **Treatment.** If the fracture is undisplaced, the recommended treatment consists of a long-arm cast with the thumb incorporated, the forearm in mid position, and the wrist at neutral extension or volar flexion, with 20 degrees of radial deviation (the second metacarpal is aligned to the long axis of the radius) for at least the first 6 weeks (10,16). The long-arm cast may then be reduced to a short-arm thumb spica cast with the wrist and hand in the same position. Immobilization for 12 weeks or more is often necessary. Several authors have advocated the use of short-arm thumb spica casts from the outset with good results, but the most conservative approach involves full immobilization of the radius initially. This can only be achieved with a long-arm thumb spica cast. If the fracture is displaced, then a reduction must be accomplished, which generally cannot be achieved by closed manipulation. Open reduction is then indicated. A short volar or transradial incision is made at the base of the thumb, and open reduction is carried out. The fracture is fixed with two 0.045-inch divergent Kirschner wires or a Herbert screw inserted across the fracture site. The fracture may also be grafted with cancellous bone, a treatment that is always appropriate in the management of fractures with marked comminution or delayed union and nonunion. Inserting a small compression Herbert screw is excellent treatment but may be more technically difficult (10,17). Aftercare includes a short-arm scaphoid cast. Internal fixation wires may be removed at 10–12 weeks if prominent, and the cast is discontinued after the fracture is healed (approximately 4 months).

4. **Complications.** Delayed union and non-union of this fracture are common. These potential complications can be minimized by good reduction and proper immobilization. If after 4 months of immobilization the frac-

ture site is freshened, Kirschner wires or Herbert screw fixation is applied, and cancellous bone grafting is performed. The short-arm thumb spica cast is continued for 3 months until union occurs (16). Radial stylectomy, proximal row carpectomy, and various intracarpal fusions have been described as treatment for scaphoid non-unions with degenerative radiocarpal disease already present.

C. **Lunate or perilunate dislocation**
   1. **Mechanism of injury.** The injury is caused by hyperextension of the wrist with the lunate pushed volarly. There can be associated carpal fractures, including the scaphoid, capitate, triquetrum, or hamate (15,22).
   2. **Examination.** Limitation of wrist motion, fullness on the volar aspect of the wrist, and wrist tenderness are apparent. Signs and symptoms of median nerve compression are frequent.
   3. **Roentgenograms.** Lunate dislocations may be diagnosed on roentgenograms by the triangular appearance of the lunate on an anteroposterior view and its volar dislocation on a lateral view.
   4. **Treatment** (22,24). This dislocation must be reduced as soon as possible to minimize additional trauma and to achieve a reduction. Reduction with closed means after 7–10 days is impossible. Reduction is accomplished under general or regional anesthesia to provide full muscle relaxation. Manipulative reduction can be accomplished by prolonged fingertrap traction with 10–20 lb of weight on the upper arm or by hyperextension of the wrist in traction with pressure directed dorsally over the volarly dislocated lunate. Pinning with percutaneous Kirschner wires to maintain the reduction may be required for more unstable injuries.
   5. **After reduction.** The wrist is immobilized in a dorsal splint, and the hand is placed in a compression dressing for the first 24–72 hours. Then the hand dressing is removed, and active exercise of the fingers is initiated. The wrist is casted for 6–12 weeks with frequent roentgenographic follow-ups.

D. **Scapholunate dissociation**
   1. **Definition.** This syndrome is a fairly common injury characterized by a displacement of the scaphoid to a vertical position relative to the lunate and by a gap between the lunate and the proximal pole of the scaphoid. This is sometimes referred to as the roentgenographic "Terry Thomas" sign. The ligaments between the radius, lunate, and capitate, as well as between the scaphoid and lunate, are ruptured (15,18). The scapholunate angle formed by the longitudinal axis of the scaphoid and the lunate on the lateral roentgenogram averages 47 degrees and ranges from 30–60 degrees in normal wrists (Fig. 19-1). An angle greater than 70 degrees indicates **carpal instability** with the lunate dorsiflexed (15, 18). This injury can occur in association with distal radius fracture (6).
   2. **Roentgenograms.** Films should include stress views of the wrist obtained in supination. The axial loading moment produced by the clenched fist view is also helpful. The normal scapholunate joint space is less than 2 mm wide. MRI scan of the wrist can be helpful.
   3. **Treatment**
      a. An **acute** scapholunate dissociation requires an anatomic reduction and meticulous ligament repair, often with fixation by Kirschner wires. A long-arm thumb spica cast is used for 8 weeks.
      b. With a **chronic** dissociation, a reduction is attempted as described in **C.4.** If this fails, a limited intracarpal or capsulodesis fusion may be indicated (30).

E. **Other carpal injuries** (15,16,18)
   1. The **lunotriquetral ligament** can rupture, leaving a gap between the lunate and triquetrum seen on posteroanterior wrist radiographs made in radial deviation. Treatment by splinting for 3–4 weeks is usually sufficient.

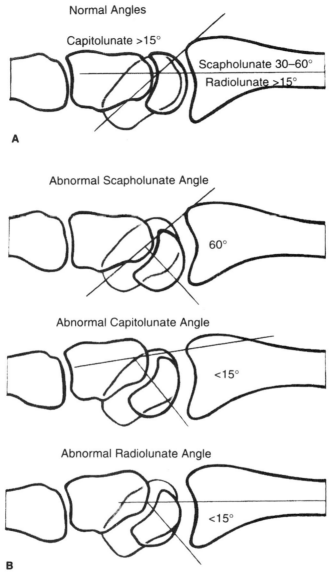

FIG. 19-1. Normal (**A**) and abnormal (**B**) carpal bone relationships seen from a lateral view. (From Hansen ST, Swiontkowski MF. *Orthopaedic trauma protocols.* New York: Raven Press, 1993:135.)

2. The **triangular fibrocartilage** (meniscus) can be torn by a torquing or twisting of the forearm. Symptoms include pain and swelling on the ulnar side of the wrist and a clicking sensation with supination. MRI or wrist arthroscopy is necessary to confirm this diagnosis (29). Initially, treatment is with splinting; repair is sometimes indicated for persistent wrist pain.

3. **Fractures of other carpal bones** are common. The so-called "dorsal chip fracture" of the wrist represents an avulsion of the ligament from the dorsal surface of the carpus, most frequently the triquetrum. Other carpal fractures occur less frequently. Because of the good blood supply, most of these fractures heal promptly with 6–8 weeks of cast or splint immobilization. If displacement is significant and the fragment large, open reduction is indicated. Of special note is the fracture of the hook of the hamate, which can be associated with an ulnar nerve motor deficit. A carpal tunnel view or CT scan is generally necessary to diagnose this fracture. Treatment consists of excision of the hook fragment (16).

F. Few **carpometacarpal dislocations** have been reported in the literature (16).

1. The **mechanism of injury** may be unclear, but such a dislocation is likely to result from both direct and indirect violence, possibly a force applied to the dorsum of the hand with the wrist in acute flexion. Volar dislocations of the fifth metacarpal probably result from a direct blow to the ulnar border of the hand.

2. **Diagnosis** may be difficult on simple examination because of the severe swelling that accompanies this injury.

3. Standard anteroposterior and lateral **roentgenograms** of the hand usually suffice to demonstrate the dislocations. Whenever a displaced or angulated metacarpal fracture is present, particularly at the proximal metaphyseal end, look carefully for a dislocation of one or more of the adjacent carpometacarpal joints.

4. The **treatment** goal is to achieve a stable anatomic reduction.

   a. **Closed reduction and cast immobilization** rarely suffice, especially if the injury is treated late. Longitudinal finger trap traction to achieve length, followed by direct pressure, should restore the normal position. The reduction is maintained by holding the fingers and wrist in extension. Postreduction roentgenograms are mandatory.

   b. If the reduction cannot be maintained, as is usually the case, then **percutaneous pin fixation** is usually the treatment of choice using fluoroscopy to judge the reduction. The wires are left in place for 6–8 weeks to prevent late subluxation. Postpinning films are mandatory.

   c. If closed reduction fails, then **open reduction** is necessary. Ligamentous reconstruction of the thumb carpometacarpal joint frequently is needed along with internal fixation (9,11). Fracture dislocations of the index and long finger carpometacarpal joint may require fusion to provide stability.

5. **Complications.** Old, unreduced dislocations that are asymptomatic do not require treatment. Symptomatic dislocations frequently require arthrodesis of the involved carpometacarpal joints using some form of internal fixation.

II. **Hand injuries**

A. **Principles.** The hand is a sophisticated, prehensile, tactile organ, unique to humans in its mobility and sensibility. Its function is based on great freedom of movement, the ability to exert a large amount of pressure on a small surface area, and sophisticated sensory feedback. Because of this sophistication, aberrations in movement, sensation, alignment, or deformity affect function, perhaps more than in other areas of the body. Therefore, accurate diagnosis and appropriate treatment are mandatory to maintain function. Most important hand functions involve the movement of the thumb against

the index and middle fingers in a variety of patterns, which is 50% of hand function and sensation.
1. **Function**
   a. **Power grasp**
   b. **Prehensile grasp** (85% of function)
      (1) **Lateral** pinch
      (2) **Tip** pinch
      (3) **Chuck** pinch
   c. **Tactile assessment** is easily made with two-point discrimination, a bent paperclip and ruler for standardization is a simple reliable tool. Normal is 3.5–5.0 mm. A braille reader can discriminate less than 1 mm. Confusion can be avoided if the adjacent digit or the contralateral uninjured hand is used for comparison.
2. **Sites for local anesthetics.** After appropriate skin preparation, a local anesthetic may be injected about a nerve with 1% lidocaine (Xylocaine) without epinephrine. The recommended sites for infiltration include the following:
   a. The **median nerve at the wrist**
   b. The **ulnar nerve at the wrist and elbow**
   c. The **superficial branch of the radial nerve as it crosses the distal radius**
3. **Management.** Hand fractures follow the same principles of management as fractures elsewhere in the body. Each fracture can be classified as stable or unstable, intraarticular or extraarticular, or open or closed. Fractures in children present special considerations (1,8).
   a. **Stable versus unstable.** Stable fractures may be reduced and then maintained in reduction with a cast or splint because of inherent stability of the fracture pattern. Unstable fractures cannot be held by splinting and, without internal fixation, lose position after reduction. Stable fractures are immobilized by means of aluminum splints, Bohler splints attached to a cast, or plaster of Paris splints. Most stable finger fractures, whether they involve a metacarpal or phalanx, should be immobilized in the same position. The metacarpophalangeal joint is placed in a minimum of 70 degrees of flexion and the interphalangeal joints are held in extension. This position is referred to as the "intrinsic plus posture" and with a few exceptions (to be noted later) is used to immobilize stable hand fractures. The most troublesome complication in closed fracture management is rotatory malalignment; the rotation of the fingernail should be checked with that of the adjacent fingers and opposite hand held in the same position. Remember that all fingers normally point to the same spot in flexion, that is, the tuberosity of the scaphoid. Stable thumb fractures are immobilized with the thumb in palmar abduction.
   b. **Intraarticular versus extraarticular.** Intraarticular fractures should be reduced anatomically if possible. Small multiple Kirschner wires or minifragment screws are usually the best method of internal fixation of hand fractures. In some cases involving the volar lip of an interphalangeal joint, immobilization in flexed posture is all that is necessary for reduction and treatment.
   c. **Open versus closed.** Open fractures are treated by careful debridement, followed by immediate loose closure, with the following general exception. If there is marked comminution or soft-tissue deficit, the wound is carefully debrided, the fracture stabilized, and delayed primary closure is performed within 3–5 days. Some fractures that, if closed, would be considered stable are best managed with internal fixation. This allows manipulation of soft tissues without compromising fracture reduction. Kirschner wires, minifragment screws or plates, or mini external fixation devices are used for stabilization and should be applied at the time of initial debridement.

4. **Hand compression dressing.** Except for open fractures, most hand fractures are best treated initially by a compression dressing. This dressing consists of a large quantity of cotton or a soft roll carefully placed about the hand, between each finger, and between the fingers and thumb so that the thumb is held in opposition. Avoid placing material proximal to the midportion of the proximal phalanx when padding between fingers, thereby avoiding constriction of the web space and creating a venous tourniquet about the digit. The padding is extended onto the wrist and forearm and incorporated into a volar or dorsal plaster of Paris splint. Compression is achieved with a loosely applied elastic bandage. The position of the hand is stated in **a;** the metacarpophalangeal joints are in a minimum of 70-degree flexion and the interphalangeal joints are extended.

B. **Treatment**

1. **Fractures of the base of the first metacarpal (Bennett's fracture).** These fractures are intraarticular fracture-dislocations of the base of the first metacarpal (27). They are unstable, and anatomic reduction is desirable. Closed reduction may be attempted by traction and full opposition of the metacarpal (full opposition can only be achieved by manipulating the thumb into full pronation relative to the fingers). It is, however, usually preferable to treat the fracture by open methods using Kirschner wires or small screws for fixation. A similar fracture at the base of the little finger metacarpal may require similar treatment; however, as a rule, it can be reduced satisfactorily by closed means and held by the insertion of percutaneous Kirschner wires.

2. **Metacarpal shaft fractures.** Despite some degree of obliquity, these fractures usually are stable because they are frequently caused by a torsional force and gain some stability from the periosteum and surrounding soft tissue. If the fractures are stable, closed reduction and immobilization may be carried out, paying particular attention to rotational alignment. If they are grossly unstable, reduction with percutaneous Kirschner wire fixation or open reduction with Kirschner wire, minifragment screw, or plate fixation is performed.

3. **Metacarpal neck fractures.** Because of the relative lack of mobility of the index and long finger metacarpals, near anatomic reduction is essential. The index finger metacarpal normally has 20 degrees of anteroposterior excursion and the little finger 30–50 degrees of excursion; hence, this amount of angulation is acceptable. Closed reduction is attempted under adequate anesthesia to allow for complete muscle relaxation. Reduction may be achieved by traction in line with the deformity, followed by dorsally directed pressure on the 90-degree flexed proximal phalanx with counterpressure volarly directed on the shaft of the metacarpal, as shown in Fig. 19-2. Great care must be taken to achieve accurate rotational alignment. The fracture is immobilized in the "intrinsic plus posture." In the past, it was recommended that these fractures be immobilized with the metacarpophalangeal and proximal interphalangeal joint flexed 90 degrees with slight counterpressure through the proximal phalanx or the metacarpal head. This method, frequently complicated with flexion contractures and skin breakdown over the dorsum of the proximal interphalangeal joint, is no longer advocated. If the fracture is unstable, then closed treatment is abandoned in favor of percutaneous Kirschner wiring or rigid internal fixation (21).

4. **Metacarpal head fractures.** These are intraarticular fractures that often have a rotational malalignment. They are treated like other intraarticular fractures with an anatomic reduction, internal fixation, and early motion.

5. **Fractures of the shaft of the middle and proximal phalanx.** Care must be taken to obtain good lateral roentgenograms to assess the degree of displacement. There usually is more dorsal angulation than is

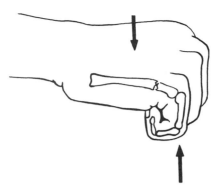

FIG. 19-2. Begin a closed reduction of a metacarpal neck fracture by placing the fully flexed finger in the operator's hand. Then exert a dorsally directed force over the proximal interphalangeal joint with the palm of the operator's hand and a palmward-directed force over the injured metacarpal shaft with the operator's fingers to complete the reduction.

originally apparent, particularly with fractures at the base of the proximal phalanx. Closed reduction should be attempted for patients with a stable fracture pattern (transverse, short oblique, and minimal comminution); the hand should be immobilized in an "intrinsic plus position" for the first 2–3 weeks. If the fracture site is pain-free after 3 weeks, then the splint is replaced with "buddy taping" of adjacent digits and the fingers mobilized. Failure to obtain or maintain satisfactory reduction is a reason for open reduction and fixation with Kirschner wires or plates and screws (21). Malunions may require corrective osteotomy (2).

6. **Volar fracture of the interphalangeal joint (Wilson's fracture).** This fairly common and notoriously sinister intraarticular fracture occurs on the volar side of the interphalangeal joint from the disruption of the distal insertion of the volar plate of the joint, as shown in Fig. 19-3 (19). The typical history is that of a proximal interphalangeal joint dislocation that was reduced by the patient or a friend at the time of injury. Radiographs usually reveal a minimally displaced joint with only a small fragment detached at the intersection of the volar plate with the middle phalanx. If this fragment represents more than 20%–30% of the articular surface, the joint invariably subluxates further, resulting in marked stiffness and pain. If the joint congruity can be maintained by flexing the proximal interphalangeal joint 30–40 degrees, then this fracture is treated with extension block splints. The amount of extension blocked is reduced by 10 degrees per week, and the joint is protected with buddy taping for 3 weeks after removing the extension block splints. If more

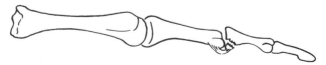

FIG. 19-3. Wilson's fracture is an intraarticular fracture on the volar aspect of an interphalangeal joint that disrupts the distal volar plate with resultant subluxation of the joint.

than 40 degrees of flexion is required to keep the acute injury reduced, then open reduction and internal fixation with an interosseus wire or small fixation screws should be considered. Ingenious methods of dynamic traction have been devised for the treatment of comminuted fractures, but these require a skilled hand surgeon for application. No matter what the method of treatment, motion is started immediately and careful postoperative follow-up with continued roentgenographic monitoring is mandatory.

7. Avulsion fracture of the distal phalanx at the insertion of the extensor tendon (**baseball fracture/mallet finger**) (31)

   a. If the fragment is small, **this fracture** may be treated with hyperextension of the joint for 6–8 weeks with an aluminum-foam splint across the distal interphalangeal joint, leaving the PIP joint free. The same treatment is used if the entire extensor tendon ruptures just proximal to its insertion (mallet finger). The splint should maintain the distal joint in hyperextension. There is no need to hold the proximal interphalangeal joint in flexion as was once thought. When the fragment is bigger than 30% of the joint surface, the joint may subluxate, in which case fixation with a small Kirschner wire or an interosseus wire should be considered. Postoperative treatment is the same as for closed treatment.

   b. With a **traumatic rupture of the central slip of the extensor expansion** near the proximal interphalangeal joint, the joint, with time, goes into a persistent flexion deformity. The lateral bands of the extensor subluxate volarly at the proximal interphalangeal joint and contract, leading to hyperextension of the distal interphalangeal joint. The combination of proximal interphalangeal joint flexion and distal interphalangeal extension is referred to as a **buttonhole or boutonniere deformity.** Making the diagnosis of an acute central slip rupture in the acute setting is difficult. Any injury resulting in pain over the dorsum of the middle phalanx base should be assumed to represent an avulsion of the central slip. In the acute setting, the proximal interphalangeal joint is immobilized in extension with an aluminum splint for 3 weeks. The metacarpophalangeal and distal interphalangeal joints are left free, and motion is encouraged. Treatment of chronic buttonhole deformities is one of the most difficult problems in hand surgery and requires overcoming joint contractures, mobilizing the extensor hood, and repairing the central slip. The key to good results after reconstruction is a well-motivated patient and a well-educated hand therapist (4). The therapist must oversee mobilization of the digit and not cause destruction of the repair.

8. **Tuft fracture.** This fracture is treated as a soft-tissue injury. An open fracture should be debrided to remove devitalized bone before closure. Reduction and Kirschner wire fixation is indicated when the tuft fracture is associated with a nailbed injury.

C. **Other hand injuries**

   1. **Ligamentous injuries and dislocations**

      a. The various collateral ligaments in the hand can rupture with or without an associated dislocation. The injured individual or a friend frequently reduces the joint before it is seen by a physician, and thus **the severity of the injury may not be appreciated.** When the history is suspect for this type of injury, one must gently test for ligamentous stability and focal tenderness.

      b. **Reduction methods**

         (1) A **metacarpophalangeal joint** dislocation frequently requires surgery to mobilize the volar plate, which becomes tightly interposed between the metacarpal head and the base of the proximal phalanx. The flexor tendons, the index lumbrical muscle,

and the superficial transverse metacarpal ligament are thought to contribute to the block in reduction. For reduction, a volar surgical approach has historically been recommended. A skin incision is made along the radial aspect of the distal palmar crease, and the neurovascular bundle is protected. The metacarpal head is freed by making a longitudinal incision through the fibrocartilaginous palmar ligament, the transverse fasciculi of the palmar aponeurosis, and the superficial metacarpal ligament. The joint can then be reduced and held in proper alignment. More recently it has become clear that the major structure preventing relocation is the palmar plate; a dorsal approach is therefore more direct and less likely to result in injury to the digital nerves.

  (2) Interphalangeal joint dislocations are identified by the orientation of the distal member to the joint. A dorsal dislocation of the **proximal interphalangeal joint** may be reduced by a closed manipulation via longitudinal manual traction with or without a local anesthetic.

  (3) A dorsal dislocation of the **distal interphalangeal joint** usually does not require a local anesthetic for successful reduction.

c. **Treatment after reduction** is different for the distal interphalangeal joint than for the proximal interphalangeal joint. Stability is the greatest functional concern, and loss of motion is well tolerated. Therefore, after reduction, the distal interphalangeal joint is immobilized with an aluminum splint for 3 weeks. A loss of 20% of motion is anticipated, but the joint is stable and no functional impairment occurs. Treatment after a proximal interphalangeal joint dislocation is determined by the stability of the joint. The proximal phalanx is the center of motion for the digit and the greatest functional concern is mobility. If the joint has a complete range of motion and does not subluxate or redislocate (as determined by radiographs), then treatment is limited to "buddy taping" or strapping the phalanges of the adjacent digit and encouraging mobilization. If the joint dislocates as extension is completed, then the lateral radiographs should be reviewed closely for the presence of a volar fracture (i.e., Wilson's fracture discussed in **II.B.6**). Treatment of these "unstable" dislocations is similar to that outlined for Wilson's fractures. Extension block splints allow mobilization of the joint while preventing dorsal subluxation. Lateral dislocations, not associated with fractures, are treated with "buddy taping" and mobilization. The patient must be warned to expect prolonged stiffness, tenderness, and generally some permanent thickening about the joint. Function will be near normal, however.

d. A special ligamentous rupture involves the ulnar collateral ligament of the thumb metacarpophalangeal joint and often is called **gamekeeper's thumb** (9).

  (1) The name is derived from an old English custom. The gamekeeper would break the neck of a hare by holding it between his or her thumb and index fingers and snapping it. After this type of repetitive motion, or after a single more severe traumatic injury, the **ulnar collateral ligament of the first metacarpophalangeal joint** becomes damaged, disrupted, or stretched and allows the joint to subluxate radially, thus weakening the pinch function. The more common mechanism of injury occurs when a skier hyperabducts the thumb during a fall.

  (2) **Treatment** of an incomplete tear is immobilization with a short-arm thumb spica splint or cast for 6–8 weeks. Treatment for a complete tear is controversial. There are strong advocates for and against a primary ligamentous repair. Complete tears

should be immobilized and the patient referred to a hand surgeon who is familiar with the pros and cons of operative intervention. The majority of surgeon's recommend repair of the acute complete tear.

2. **Extensor tendon lacerations** may be repaired primarily with nonabsorbable suture. The repair is protected with either dynamic extension assist splinting or prolonged immobilization. The choice of postoperative management is determined by the patient's ability to cooperate with rehabilitation and the availability of a hand therapist.

3. **Flexor tendon injuries** (7,20,26)
   a. These are divided into five zones:
      (1) **Zone I** extends from the distal half of the middle phalanx to the fingertip (green zone).
      (2) **Zone II** (no-man's land) extends from the distal palmar crease to the proximal half of the middle phalanx (red zone).
      (3) **Zones III, IV, and V** are the regions from the proximal end of the flexor sheath to the distal end of the carpal tunnel, the carpal tunnel, and the forearm, respectively. These regions constitute the yellow zone.
   b. **Treatment**
      (1) **Zone I** lacerations are repaired primarily. If the tendon is lacerated less than 1 cm from its insertion, the distal stump is excised, and the proximal portion is reattached to a periosteal flap with a pullout wire or suture secured over a button or a cotton pledget. If the laceration is more than 1 cm from the tendon insertion, it should be handled as a zone II injury.
      (2) **Zone II** lacerations should be treated only by surgeons who specialize in hand surgery. Specialized, atraumatically placed locking suture techniques, such as the Kessler suture, are used to provide internal strength. A running epitenon suture assists tendon gliding. Acute tendon injuries require urgent care, ideally within 24 hours of injury. If treatment is to be delayed longer then this, the wound should be closed loosely. Attempts to "tag" tendon ends are harmful and should be avoided.
      (3) **Zones III, IV, and V** lacerations are repaired primarily but require a skilled surgeon for a good result.

4. **Definitive treatment of fingertip lacerations** may be delayed up to 10–12 hours if the wound is clean and if the patient is taking prophylactic antibiotics. For simple fingertip amputations, follow the treatment guidelines in Fig. 19-4. Tip amputations that result in loss of skin, but not fat or bone, are best managed with daily cleansing and application of a nonadherent dressing. Amputations that involve bone loss, soft-tissue defects, and nail injuries may require local or regional flaps for coverage (5). Such repairs should be done by a knowledgeable hand surgeon.

D. **Noninfective tenosynovitis**

1. The hand and wrist are frequent sites of **acute** and **chronic tenosynovitis.** Acute tenosynovitis is usually an infectious process of insidious onset that manifests with swelling along the length of the digit, severe pain with passive motion (especially extension), increased warmth, and slight redness. Point tenderness and occasionally crepitus on tendon movement are elicited. The differential diagnosis is between an acute noninfectous process and septic tenosynovitis. Roentgenograms may reveal calcification in the tendon or sheath, which is diagnostic of the degenerative or noninfective type. If the etiology remains questionable, then it is best to assume that the sheath is infected and proceed with drainage.

2. **Chronic tenosynovitis** presents itself as a catching or **trigger phenomenon** of the flexor tendons. It occurs when there is a disproportionate size between the tendon sheath and the tendon and is associated with degenerative phenomenon or rheumatoid arthritis. The patient

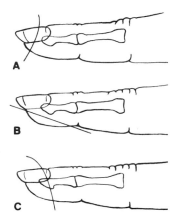

FIG. 19-4. Treatment of fingertip amputations. **A:** Small areas of skin loss require dressing only, but for larger areas, a split-thickness skin graft from the forearm or hypothenar area can be used to repair the defect. The graft will contract, thus decreasing the area of anesthetic skin. **B:** When the nail is not involved, a full-thickness skin graft is used, which gives a thicker pad of skin over the bone. Be sure to remove all fat from the base of the skin graft. **C:** With a rongeur, cut bone proximally to clean, healthy tissue, and close primarily. In children and in adults who require finer finger sensation, an appropriate skin flap may be considered.

may complain of pain in the digit, stiffness, and, in the classic case, is unable to extend the distal interphalangeal joint once it has been actively flexed. In the degenerative process, a nodule is usually palpable just proximal to the flexor tendon sheath. Passive motion is not affected. In rheumatoid disease there is diffuse synovial infiltration of the tendon, which leads to the sensation of crepitance as the finger is actively flexed. Passive motion is affected by joint disease as well.

3. The common sites for wrist tenosynovitis are the abductor pollicis longus and extensor pollicis brevis. Tenosynovitis of this tendon group is referred to as **de Quervain's tenosynovitis** (see Chap. 20, **III.B.**) (1).

4. **Treatment** of tenosynovitis is rest with immobilization and antiinflammatory drugs. If this treatment is unsuccessful, injection of steroid into the tendon sheath usually brings relief of symptoms. The patient should be warned of the danger of tendon rupture when steroids are placed in the tendon or tendon sheath. Occasionally, it is necessary to incise the tendon sheath to reduce the triggering phenomenon or to relieve the symptoms of de Quervain's disease. Great care must be used in this latter situation to prevent injury of the superficial branch of the radial nerve. Rheumatoid patients who do not respond to injection are treated with synovectomy, taking care to preserve annular pulleys of the flexor sheath.

E. A **human bite** or a puncture wound from a tooth injury, with or without an associated metacarpal fracture, is a serious injury. The offending tooth passes through the skin, tendon, and joint capsule of a clenched fist, and comes to rest on the metacarpal head. When the hand is removed from the mouth and the digit extended, the skin, the tendon, and the joint capsule come to rest at different levels, thus trapping the mouth flora inside the joint. Treatment must include skin debridement and joint exploration in an operating room. The wound is left open, and broad-spectrum antibiotics are used until culture results are available (25). Great care must be taken in patients with diabetes who have acute hand infections because they can be especially aggressive (13,14).

F. Injection injuries. High-velocity injection from a paint gun, hydraulic valve leak, or the like is a serious condition requiring emergency treatment. An injection injury occurs when a stream of fluid, often highly necrotizing hydrocarbons, enters a subcutaneous area of the hand and disseminates widely and deeply. A puncture wound to the fingertip from such an injury can present as a mildly painful, swollen tip, but the entire hand is involved within 30 minutes. Immediate decompression and extensive, serial debridement are essential.

G. Complications of hand injuries. Complications in the treatment of hand fractures frequently are iatrogenic and usually can be avoided. The excellent vascularity of the hand, small size of the bones, and relative amount of vascular cancellous bone make it possible to treat fractures of the hand with short periods of immobilization followed by gentle active movement. Slings must be avoided because the hand then rests in a dependent position. Careful follow-up, often employing the therapist of the hand (occupational therapist), and attention to detail obviate many of the complications of trauma to the hands.

H. Nerve injuries should be treated as outlined in Chap. 1, **V.E.**

I. Traumatic amputations are discussed in Chap. 1, **V.H.** (3,12,23,28). Replantation is the treatment of choice for thumb and multiple digits on the same hand.

HCMC Treatment Recommendations
Scaphoid Fractures
   Diagnosis: Anteroposterior, lateral, and scaphoid views plus clinical examination
   Treatment: Long arm thumb spica cast 4–6 weeks followed by a short arm thumb spica for 8–12 weeks until clinically and radiographically united
   Indications for surgery: Displaced fracture or non-union in an active adult
   Recommended technique: Herbert or similar small cannulated screw with bone graft for significant comminution—add K-wire for rotational instability

---

HCMC Treatment Recommendations
Carpal Fractures
   Diagnosis: Anteroposterior, lateral, and anteroposterior with radial and ulnar deviation radiographs, physical examination
   Treatment: Short arm splint followed by short arm cast for 6 weeks for minor avulsion fractures
   Indications for surgery: Marked displacement of main body of carpal bone
   Recommended technique: Minifragment screws, K-wires, or both

---

HCMC Treatment Recommendations
Wrist Ligament Injuries
   Diagnosis: Anteroposterior, lateral, and anteroposterior with radial and ulnar deviation—MRI can be helpful.
   Treatment: Short arm splint followed by short arm cast 4–6 weeks.
   Indications for surgery: Major instability in active, high-demand wrist
   Recommended technique: Primary ligament repair with or without temporary K-wire stabilization.

HCMC Treatment Recommendations
Metacarpal Fractures
  Diagnosis: Anteroposterior, lateral hand radiographs, physical examination
  Treatment: Closed reduction and splinting—casting at 1–2 weeks; total immobilization 6–8 weeks
  Indications for surgery: Open fractures, multiple metacarpal shaft fractures, shortening more that 4–6 mm or malrotation that is not correctable by closed methods
  Recommended technique: K-wires for metaphyseal fractures, minifragment plates for shaft fractures

HCMC Treatment Recommendations
Thumb Metacarpal Fractures
  Diagnosis: Anteroposterior and lateral radiographs of the thumb, physical examination
  Treatment: Short arm thumb spica splint 1–2 weeks followed by thumb spica casting for 6–8 weeks
  Indications for surgery: Intraarticular fractures with subluxation of the metacarpal shaft or major articular (>2 mm) displacement; ulnar collateral ligament injury with instability (Gamekeeper's thumb, Skier's thumb).
  Recommended technique: K-wires or minifragment plates

HCMC Treatment Recommendations
Phalangeal Fractures
  Diagnosis: Anteroposterior and lateral radiographs of the affected digit, physical examination
  Treatment: Splint for 3 weeks followed by AROM
  Indications for surgery: Articular fractures with major (>2 mm) displacement or shaft fractures with nonreducible shortening greater than 4–5 mm or rotatory deformity
  Recommended technique: K-wires or minifragment screws/plates

HCMC Treatment Recommendations
Interphalangeal Dislocations
  Diagnosis: Anteroposterior and lateral radiographs of the affected digit, physical examination
  Treatment: Closed reduction, splinting for 2-3 days, then AROM with buddy taping
  Indications for surgery: Intraarticular fractures with displacement greater than 1 mm, irreducible dislocation
  Recommended technique: Intraosseous wire suture or small K-wires for fractures

---

HCMC Treatment Recommendations
Mallet Finger
   Diagnosis: Anteroposterior and lateral radiographs of the affected digit, physical examination (active extensor lag of the DIP joint)
   Treatment: Splint in hyperextension for 6-8 weeks with Stack or Alumina-foam splint, PIP joint should be left free to move
   Indications for surgery: Displaced large dorsal intraarticular fragment with DIP joint subluxation.
   Recommended technique: Intraosseous suture (wire) with optional K-wire joint pinning

---

References
 1. Baker GL, Kleinert JM. Digit replantation in infants and young children: determinants of survival. *Plast Reconstr Surg* 1994;84:139–145.
 2. Buchler U, Gupta A, Ruf S. Corrective osteotomy for post-traumatic malunion of the phalanges in the hand. *J Hand Surg (Br)* 1996;21:33–42.
 3. Chiu HY, Shieh SJ, Hsu HY. Multivariate analysis of factors influencing the functional recovery after finger replantation or revascularization. *Microsurgery* 1995; 16:713–717.
 4. Evans RB. Immediate active short arc motion following extensor tendon repair. *Hand Clin* 1995;11:483–512.
 5. Foucher G, Dallaserra M, Tilquin B, et al. The Hueston flap in reconstruction of fingertip skin loss: results in a series of 41 patients. *J Hand Surg (Am)* 1994; 19:508–515.
 6. Geissler WB, Freeland AE, Savoie FH, et al. Intracarpal soft-tissue lesions associated with an intra-articular fracture of the distal end of the radius. *J Bone Joint Surg (Am)* 1996;78:357–365.
 7. Grobbelaar AO, Hudson DA. Flexor tendon injuries in children. *J Hand Surg (Br)* 1994;19:696–698.
 8. Hastings H, Simmons BP. Hand fractures in children: a statistical analysis. *Clin Orthop* 1984;188:120.
 9. Helm RH. Hand function after injuries to the collateral ligaments of the metacarpophalangeal joint of the thumb. *J Hand Surg (Br)* 1987;12:252.
10. Herbert TJ, Fisher WE. Management of the fractured scaphoid using a new bone screw. *J Bone Joint Surg (Br)* 1984;66:114.
11. Heyman P. Injuries to the ulnar collateral ligament of the thumb: metacarpophalangeal joint. *J Am Acad Orthop Surg* 1997;5:224–229.
12. Janezic TF, Arnez ZM, Solinc M, et al. Functional results of 46 thumb replantations and revascularizations. *Microsurgery* 1996;17:264–267.
13. Kann SE, Jacquemin JB, Stern PJ. Simulators of hand infections. *J Bone Joint Surg (Am)* 1996;78:1114–1128.
14. Kour AK, Looi KP, Phone MH, et al. Hand infections in patients with diabetes. *Clin Orthop* 1996;331:238–244.
15. Mayfield JK. Patterns of injury to carpal ligaments. *Clin Orthop* 1984;187:36.
16. Meals RA, ed. Problem fractures of the hand and wrist. *Clin Orthop* 1987;214: 2–152.
17. Mintzer CM, Waters PM, Simmons BP. Nonunion of the scaphoid in children treated by Herbert screw fixation and bone grafting: a report of five cases. *J Bone Joint Surg (Br)* 1995;77:98–100.
18. Moneim MS, Bolger JT, Omer GE. Radiocarpal dislocation—classification and rationale for management. *Clin Orthop* 1985;192:199.
19. Morgan JP, Gordon DA, Klug MS, et al. Dynamic digital traction for unstable comminuted intra-articular fracture-dislocations of the proximal interphalangeal joint. *J Hand Surg (Am)* 1995;20:565–573.
20. O'Connell SJ, Moore MM, Strickland JW, et al. Results of zone I and zone II flexor tendon repairs in children. *J Hand Surg (Am)* 1994;19:48–52.

21. Ouellett EA, Freeland AE. Use of the minicondylar plate in metacarpal and phalangeal fractures. *Clin Orthop* 1996;327:38–46.
22. Panting AL, et al. Dislocations of the lunate with and without fracture of the scaphoid. *J Bone Joint Surg* 1984;66B:391.
23. Povlsen B, Nylander G, Nylander E. Cold-induced vasospasm after digital replantation does not improve with time: a 12-year prospective study. *J Hand Surg (Br)* 1995;20:237–239.
24. Sotereanos DG, Mitsionis GJ, Giannakopoulos PN, et al. Perilunate dislocation and fracture dislocation: a critical analysis of the volar-dorsal approach. *J Hand Surg (Am)* 1997;22:49–56.
25. Spiegel JD, Szabo RM. A protocol for the treatment of severe infections of the hand. *J Hand Surg (Am)* 1988;13:254.
26. Strickland JW. Flexor tendon injuries: 1. Foundations of treatment. *J Am Acad Orthop Surg* 1995;3:44–54.
27. Timmenga EJ, Blokhuis TJ, Maas M, et al. Long-term evaluation of Bennett's fracture: a comparison between open and closed reduction. *J Hand Surg (Br)* 1994;19:373– 377.
28. Wang WZ, Crain GM, Baylis W, et al. Outcome of digital nerve injuries in adults. *J Hand Surg (Am)* 1996;21:138–143.
29. Weiss AP, Akelman E, Lamiase R. Comparison of the findings of triple-injection cinearthrography of the wrist with those of arthroscopy. *J Bone Joint Surg (Am)* 1996;78:348–356.
30. Winman BI, Gelberman RH, Katz JN. Dynamic scapholunate instability: results of operative treatment with dorsal capsulodesis. *J Hand Surg (Am)* 1995;20: 971–979.
31. Wehbe MA, Schneider LH. Mallet fractures. *J Bone Joint Surg (Am)* 1984;66:658.

Selected Historical Readings

Bowers WH, Hurst LC. Gamekeeper's thumb. *J Bone Joint Surg (Am)* 1977;59:519.
Chuinard RG, D'Ambrosia RD. Human bite infections of the hand. *J Bone Joint Surg (Am)* 1977;59:416.
Cooney WP, Dobyns JH, Linscheid RL. Fractures of the scaphoid: a rational approach to management. *Clin Orthop* 1980;149:90.
Kaplan EB. Dorsal dislocation of the metacarpophalangeal joint of the index finger. *J Bone Joint Surg (Am)* 1957;39:1081.
Linscheid RL, et al. Traumatic instability of the wrist. *J Bone Joint Surg (Am)* 1972;54:1612.
Souter WA. The boutonniere deformity. A review of 101 patients with division of the central slip of the extensor expansion of the fingers. *J Bone Joint Surg (Am)* 1967;49:710.
Stark HH, et al. Fracture of the hook of the hamate in athletes. *J Bone Joint Surg (Am)* 1977;59:575.
Thomaidis VT. Elbow-wrist-thumb immobilization in the treatment of fractures of the carpal scaphoid. *Acta Orthop Scand* 1973;44:679.
Wilson JN, Rowland SA. Fracture-dislocation of the proximal interphalangeal joint of the finger. *J Bone Joint Surg (Am)* 1966;48:493.

20. NONACUTE ELBOW, WRIST, AND HAND CONDITIONS

I. Basic examination
A. History.
As with any medical problem, the history of events leading up to the patient's visit to the physician with an upper extremity problem is critical. The history should contain family history, social history, personal medical history unrelated to the musculoskeletal system, infectious disease history and risk behavior history. Some additional key facts to record include the following:

1. **Handedness.** Is the patient right or left handed?
2. **Work-relatedness.** If the patient believes a problem is related to work or a series of events, it is the physician's job to document the patient's beliefs. The physician can do this by "quoting" the patient exactly. It **is not** the physician's job or duty to question the veracity of a patient's complaint.
3. **Mechanism of injury.** Record the details of the incident or accident as completely as possible. This is particularly relevant for motor vehicle accidents. Record details such as whether the patient was in the car, whether the air bags deployed, whether the steering wheel was bent (particularly if the injured person was the driver), and the amount of damage done to the car.
4. **Date of most recent tetanus booster.** This is important with any direct trauma. **Do not** assume that another first examiner has resolved this issue.

B. Physical examination
1. **General.** At first glance, the upper extremity is a mirror of the lower. But, several key differences are obvious:
   a. The **shoulder** has more freedom of motion and is consequently less stable than the hip.
   b. The "patella" of the elbow is fused to the ulna as the **olecranon.** However, it performs a similar function to the patella in that it increases the "lever-arm" for the attached muscle (triceps in the arm, quadriceps in the leg).
   c. The **elbow and wrist** participate equally in guiding forearm rotation (supination and pronation). A similar motion is not available in the lower extremity.
   d. The **wrist** has more motion and less bony stability than the ankle.
   e. The **fingers** are longer in proportion to the palm than the toes in relationship to the midfoot.
   f. The **thumb** is longer and is opposable to the digits.
2. **Region specifics**
   a. **Elbow**
      (1) The elbow joint moves in a hinge manner at its articulation between the humerus and ulna. Thus, the ulnar-humeral articulation is uniaxial. In addition to its critical role in forearm rotation, the radius can transmit load to the humerus in "high-strength" situations. This issue is even more important if the elbow ligaments are injured. In general, the elbow gains minimal stability from muscle support and is reliant upon ligament support to guide joint motion.
      (2) Examination of this joint should document the active and passive arc of flexion and extension. Varus (lateral ligament loading) and valgus (medial ligament loading) should be assessed.
      (3) Standard radiographs include anteroposterior (AP) and lateral views.
   b. **Forearm**
      (1) Rotation of the forearm is guided by bone support at the proximal and distal radioulnar joints (PRUJ and DRUJ, respec-

tively). Additional stability and guidance for this motion is provided by the interosseous membrane.

(2) Examination should record the active and passive arc of supination and pronation. Crepitance or pain at the PRUJ or DRUJ should be noted. Pain or swelling in the mid-forearm should be assessed.

(3) Standard radiographs include AP and lateral views.

c. Wrist

(1) The **wrist moves in a multiaxial manner.** The carpus is divided into a proximal (scaphoid, lunate, triquetrum) and distal (hamate, capitate, trapezoid, trapezium) row. Some of the key intercarpal articulations have more easily described relationships (the scaphoid moves relative to the lunate in flexion and extension). However, taken as a whole, the wrist is multiaxial and its motion is highly dependent on ligament function. There is no direct attachment of an extrinsic (forearm based) muscle or tendon to the bones of the proximal wrist. Thus, these bones (scaphoid, lunate, and triquetrum) are 100% dependent on ligament integrity for function.

(2) **Examination** should record passive and active arcs of flexion, extension, radial deviation, and ulnar deviation. Obvious pain or crepitance should be recorded as specifically as possible.

(3) **Standard radiographs** include posteroanterior (PA) or AP and lateral views. If the scaphoid is the focus of attention, AP and lateral views of the scaphoid should be specifically requested. These are oblique to the normal PA and lateral views of the wrist.

d. Hand

(1) The **hand** contains uniaxial (interphalangeal), multiaxial-stabilized (metacarpal phalangeal), and multiaxial-unstabilized (first and fifth carpometacarpal) articulations. Thus, these joints have varying degrees of ligamentous or muscle stability requirements. For example, the proximal interphalangeal joint of the index finger is dependent on ligament support. Whereas, the same finger metacarpophalangeal joint can be partially stabilized by hand intrinsic muscle support.

(2) **Examination** should record active and passive arcs of flexion and extension for all joints. Thumb examination should additionally include ability to abduct (palmar and radial), adduct, retropulse (extend), and oppose. Joint stability should be tested and any masses or tenderness noted.

(3) **Standard radiographs** include PA and lateral views. Note: To obtain a lateral view of a finger, the adjacent digits need to be moved aside. Similar to the scaphoid, "normal" thumb views are oblique to the hand.

(4) **Note:** Always examine the opposite or unaffected side. This is particularly important when assessing stability.

II. Developmental differences

A. Developmental birth conditions

1. **Radial agenesis.** Absence of the radius can be full or complete. Occasionally, this longitudinal deficiency is accompanied by thumb agenesis. An even more rare condition is presence of the radius and absence of the ulna. In either event, stability of the wrist is compromised. The deformity is often characterized with a "club hand." The absence of the radius would then be termed a radial club hand. Full assessment of this condition requires complete assessment of the child to include renal, cardiovascular, neural, and other musculoskeletal regions (shoulder, elbow, and hand). If the child has associated anomalies, correction of the deformity at the forearm carpal articulation may actually compromise

function. Thus, any direct treatment must consider the whole forearm and carpal articulation.

2. **Syndactyly**

   a. This is the most common congenital hand condition (1 in 2,000 live births). The cause is not known. It is divided into **simple** (soft-tissue joining of two or more digits with no associated bone or joint anomaly) and **complex** (joining of two or more digits to include soft tissue and bones or joints) categories. Further subdivision is possible based on the length of the syndactyly. **Complete** syndactyly involves the whole length of the finger, whereas **incomplete** syndactyly does not. Simple syndactyly differences are often completely correctable. The complex differences, however, can occur in combination with other congenital differences (Apert's syndrome).

   b. In general, surgical correction of this difference should be performed as soon as is anesthetically feasible. Correction of a multiple finger difference is done in stages. Limitations of correction are often related to digital blood supply; usually, full-thickness skin grafts are required at surgery.

3. **Polydactyly**

   a. This difference is classified into **preaxial duplication** (involvement of the thumb), central duplication (index, middle, or ring involvement), and postaxial duplication (small finger involvement). **Post axial duplication** has a clear genetic component and is seen in as many as 1 in 300 live births. Correction of this difference usually involves excision. The degree of duplication and joint involvement determines the complexity of the procedure.

   b. **Treatment methods** for thumb duplication generally focus on excision of an unstable duplicate thumb. Duplication of the thumb has been characterized to occur in at least seven different patterns. The outcome of thumb reconstruction depends on the ability to create a thumb of appropriate length, rotation, stability, and mobility and to integrate the thumb into the child's daily routine. It is on this basis that earlier correction is generally recommended.

4. **Madelung's deformity.** First described by Malgaigne in 1855 and later by Madelung in 1878, this difference of growth related to the distal epiphysis of the radius is believed to be congenital in nature, although it is usually not noted before adolescence. It is a rare, genetic condition transmitted in an autosomal dominant pattern. Because of incomplete growth of the radius, the clinical presentation may be prominence of the ulnar head (distal ulna). Alternatively, abnormal forearm rotation may be the presenting complaint. At present, pain may not be a component. The method of surgical correction (shortening of the ulna versus lengthening of the radius) is less important than the goal of obtaining and preserving stable, painless forearm rotation with full and unrestricted use of the wrist.

5. **Brachial plexus**

   a. The brachial plexus comprises a coalescence of cervical and upper thoracic spine nerve roots. It traverses the space between neural foramina and the infraclavicular region where it again separates into individual nerves. Birth injuries relating to the brachial plexus are thought to represent an avulsion or stretch of the upper **(Erb's),** lower **(Klumpke's),** or both aspects (combined) of the brachial plexus. These injuries occur generally in the process of vaginal delivery of the child.

   b. Critical to the **examination** of any child with a presumed brachial plexus lesion is verification of normal shoulder bony anatomy. The physician should document this by way of physical examination and shoulder radiographs confirming the shoulder (glenohumeral joint) is located.

   c. Occasionally a child with nothing more than **a fractured clavicle (birth related)** will be mistaken to have a brachial plexus injury. Thus, it is important to include the clavicle in the physical examination of the infant. Generally speaking, a single AP radiograph suffices to detect such a fracture in the neonate.

   d. **Management** of brachial plexus injuries at birth should include the following:

      (1) Documentation of glenohumeral joint status (located)

      (2) Documentation of passive mobility of all upper extremity joints, including cervical spine mobility

      (3) Documentation of observed active motion in shoulder, upper arm, elbow, forearm, wrist, and hand

      (4) Initiation of twice-daily active assisted "whole-arm" mobilization program to be completed by the **care team** or parents

      (5) Plan for follow-up examination on a frequent interval to verify understanding and completion of passive and active-assisted exercises and available joint motion (both passive and active— looking for change or improvement)

   e. The **prognosis** for most brachial plexus injuries is for complete or near complete recovery. Children whose function remains compromised are evaluated and occasionally operated upon within the first 6 to 18 months of age. The treating physician who cannot document substantial improvement early (less than 6 months of age) should arrange further evaluation by an upper extremity specialist.

B. Delayed presentation of developmental differences

  1. Cerebral palsy

   a. Patients with cerebral palsy constitute the largest group of pediatric patients with neuromuscular disorders. The frequency varies from 0.6 to 5.9 patients per 1,000 live births. Difficulties related to this problem persist into adulthood. However, unlike many neuromuscular disorders, this condition does not progress. Relative progression of the disorder may occur in relation to growth, weight gain, or onset of degenerative change. However, any real progression should cause review of the original diagnosis. Generally, the problem relates to prenatal, natal, or early postnatal brain injury. The injury can express itself in a wide pattern, ranging from single limb to whole body involvement. Two clinical types of injury are seen:

      (1) **Spastic type**—represents an injury to pyramidal tracts in the brain. Exaggerated muscle stretch reflex and increased tone are seen.

      (2) **Athetoid type**—probably a lesion in the basal ganglia. Continuous motion of the affected part is present; this type is more rare.

   b. **Diagnosis** is the first component of treatment. In cases with lesser involvement, diagnosis may not be obvious until the child fails to reach normal motor milestones or has difficulty with coordinated tasks. In some cases, the diagnosis is suspected because of early "underuse" of a part. For example, a child should not have a hand preference before 18 months of age.

   c. **Treatment** of cerebral palsy should always focus on functional improvement. Surgery generally has a cosmetic benefit, but the initial goal should be to improve a specific function. Intelligence and sensory awareness of the child are the two biggest determinants for functional improvement after surgery. Improvements of arm function are possible by improvement in the position of the shoulder, elbow, forearm, wrist, hand, and thumb. Three of the more successful surgeries are release of an internal rotation/adduction spastic contracture involving the shoulder, release/rebalancing of a flexed and pronated spastic wrist/forearm, and release/rebalancing of a thumb into palm deformity.

III. Acquired nonacute dysfunction of the elbow, wrist, and hand

A. Nerve. Nerve tissue is responsible for communication in two directions between the brain and the external environment (peripheral). Like the brain, nerve function is highly dependent on oxygen. Although depolarization of a single axon is energy independent, repolarization of the axon is dependent on adenosine triphosphate to run the Na^+/K^+ pump to "recharge" the axon potential. Thus, although local loss of O_2 will not cause death of the peripheral axon cell body, local loss of O_2 will affect the ability of the axon to conduct **information.** This change in conduction is generally transient, depending on O_2 availability. However, frequent episodes of reduced O_2 can produce permanent change in function. Common sites for nerve dysfunction to occur in the arm are the carpal canal (median nerve), the cubital tunnel (ulnar nerve), and the arcade of Froshe (posterior interosseous branch of the radial nerve).

1. Carpal tunnel syndrome (CTS)

a. Figure 20-1 depicts the carpal tunnel as seen from end on. The carpal tunnel is seen to be formed by the three bony borders of the carpus (trapezium, lunate, hook of hamate) and the transverse carpal ligament. As such, it is a defined space with a fixed volume. Changes in the fixed volume can occur as a result of actual changes in the bony outline resulting from late effects of trauma or arthritis. Also, rela-

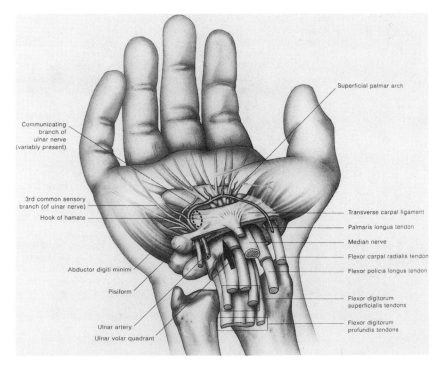

FIG. 20-1. The carpal tunnel is bounded by bone on three sides and by the ligament (transverse carpal) on one side. Guyon's canal overlies the ulnar side of the carpal tunnel. The median nerve lies in the radial volar quadrant of the carpal canal. Generally, it is immediately below or slightly radial to the palmaris longus.

tive change in volume available can be the result of mass effect occurring from tendon or muscle swelling or synovitis, presence of an anomalous muscle, or presence of an actual mass (e.g., lipoma). The patient with reduction in available volume is less able to tolerate or accommodate increases in pressure within the carpal canal. Thus, in patients with reduced carpal canal volume, provocative maneuvers such as Tinel's (tapping or percussion of a nerve in a specific location), Phalen's (flexion of the wrist causing indirect nerve pressurization), or Durkin's compression test (manual pressure by examiner upon the median nerve) are more likely to be positive.

b. **Presenting complaint** is most commonly pain in the median nerve distribution. Pain is often exacerbated at night or by specific activities (1). As the syndrome advances, numbness occurs in the distribution of the median nerve. Weakness of the thenar muscles with associated wasting is a late stage event.

c. **Laboratory testing** (thyroid levels and rheumatoid factor) and radiographs to check for degenerative joint disease (DJD) or old fractures are occasionally of benefit. The most widely accepted diagnostic method is electrodiagnostic testing (electromyogram/nerve conduction velocity [EMG/NCV]). This test can document slowing of nerve conduction and early muscle denervation.

d. **Treatment** of CTS focuses on relief of pain. Initial therapy can include medication to relieve pain and swelling (NSAIDs), splint support, and exercises to increase mobility. No test or study has shown definite value for NSAIDs in management of CTS, except as they are related to relief of pain. An injection of corticosteroid into the carpal tunnel may be effective. There is some benefit from vitamin B6 and C oral therapy.

e. **Surgery** for relief of CTS symptoms is successful, with patient satisfaction exceeding 95% and complications less than 1%. The surgery can be completed by a variety of methods (open surgery versus percutaneous or arthroscopic-assisted release) without a clear benefit to one method versus another, as long as complete longitudinal division of the transverse carpal ligament is achieved along the ulnar half (1,4–6). Return to unrestricted activity after CTS surgery requires 4–8 weeks.

2. **Cubital tunnel syndrome**
   a. The **cubital tunnel** is formed by the bony borders of the medial epicondyle and medial ulna and overlying soft-tissue constraints including the entrance between the ulnar and humeral head of the bipennate flexor carpi ulnaris. It is a defined space with a fixed volume. Changes in the fixed volume can occur as a result of actual changes in the bony outline as a result of late effects of trauma or arthritis (osteoarthritis or rheumatoid arthritis). Relative change in volume available can be the result of mass effect occurring from tendon and muscle swelling or synovitis. Laxity of the soft-tissue–supporting structures can allow the ulnar nerve to migrate out of the cubital tunnel and over the medial epicondyle during flexion. This motion is often referred to as subluxation of the ulnar nerve and produces a "Tinel-like" distal sensory disturbance.

   b. **Presenting complaint** is most commonly pain in the distribution of the ulnar nerve distribution (10). Pain is often exacerbated at night or by specific activities. As the syndrome advances, numbness occurs in the distribution nerve. Weakness or atrophy of the hypothenar muscles is a late stage event.

   c. **Laboratory testing** (thyroid function tests and rheumatoid factor) and radiographs (DJD, old fractures) are occasionally of benefit. The most widely accepted diagnostic test method is electrodiagnostic testing (EMG/NCV). This test can document slowing of nerve conduction and early muscle denervation.

    d. Treatment of cubital tunnel syndrome focuses on relief of pain (8). Initial therapy can include medication (NSAIDs) to relieve pain and swelling, provision of anti–elbow flexion splint support or pad, and exercises to increase mobility. No test or study has shown definite value for NSAIDs in management of cubital tunnel syndrome, except as related to relief of pain.

    e. Surgery for relief of cubital tunnel symptoms is substantially less successful than surgery for relief of CTS. The surgery can be completed by a variety of methods (small versus large surgical exposure) without a clear benefit to one method versus another as long as the point of observed nerve compression is released (7). The patient returns to unrestricted activity after surgery after 12–24 weeks.

  2. PIN compression/other

    a. The **PIN (posterior interosseous)** branch of the radial nerve travels through a defined space with a fixed volume. The tightest region of this space is formed by a fascial connection at the proximal margin of the two heads of the supinator muscle in the proximal forearm (arcade of Froshe). Changes in the fixed volume can occur as a result of actual changes in the bony outline that result from late effects of trauma or arthritis. Relative change in volume available can be the result of mass effect occurring from tendon and muscle swelling or synovitis, presence of an anomalous muscle, or presence of an actual mass (e.g., lipoma). The most common cause of nerve irritation in this region is believed to be the result of thickening of the facial margin in response to time (age) and stress.

    b. Presenting complaint is most commonly pain in the general region of the supinator muscle. Pain is often exacerbated at night or by specific activities. As the syndrome advances, numbness does not occur. Weakness of the PIN innervated muscles with associated wasting is a late stage event. NSAIDs are currently of benefit.

    c. The most widely accepted **diagnostic test** method is electrodiagnostic testing (EMG/NCV). PIN compression with this test is of substantially less benefit when compared with other nerve compression syndromes. Nonetheless, it shows muscle denervation in some cases.

    d. Treatment of PIN syndrome focuses on relief of pain. Initial therapy can include medication to relieve pain or swelling (NSAIDs) and exercises to increase mobility. Splints may exacerbate the problem if placed over the nerve. Wrist splints to reduce load on wrist extensors (the wrist extensors cross over the supinator) are occasionally helpful. As with the other nerve compression syndromes, no test or study has shown definite value for NSAIDs in management of PIN syndrome.

    e. Surgery for relief of PIN symptoms is substantially less successful than surgery for relief of CTS. The surgery can be completed by a variety of approaches, the arcade of Froshe is identified and released. Return to unrestricted activity after surgery requires 12–24 weeks.

  3. Other. Nerve compression can essentially occur wherever a nerve exits or enters a fascial plane/transition zone. The foregoing are the most common sites. A knowledge of extremity anatomy will aid the student in assessing other sites of suspected nerve entrapment.

B. Muscle and tendon. Muscles and tendons work together to generate and transmit force. The effect of load transfer depends on stable points of origin and insertion. Thus, at least **three locations of function failure** are apparent: (1) bone-muscle origin, (2) muscle-tendon junction, (3) tendon-bone insertion. An example of each is provided.

  1. Bone–muscle origin interface failure: lateral epicondylitis (Fig. 20-2)

    a. Failure of the muscle origin of forearm extensors (lateral) or flexors (medial) is a common condition. The condition is uncommon

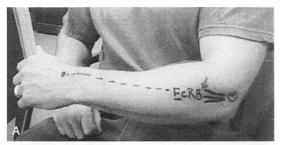

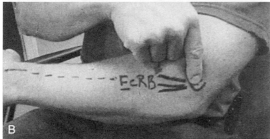

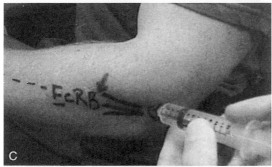

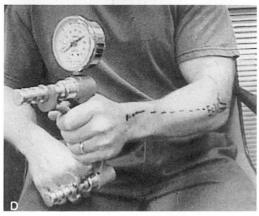

FIG. 20-2. A: The path of the extensor carpi radialis brevis (ECRB) from lateral epicondyle to the base of the third metacarpal. **B:** The center of the epicondyle is the usual pain foci. **C:** Injection of lidocaine at the painful site. This should eliminate the pain. The injection is into the muscle origin, below the fascia. **D:** Postinjection strength testing usually reveals greater strength after pain is eliminated (successful injection). (From Putnam MD, Cohen M. Painful conditions around the elbow. *Orthop Clin North Am* 1999;30(1): 109–118.)

in youth or persons of advanced age. It is occasionally seen in conjunction with working activities. Most often, the condition begins after a period of repetitive stress.

b. Presenting complaint is usually pain focused at the muscle origin. Resisted use of the muscle aggravates the condition. The pain usually subsides with rest. Swelling is rarely present; no mass is seen with this condition. Range of motion may be uncomfortable; but, a full active or active-assisted range of motion should be possible.

c. Laboratory testing is of no particular value. Screening roentgenograms may be obtained but are generally normal for age. An injection test is of confirmatory benefit. This is performed as outlined in Fig. 20-2. In this situation, the hope is that a precise injection of lidocaine with steroid into the area of extensor origin will eliminate or significantly alleviate the pain.

d. Treatment of epicondylitis focuses on reducing the stress at the "inflamed" interface. Theoretically, if the stress is low enough, the healing process can succeed in healing the injured interface. Thus, use of splints (Froimson barrel or forearm band) to reduce the load on the injured muscle origin, massage to increase the blood supply for healing, and stretching exercises to increase muscle excursion are all measures that are likely to provide success. The value of injections versus oral NSAIDs, rest, and splint support has not been clarified.

2. **Muscle–tendon pathway failure** results in trigger finger, trigger thumb, and de Quervain's tenosynovity.

a. The **junction** between a specific muscle and its tendon is a potential site of failure. However, failure or pain at this location is uncommon in the upper extremity. Achilles tendinitis represents a condition occurring in the lower extremity. A similar condition does not occur in the upper extremity with any frequency. Problems along the tendon pathway, however, do occur.

b. Commonly referred to as **trigger digits,** snapping of flexor tendon function caused by bunching of the flexor synovium at the annular one (A1) pulley does occur. This condition is seen more often in older patients, although a congenital version is also common. The condition occurs more often in patients with diabetes. Patients with active tenosynovitis (rheumatoid arthritis) may have a condition that is often confused for tendon triggering. But, rheumatoid arthritis and synovitis in other patients can be distinguished from true trigger digit by the inability to obtain complete active flexion. This is the result of too much synovium "blocking" the active flexion of the digit (the excursion of the flexor tendon is blocked). In the case of de Quervain's tenosynovitis, the problem is focused within the first dorsal extensor compartment of the wrist. The pathophysiology is the same, but this condition results in pain and crepitus along the tendon rather than triggering. The problem and degree of discomfort varies with time of day and activity.

c. Clinical diagnosis of trigger dysfunction is made based on pain or tenderness, crepitance, and locking focused at the A1 pulley of a specific digit.

d. Laboratory studies are essentially within normal limits. Radiographic studies are not generally useful. In the case of de Quervain's tenosynovitis, a special clinical test (Finkelstein's) is routinely performed. Finkelstein's test is positive if ulnar wrist deviation combined with thumb adduction and flexion of the metacarpal phalangeal joint reproduces the patient's complaint of pain.

e. Treatment of trigger digit and de Quervain's synovitis includes rest, stretching exercises, steroid injection into the tendon sheath, and surgical release of the tendon sheath (5,11). If conservative care fails response to supportive modalities is variable. In up to 60% of patients, the condition resolves after steroid injection (13). Surgical release of the sheath is thought to be 95% effective in those who fail to respond to lesser treatments (12).

3. **Tendon–bone insertion failure** results in mallet finger and biceps rupture.

   a. **Failure** at the distal point of muscle action can occur as a result of attrition or age-related change, or excessive load. Occasionally, both methods are involved. Patients are usually seen for diagnosis soon after the failure occurs. Pain is usually less an issue than is weakness or dysfunction.

   b. These conditions are **diagnosed** based on findings observed on clinical examination. Laboratory studies and roentgenographic findings are normal. Larger tendon ruptures can be further clarified using magnetic resonance imaging (MRI) if there are unclear physical findings.

   c. **Treatment** is based on the ability to reposition the specific insertion and maintain this in a resting position. For the terminal extensor–mallet finger, conservative hyperextension splint treatment is possible (2,3). Conversely, distal biceps ruptures will not heal without surgery because the tendon cannot be reliably positioned. However, because the muscle is a supporting elbow flexor (not the only elbow flexor), patients who do not require forceful supination (the biceps is the prime supinator) may choose to forego repair (and tolerate the functional limitations).

C. **Joint.** Painless, stable joint function is maintained by a combination of healthy cartilage, retained shape of the joint surface, ligamentous integrity, and muscle/tendon strength. Change in any of these four factors begins a process of increasing joint wear and dysfunction. Aging alone causes changes in the surface of the joint that accelerate wear. Most **arthritic conditions** of the arm are a combination of load, genetics, and history. However, it is occasionally possible to point to a single event many years earlier that has gradually led to joint dysfunction. Processes such as rheumatoid arthritis are usually the sole cause of dysfunction. Even in these diseases, isolated or cumulative trauma can play a role.

   1. **Thumb carpometacarpal (CMC)** (Fig. 20-3), wrist, and elbow DJD occur with decreasing frequency. Thumb CMC DJD may be the most common site of arthritic presentation. In any of the upper extremity sites, the most common presenting complaint is pain. To the degree that a specific joint is unstable, incongruous, or both, motion and stress aggravate symptoms. Certain activities and prior injury may predispose to arthritis, but underlying genetics is likely the most predominant cause.

   2. **Diagnosis** is a combination of history, examination, laboratory study, and plain radiographs. MRI or computed tomography (CT) methodology is rarely useful. Most patients complain of pain after activity that is relieved by rest. Oral NSAIDs are of some benefit. However, care must always be taken with long-term administration of these medications, particularly in elderly patients.

   3. **Treatment** begins with supportive splints and hot/cold modalities. Hand-based flexible splints are particularly helpful for thumb CMC.

   4. At some point, many patients can no longer "tolerate" the pain. This is the time to consider **surgery**. Unlike the lower extremity, upper extremity arthritic surgery can offer patients reliable joint rebuilding procedures without resorting to joint replacements. An example of such an excisional arthroplasty is shown in Figure 20-4. Such procedures report greater than 90% success rate relative to pain relief.

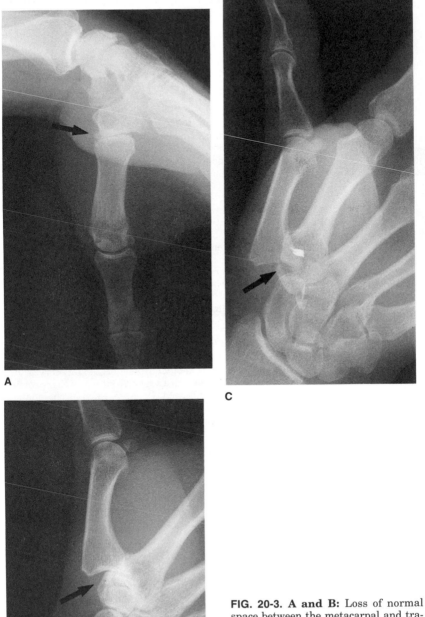

FIG. 20-3. A and B: Loss of normal space between the metacarpal and trapezium typical of basilar joint thumb arthritis. **C:** After trapezial resection and stabilization of the first to second metacarpal, a new space for thumb carpometacarpal motion has been "created."

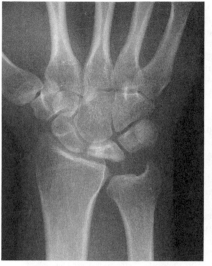

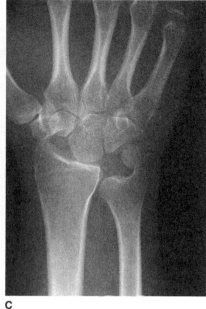

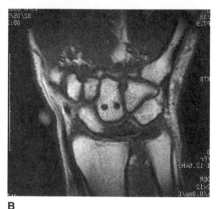

A

B

C

FIG. 20-4. A: Posteroanterior (PA) wrist radiograph showing "collapse" of the lunate. B: Magnetic resonance imaging study of the same wrist from the same point in time showing essentially no vascular signal within the lunate marrow. C: PA wrist radiograph showing the capitate "seated" in the lunate fossae after excision of the lunate.

   5. In the event that first-stage arthritic procedures do not work, newer and increasingly durable total **joint replacement** options are becoming available for the elbow, wrist, and the proximal interphalangeal joints.
D. **Bone.** Skeletal support is essential for function of the legs and arms. As such, immediate change (fracture) or gradual change (e.g., avascular necrosis, tumor) will alter the function of the arm or leg. Gradual change is rarely as painful as acute or fracture change in bone support. This may explain the late presentation for treatment of patients whose slow change process has progressed to the point at which curative or reconstructive treatment is no longer an option. Avascular necrosis of bone is a condition in which presentation and diagnosis are often delayed. As such, it is a good model to discuss the workup of bone pain.
   1. **Avascular necrosis, Kienböck's (lunate)** (Fig. 20-4), **Presiser's (scaphoid), and Panner's (humeral capitellum)** are focal avascular lesions of bone seen in the upper extremity. Genetics, overload, endocrine and systemic illness, and steroid use may play contributory

roles. Patients usually have pain in the focal area and, on testing, it is usually possible to document a reduction in motion. Age of presentation varies from adolescence to late adulthood. Plain radiographs may reveal a change in bone density. In more advanced cases, the shape of the bone is altered. Change in shape is a precursor to diffuse arthritis.

    a. Conservative treatment starts with making a definite diagnosis. This is true for any unexplained pain in bone. If the diagnosis confirms a focal change in bone vascularity without change in bone shape, initial treatment may focus on joint support. However, many patients, particularly those with Kienböck's disease, do not gain sufficient pain relief from splints, and other joint "unloading" treatments are sought.

    b. Surgical treatments for these processes can be broken down into treatments that reduce load on the injured bone segment, debride the injured bone segment, or replace/excise the injured bone segment. These treatments are likely to relieve pain in more than 80% of patients; however, full functional recovery rarely occurs.

2. Tumors. The upper extremity is the site of a variety of tumors, many of which are rare, some appearing almost exclusively on the hand and the arm, and still others are common to all regions of the body. Although most tumors of the upper extremity are benign, few present simple therapeutic problems. The close anatomic relation of the tumor to the nerves, vessels, and muscles in the upper extremity presents a great challenge to the treating surgeon.

    a. Surgeons who treat hand and upper extremity tumors must be familiar with the wide range of **possible diagnoses.** Tumors that look innocent may not be; every mass should be considered potentially dangerous. This section focuses on primary malignant bony tumors of the upper extremity: diagnosis, evaluation, pathology, and treatment recommendations.

    b. Symptomatic tumors, especially those that have increased in size, must be diagnosed and then classified as to stage. The patient's clinical and family history, the physical characteristics of the lesion, and diagnostic images provide information to determine whether the growth is aggressive and should be "staged."

    c. Diagnostic strategies to accurately stage the lesion should be pursued before obtaining a biopsy. Appropriate evaluation includes a detailed history and proficient physical examination, imaging, and laboratory studies. The history should determine the length of time a lesion has been present, associated symptoms, and any incidence of family history. Physical examination requires detailed evaluation of the entire limb and testing, especially for sensibility, erythema, fluctuant, range of motion, tenderness, and adenopathy.

    d. There are a few lesions that have significant associated **blood chemistry changes.** These include the elevated sedimentation rate of Ewing's sarcoma and the serum protein changes in multiple myeloma. Serum alkaline phosphatase is elevated in metabolic bone disease and in some malignancies. A serum immunoelectrophoresis determines whether multiple myeloma is present.

    e. Imaging further aids in determining the location of the tumor and the presence or absence of tumor metastasis. There are a variety of imaging techniques that are useful tools.

        (1) Plain films and tomography. Radiographs are of great importance in the diagnosis of bone tumors. Excellent technique is required to ensure good resolution of bone and adequate soft tissue surrounding the lesion. Plain films are the benchmark in predicting presence and location of bone involvement. Tomography or CT affords improved resolution.

(2) **MRI** has recently developed as one of the more important tools for diagnosing bone tumors. It offers excellent delineation of soft-tissue contrast as well as the ability to obtain images in axial, coronal, and sagittal planes. Additionally, MRI can visualize nerve, tendon, and vessels and, with advanced protocols, cartilage can also be evaluated.

f. **Classification of lesions.** Correct treatment must always take into consideration the location and size of the tumor, the histologic grade and clinical behavior, and the potential for metastasis. If a lesion increases in size or becomes symptomatic, or if the physical or radiographic appearance suggests an aggressive lesion, appropriate staging studies including a tissue diagnosis (biopsy) must be obtained.

g. **Specific tumors**
   (1) **Benign**
      (a) **Lipoma.** This common tumor occasionally presents in the hand or wrist as a firm mass within a nerve or vascular passageway. As such, it may be associated with carpal tunnel syndrome. Its nature may be suspected based on clinical examination alone (mass). To understand its dimensions and relationship to adjacent tissues, an MRI scan is usually obtained. Excision (marginal) is the treatment of choice.
      (b) **Enchondromas** (Fig. 20-5) of the hand are common; they are sometimes multiple and often present after a fracture. Initial treatment in this circumstance is aimed at satisfactory fracture healing. They can clinically be confused with osteochondromas. Radiographic examination easily differentiates the two processes. Most randomly identified lesions can be observed; any lesion associated with pain or increasing size in adulthood should be more carefully studied. Treatment is either observation or intralesional excision. Occasionally, previously benign lesions recur or undergo malignant transformation (Fig. 20-5). Any such lesion should be biopsied and carefully considered for wide excision.
   (2) **Malignant**
      (a) **Melanoma.** The hand, wrist, and forearm are common sites of melanoma. Any change in a pigmented lesion warrants biopsy.
      (b) **Osteosarcoma and chondrosarcoma.** Malignant bone lesions do occur in the arm. Most distal lesions are likely to represent degenerative change of benign processes (Fig. 20-5). Any bone or enlarging soft-tissue mass must always receive a complete evaluation (staging and biopsy) leading to a definitive diagnosis.

h. **Metastasis.** Lesions from elsewhere appearing as metastasis are the most common form of malignancy in the hand. This should be kept in mind, particularly for the patient who is not known to have a malignancy and whose lesion is not in keeping with local origin. A search for the primary tumor is appropriate.

E. **Other factors: Workmen's Compensation.** The hand is often the first tool in and last tool out of a dangerous situation. As such, it is the frequent site of workplace injuries (9). Not all injuries are clearly documented. It is the physician's responsibility to remain the patient's advocate while at the same time remaining an objective observer. Occasionally, these tasks are in conflict. Three simple rules apply in these situations:
   1. Remain a dispassionate recorder of medical facts.
   2. Search for an accurate diagnosis.
   3. Offer no treatment without a specific diagnosis.

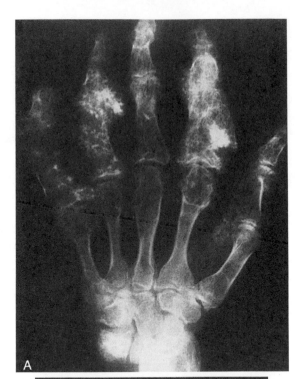

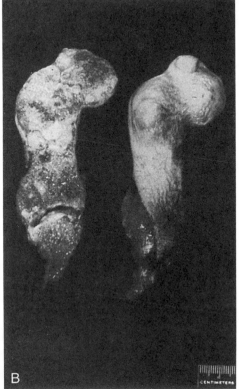

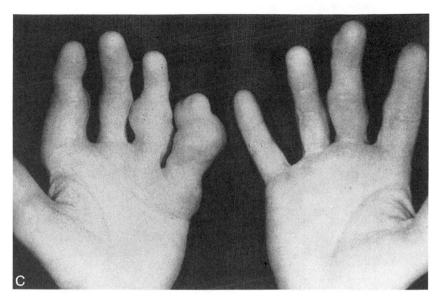

FIG. 20-5. A: Posteroanterior radiograph showing bone changes consistent with multiple enchondromas. **B:** Longitudinal section of the small finger. Pathology seen was consistent with low-grade chonorosarcoma. **C:** Preoperative clinical photo showing multiple digit enlargements. In this case, the patient noted rapid enlargement of the small finger during several months before surgery. (From Putnam MD, Cohen M. Malignant bony tumors of the upper extremity. **Hand Clin** 1995;11(2):265–286.

References

1. D'Arcy CA, McGee S. Does this patient have carpal tunnel syndrome? *JAMA* 2000;283(23):3110–3117.
2. Foucher G, Binhamer P, Cange S, et al. Long-term results of splintage for mallet finger. *Int Orthop* 1996;20(3):129–131.
3. Geyman JP, Fink K, Sullivan SD. Conservative versus surgical treatment of mallet finger: a pooled quantitative literature evaluation. *J Am Board Fam Pract* 1998;11(5):382–390.
4. Katz JN, Keller RB, Simmons BP, et al. Maine carpal tunnel study: outcomes of operative and nonoperative therapy for carpal tunnel syndrome in a community-based cohort. *J Hand Surg (Am)* 1998;697–710.
5. Kay NR. De Quervain's disease. Changing pathology or changing perception. *J Hand Surg (Br)* 2000;25(1):65–69.
6. Keller RB, Largay AM, Soule DN, et al. Maine carpal tunnel study: small area variations. *J Hand Surg (Am)* 1998;23(4):692–699.
7. Kleinman WB. Cubital tunnel syndrome: anterior transposition as a logical approach to complete nerve decompression. *J Hand Surg (Am)* 1999;24(5):886–897.
8. Mowlavi A, Andrews K, Lille S, et al. The management of cubital tunnel syndrome: a meta-analysis of clinical studies. *Plast Reconstr Surg* 2000;106(2):327–334.
9. Piligian G, Herbert R, Hearns M, et al. Evaluation and management of chronic work-related musculoskeletal disorders of the distal upper extremity. *Am J Ind Med* 2000;37(1):75–93.
10. Posner MA. Compressive neuropathies of the ulnar nerve at the elbow and wrist. *Instr Course Lect* 2000;49:305–317.

11. Rankin ME, Rankin EA. Injection therapy for management of stenosing tenosynovitis (de Quervain's disease) of the wrist. *J Natl Med Assoc* 1998;90(8):474–476.
12. Ta KT, Eidelman D, Thomson JG. Patient satisfaction and outcomes of surgery for de Quervain's tenosynovitis. *J Hand Surg (Am)* 1999;24(5):1071–1077.
13. Zingas C, Failla JM, Van Holsbeeck M. Injection accuracy and clinical relief of de Quervain's tendinitis. *J Hand Surg (Am)* 1998;23(1):89–96.

Selected Historical Readings
De Quervain F. On a form of chronic tendovaginitis by Dr. Fritz de Quervain in a la Chaux-de-Fonds. 1895. *Am J Orthop* 1997;26(9):641–644.

21. FRACTURES OF THE PELVIS

I. **Incidence and mechanism of injury. Pelvic fractures are a common cause of death associated with trauma;** head injuries are the most common cause (2,6,15). Approximately two thirds of pelvic fractures are complicated by other fractures and injuries to soft tissues. The fatality rate from pelvic hemorrhage with current management techniques ranges from 5% to 20% (2,6). Pelvic fractures generally are the result of direct trauma or of transmission of forces through the lower extremity. The importance of these fractures lies more in the associated soft-tissue injury and hemorrhage than in the fracture per se (2,13).

II. **Classification of pelvic fractures.** Numerous systems have been proposed, but the **Tile system,** which expands on Pennel's work, is the most widely used (17). Burgess has expanded on this work by adding a combined mechanism notion (2).
   A. **Types**
      1. **Type A:** stable
      2. **Type B:** rotationally unstable, but **vertically** and **posteriorly** stable
      3. **Type C: rotationally** and **vertically unstable**
   B. **Subtypes,** which have important influences on treatment, are presented in Table 21-1 and illustrated in Figs. 21-1, 21-2, and 21-3.
   C. **Fractures of the acetabulum** are discussed in Chap. 22.
   D. Note for historical purposes that a **Malgaigne fracture** is a vertical fracture or dislocation of the posterior sacroiliac joint complex involving one side of the pelvis.

III. **Examination**
   A. Pelvic fractures are suspected because of pain, crepitus, or **tenderness over the symphysis pubis, anterior iliac spines, iliac crest, or sacrum,** but a good roentgenographic examination is essential for diagnosis. Patients with these injuries are often unconscious or intubated, so the examination for stability is helpful. The iliac wings are grasped and force-directed to the midline; instability can be detected with this maneuver. Gentle handling of the patient minimizes further bleeding and shock.
   B. **Specific studies.** Patients with all but minimal trauma should have an indwelling urinary catheter for the dual purposes of measuring urine output while the associated shock is being treated and investigating possible bladder trauma. If there is blood at the penile meatus, then a retrograde urethrogram should be performed before passage of the catheter (2,6,13). This prevents completion of a partial urethral tear. Intravenous pyelography and cystography document renal function, bladder anatomy, and help delineate the size of any pelvic or retroperitoneal hematoma. Despite the difficulties involved, a pelvic (in women) and rectal examination should be done to check for fresh blood and open wounds, perineal sensation in a conscious patient, a displaced unstable prostate, and sphincter tone. These fractures frequently are associated with neurologic damage, so a careful neurologic evaluation should be done in all patients.

IV. **Pelvic hemorrhage** (3)
   A. **Symptoms and signs.** At presentation, approximately 20% of patients are in shock. Severe backache can help differentiate the pain of retroperitoneal bleeding from the pain of intraabdominal bleeding.
   B. **Treatment.** Pneumatic antishock garments (MAST trousers) help reduce the pelvic volume by compression of the iliac wings. MAST trousers are not useful as a routine transfer aid for patients with blunt trauma (12). These garments are useful in patient transport but should be removed as soon as resuscitation is underway because they are associated with compartment syndrome in the legs (1). Most causes of hemorrhage are adequately handled by rapid replacement and maintenance of blood volume, followed by reduction (when appropriate) and stabilization of the fractures as described

Table 21-1. Substances of pelvic fractures

Type A: Stable
 A1 Fractures not involving ring; avulsion injuries
   A1.1 Anterior superior spine
   A1.2 Anterior inferior spine
   A1.3 Ischial tuberosity
 A2 Stable, minimal displacement
   A2.1 Iliac wing fractures
   A2.2 Isolated anterior ring injuries (four-pillar)
   A2.3 Stable, undisplaced, or minimally displaced fractures of the pelvic ring
 A3 Transverse fractures of sacrum and coccyx
   A3.1 Undisplaced transverse sacral fractures
   A3.2 Displaced transverse sacral fractures
   A3.3 Coccygeal fracture
Type B: Rotationally unstable; vertically and posteriorly stable
 B1 External rotation instability; open-book injury
   B1.1 Unilateral injury
   B1.2 Less than 2.5-cm displacement
 B2 Internal rotation instability; lateral compression injury
   B2.1 Ipsilateral anterior and posterior injury
   B2.2 Contralateral anterior and posterior injury; bucket-handle fracture
 B3 Bilateral rotationally unstable injury
Type C: Rotationally, posteriorly, and vertically unstable
 C1 Unilateral injury
   C1.1 Fracture through ilium
   C1.2 Sacroiliac dislocation or fracture-dislocation
   C1.3 Sacral fracture
 C2 Bilateral injury, with one side rotationally unstable and one side vertically
    unstable
 C3 Bilateral injury, with both sides completely unstable

From Tile M. Pelvic ring fractures: should they be fixed? *J Bone Joint Surg* 1988;70B:I.

in **VI.** Adequate blood replacement is the first priority, and its effectiveness is monitored by the patient's pulse, blood pressure, central venous pressure, urine output, and so on, as described in Chap. 1. Blood loss of 2500 mL is common, and blood replacement is usually necessary even without evidence of an open hemorrhage. Diagnostic peritoneal lavage is a useful test to rule out intraabdominal injury at the site of hemorrhage (13). Abdominal computed tomography (CT) scan is being used increasingly as a screening test for this condition (6). The surgeon must follow the patient's platelet count and coagulation studies after 4 units of blood have been given because disseminated intravascular coagulation can result from dilution of these components. The use of angiography and embolization of distal arterial bleeding points with blood clot, Gelfoam, or coils has recently been popularized (2,6). Because only 10% of patients have identifiable arterial bleeding, the authors prefer to stabilize the pelvis with internal or external fixation first (2,6,9,11,16). Anterior external fixation with one or two pins in each iliac wing is an effective means of stabilizing the pelvis when the traumatic pattern allows its use (8,9,14). If the pelvic injury involves the posterior wing with a sacral fracture or unstable sacroiliac joint injury, the antishock clamp can be life saving. It requires skill, familiarity with the device, and fluoroscopic control (5). Spica casting can also be used if the necessary expertise or equipment is not available (4). Distal femoral pins must be incorporated into the cast. If this does not control the bleeding, then arteriography and embolization are indicated (6).

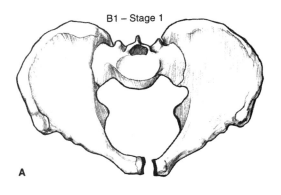

B1 – Stage 1

A

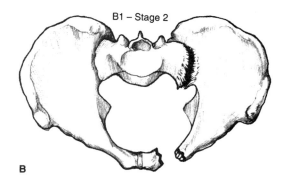

B1 – Stage 2

B

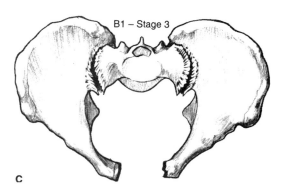

B1 – Stage 3

C

FIG. 21-1. A: Type B1, stage 1 symphysis pubis disruption. **B:** Type B1, stage 2 symphysis pubis disruption. **C:** Type B1, stage 3 symphysis pubis disruption. (From Hansen ST, Swiontkowski MF. *Orthopaedic trauma protocols.* New York: Raven, 1993:228.)

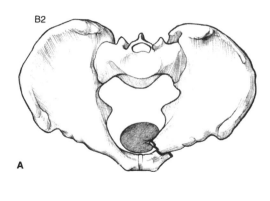

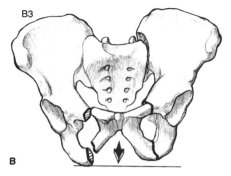

FIG. 21-2. A: Type B2 lateral compression injury (ipsilateral). **B:** Type B3 lateral compression injury (contralateral). (From Hansen ST, Swiontkowski MF. *Orthopaedic trauma protocols.* New York: Raven, 1993:228.)

V. **Roentgenograms**
   A. **An anteroposterior view of the pelvis** is made routinely in all patients who have suffered severe trauma or who complain of pain in and around the pelvic region. After the patient's general condition has stabilized following a pelvic fracture, special films are indicated, including a 60-degree caudad-directed inlet view and a 40-degree cephalad-oriented tangential (or outlet) view (11,17). The former helps visualize the posterior pelvic ring, and the latter is for the anterior ring.
   B. **CT scans** can be most useful in defining posterior ring fractures (2,6,16). Fifty percent of sacral fractures are missed on plain roentgenograms, but they are well visualized on CT scans.
VI. **Treatment**
   A. **Stable A type fractures** are treated symptomatically. Turn the patient by logrolling or begin treatment on a Foster frame until the severe pain subsides. As soon as the patient can move comfortably in bed, he or she can ambulate in a walker and progress to walking with crutches. The fractures are through cancellous bone that has good blood supply, and stability of the fracture usually is present in 3–6 weeks, with excellent healing expected within 2 months. Because of the dense plexus of nerves about the

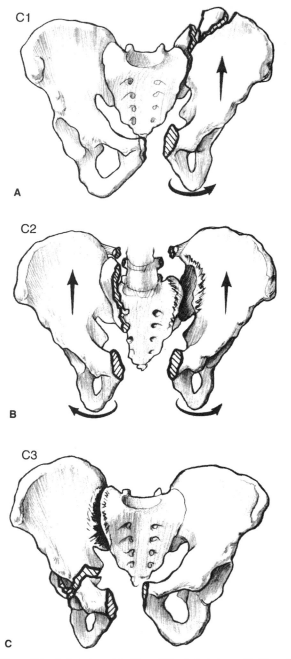

FIG. 21-3. A: Type C1 pelvic injury. **B:** Type C2 pelvic injury. **C:** Type C3 pelvic injury. (From Hansen ST, Swiontkowski MF. *Orthopaedic trauma protocols.* New York: Raven, 1993:229.)

sacrum and coccyx, injuries to this area may produce chronic pain, especially if the patient is not encouraged to accept some discomfort and start an early active exercise program.

B. **Type B fractures** (rotationally unstable, but vertically and posteriorly stable) must be treated on an individual basis. Fracture displacements, associated injuries, age of the patient, and functional demands should be taken into account (2,16). In open-book fractures, disruption of the anterior sacroiliac joints occurs if the displacement is more than 2.5 cm. These may be reduced and stabilized by external fixation or plate fixation across the symphysis (9,11). The authors generally prefer plate fixation because of the problems with patient comfort, pin tract infection, and loosening and loss of reduction with external fixation (6,8,10). Minimally displaced B1, B2, and B3 injuries may be treated conservatively with bed to wheelchair mobilization for 6–8 weeks, followed by crutch ambulation with weight bearing to tolerance on the side of the pelvis where the posterior ring is uninjured or more stable. Internal fixation is used for more widely displaced and unstable injuries (6,11,16). Traction is not recommended because of patient morbidity and the inability to improve fracture displacements.

C. **Type C** minimally displaced isolated injuries, especially those involving the ilium, may be treated conservatively as in **B.** However, patients need to be followed up closely roentgenographically and, if fracture displacement is increasing, reduction and fixation treatment is indicated. Improved results with internal fixation over traction treatment have been documented (11). If seen early on, then fractures of the sacrum and sacroiliac joints can be managed with closed reduction and percutaneous lag screw fixation (6,16). Because of the complexity of reduction and fixation techniques as well as the potential for high morbidity resulting from adjacent neurovascular structures, patients with type C injuries should be referred to an experienced pelvic and acetabular surgeon.

VII. Complications

A. Complications from **associated injuries** (e.g., of the bladder, cranium, chest)

B. **Persistent symptoms from sacroiliac joint instability,** including pain and leg length inequality

C. **Chronic pain patterns** from injuries around the coccyx and sacrum and sacroiliac joint (3,14), including dyspareunia

D. **Persistent neurologic deficit** from nerve root injury with L5, S1, and distal sacral root injuries most common; erectile dysfunction is common in males

E. **Pulmonary and fat emboli**

F. **Infection** from bacterial seeding of the large hematomas or from open pelvic fractures (7). Injuries to the large bowel are not uncommon.

HCMC Treatment Recommendations

Pelvic Ring Fractures

   Diagnosis: Anteroposterior pelvic radiograph, inlet-outlet views, physical examination, CT scan

   Treatment: Management of hemorrhage, limited weight bearing (6–8 weeks) for lateral compression fractures that do not have significant deformity, non–weight bearing for other nondisplaced patterns for 8–12 weeks, follow-up radiographs to check for late instability

   Indications for surgery: Ongoing hemorrhage (external fixation or posterior pelvic clamp), displaced posterior pelvic injury, symphysis widening more than 2.5 cm, unacceptable pelvic deformity

   Recommended technique: Symphysis plating, posterior iliosacral screws. Open reduction and iliosacral screw placement is safest; consider percutaneous iliosacral screws in thin patient with minimal deformity. Occasionally, anterior sacroiliac joint fixation is performed if posterior skin is not safe or if the injury is associated with an ipsilateral acetabular fracture.

References

1. Apprahamian C, Gessert G, Bandyk D, et al. MAST–associated compartment syndrome (MACS): a review. *J Trauma* 1989;29:549–555.
2. Burgess AR, Eastridge BJ, Young JWR, et al. Pelvic ring disruptions: effective classification system and treatment protocol. *J Trauma* 1990;30:848–856.
3. Copeland CE, Bosse MJ, McCarthy ML, et al. Effect of trauma and pelvis fracture on female genitourinary, sexual and reproductive function. *J Orthop Trauma* 1997; 11:73–81.
4. Cotler HB, LaMont JB, Hansen ST. Immediate spica cast for pelvic fractures. *J Orthop Trauma* 1988;2:222.
5. Ganz R, Krushell RJ, Jakob RP, et al. The antishock pelvic clamp. *Clin Orthop* 1991;267:71–78.
6. Gruen GS, Leit ME, Gruen RJ, et al. The acute management of neurodynamically unstable multiple trauma patients with pelvic ring fractures. *J Trauma* 1994; 36:706–713.
7. Hak DJ, Olson SA, Matta JM. Diagnosis and management of closed internal degloving injuries associated with pelvic and acetabular fractures: the Morel-Lavallee lesion. *J Trauma* 1997;42:1048–1051.
8. Hupel TM, McKee MD, Waddell JP, et al. Primary external fixation of rotationally unstable pelvic fractures in obese patients. *J Trauma* 1998;45:111–115.
9. Kellam JF. The role of external fixation in pelvic disruptions. *Clin Orthop* 1989; 241:66.
10. Lindahl J, Hirvensalo E, Bostman O, et al. Failure of reduction with an external fixator in the management of injuries of the pelvic ring—long-term evaluation of 110 patients. *J Bone Joint Surg (Br)* 1999;81:955–962.
11. Matta JM, Sacedo T. Internal fixation of pelvic ring fractures. *Clin Orthop* 1989; 242:83.
12. Mattox KL, Bickell W, Pepe PE, et al. Prospective MAST study in 911 patients. *J Trauma* 1989;29:1104–1112.
13. Mendez C, Grubler KD, Maier RV. Diagnostic accuracy of peritoneal lavage in patients with pelvic fractures. *Arch Surg* 1994;129:477–481.
14. Nepola JV, Trenhaile SW, Miranda M, et al. Vertical shear injuries: is there a relationship between residual displacement and functional outcome? *J Trauma* 1999; 46:1024–1030.
15. Poole GV, Ward EF, Muakkassa FF, et al. Pelvic fractures from major blunt trauma; outcome is determined by associated injuries. *Ann Surg* 1991;213:532–539.
16. Routt ML Jr, Kreger PI, Simonian PT, et al. Early results of percutaneous iliosacral screws placed with the patient in the supine position. *J Orthop Trauma* 1995; 9:207–214.
17. Tile M. Pelvic ring fractures: should they be fixed? *J Bone Joint Surg* 1988;70B:1.

Selected Historical Readings

Bucholz RW. The pathological anatomy of the Malgaigne fracture-dislocation of the pelvis. *J Bone Joint Surg* 1981;63A:400.
Peltier LF. Complications associated with fractures of the pelvis. *J Bone Joint Surg* 1965;47A:1060.
Rafii M, et al. The impact of CT in clinical management of pelvic and acetabular fractures. *Clin Orthop* 1983;178:228.
Saibil EA, Maggisano R, Witchell SS. Angiography in the diagnosis and treatment of trauma. *Can Assoc Radiol J* 1983;34:218.

22. HIP DISLOCATIONS, FEMORAL HEAD FRACTURES, AND ACETABULAR FRACTURES

I. **Introduction.** A hip dislocation, with or without associated acetabular fracture, is a major injury. The forces needed to cause hip dislocation are considerable, and, in addition to the disruption noted on roentgenography, soft-tissue injury is significant. Occasionally, small osseous or cartilaginous fragments become loose in the joint. The injury is most frequently caused by an automobile or automobile-pedestrian accident, so significant injury elsewhere in the body is likely. A fracture or fracture-dislocation at the hip can easily be missed when associated with an ipsilateral extremity injury. Such an injury emphasizes the rule: always visualize the joint above and the joint below the diaphyseal fracture. Because injuries about the pelvis can be missed in a seriously traumatized patient, most authorities advocate a routine pelvic roentgenogram for all patients involved in severe trauma. The condition is viewed as an orthopaedic emergency. In general, the sooner the reduction is achieved, the better is the end result (2,20).

II. **Classification of dislocations**
   A. **Anterior dislocations**
      1. **Obturator**
      2. **Iliac**
      3. **Pubic**
      4. **Associated femoral head fractures** (see **V**)
   B. **Posterior dislocations**
      1. **Without fracture**
      2. **With posterior wall fracture** (see **IV**)
      3. **With femoral head fracture** (see **V**)

III. **Anterior dislocations**
   A. This injury usually occurs in an automobile accident, in a severe fall, or from a blow to the back while squatting. The **mechanism of injury** is forced abduction. The neck of the femur or trochanter impinges on the rim of the acetabulum and levers the femoral head out through a tear in the anterior capsule. If in relative extension, an iliac or pubic dislocation occurs; if the hip is in flexion, an obturator dislocation occurs. In many instances, there is an associated impaction or shear fracture of the femoral head as the head passes superiorly over the anteroinferior rim of the acetabulum. These injuries are associated with poor long-term results (1,9,18).
   B. On **examination** with an **obturator dislocation,** the hip is abducted, externally rotated, and flexed, but in the **iliac or pubic dislocation,** the hip may be extended. The femoral head can usually be palpated near the anterior iliac spine in an iliac dislocation or in the groin in a pubic dislocation. In all patients, carefully assess the circulatory and neurologic status before attempting a reduction. The diagnosis is readily apparent on roentgenogram, which shows the femoral head out of the acetabulum in an inferior and medial position.
   C. **Treatment** (1, 20). Early closed reduction is the treatment of choice, but open reduction may be necessary. Reduction is optimally attempted under spinal or general anesthesia, which ensures complete muscle relaxation. In the multiply injured patient, reduction may be attempted in the emergency department with sedation or paralysis after the airway is controlled. Initiate strong but gentle traction along the axis of the femur while an assistant applies stabilization of the pelvis by pressure on the anterior iliac crests. For the **obturator dislocation,** the traction is continued while the hip is gently flexed, and the reduction is accomplished usually by gentle internal rotation. A final maneuver of adduction completes the reduction but should not be attempted until the head has cleared the rim of the acetabulum with traction in the flexed position. For the **iliac or pubic dislocation,** the head should be

pulled distal to the acetabulum. The hip is gently flexed and internally rotated. No adduction is necessary. If the hip does not reduce easily, forceful attempts are not indicated. Failure to obtain easy reduction with the above maneuvers usually indicates that traction is increasing the tension on the iliopsoas or closing a rent in the anterior capsule, producing a "buttonhole" effect. Forced maneuvers only increase the damage. Because the closed reduction may fail, the patient is initially prepared for an open procedure. The open reduction can be accomplished through a muscle-splitting incision, using the lower portion of the standard anterior approach. The structures preventing the reduction are released. The postreduction treatment is the same as for a posterior dislocation of the hip, except it is important to avoid excessive abduction and external rotation.

D. Prognosis and complications. Excellent reviews of hip dislocations are recorded, and they report anterior dislocations occurring in approximately 13% of some 1,000 hip dislocations. Early reduction is necessary if a satisfactory result is to be obtained, and although the end result is frequently excellent in the child, traumatic arthrosis and, occasionally, avascular necrosis make the prognosis guarded in the adult. Recurrent dislocation is rare in an adult (1,2,20).

IV. Posterior dislocations

A. The **mechanism of injury** is usually a force applied against the flexed knee with the hip in flexion, as occurs most commonly when the knee strikes the dashboard of an automobile during a head-on impact. If the hip is in neutral or adduction at the time of impact, a simple dislocation is likely, but if the hip is in slight abduction, an associated fracture of the posterior or posterosuperior acetabulum can result. As the degree of hip flexion increases, it is more probable that a simple dislocation is produced.

B. Physical examination reveals that the leg is shortened, internally rotated, and adducted. A careful physical examination should be carried out before reduction. Sciatic nerve injury is associated with 10%–13% of these injuries (16). Associated bony or ligamentous injury to the ipsilateral knee, femoral head, or femoral shaft is not uncommon. When associated with a femoral shaft fracture, a dislocation may go unrecognized because the classic position of flexion, internal rotation, and adduction is not apparent. In this situation, the diagnosis is confirmed by a single anteroposterior roentgenogram of the pelvis as part of the initial trauma roentgenographic series. This single examination does not allow adequate assessment of any associated acetabular fracture (10,11,12), however, so more roentgenograms are needed for treatment planning before carrying out a reduction if an acetabular fracture is suspected. The patient, not the x-ray beam, is moved to obtain the following films: the anteroposterior obturator oblique and the iliac oblique views (10,13). This is best accomplished by keeping the patient on a backboard and using foam blocks to support the oblique position of the board (Fig. 22-1). If necessary, computed tomography (CT) scanning can also be performed; optimally, this is done after the closed reduction to reestablish femoral head circulation. Although some authors question its routine use after uneventful closed reduction, others report a 50% incidence of bony fragments being identified with CT (3,7,13,17).

C. Treatment

1. Posterior dislocation without fracture. This dislocation is reduced as soon as possible and always within 8–12 hours when possible. Reduction is accomplished with the Allis maneuver under spinal or general anesthesia to overcome the significant muscle spasm. The essential step in a reduction is traction in the line of the deformity, followed by gentle flexion of the hip to 90 degrees while an assistant stabilizes the pelvis with pressure on the iliac spine. With continued traction, the hip then is gently rotated into internal and external rotation, which usually brings about a prompt restoration of position. Be-

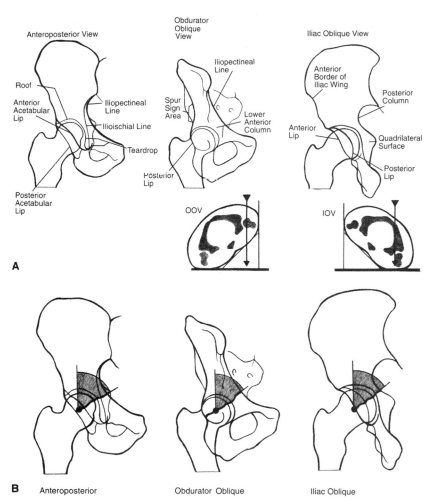

FIG. 22-1. Radiographic assessment of acetabular fractures. **A:** The anteroposterior, obturator oblique, and iliac views are essential for the definition of the fracture. **B:** The "roof arc" measurement is made between a vertical line and the angle of the fracture. Angles greater than 40° on all 3 views indicate a fracture which may be treated non-operatively. (From Hansen ST, Swiontkowski MF. *Orthopaedic trauma protocols.* New York: Raven, 1993:249.)

cause considerable traction is required, even with good muscle relaxation, the alternative method of Stimson may be attempted. The patient is placed prone with the hip flexed over the end of the table, and an assistant fixes the pelvis by extending the opposite leg. The same traction maneuvers described earlier are completed, but the pull is toward the floor with pressure behind the flexed knee. Although considerable traction is necessary, under no circumstances should rough or sudden manipulative movement be attempted. Postreduction stability should be confirmed on physical examination and by a roentgenogram obtained in the operating room to be sure there are no fractures around the femoral head or neck.

a. **Postreduction treatment.** Isometric exercises for the hip musculature are instituted as soon as pain subsides sufficiently. Continuous passive motion (CPM) may be useful to maintain joint motion but is not essential. There is no consensus in the literature as to the length of time the patient should be restricted from weight bearing. The authors favor bed rest until the patient is pain-free and has established near-normal abduction and extension muscle power. The patient then is allowed to move around, using crutches for protective weight bearing until it is determined that he or she can ambulate without pain or an antalgic limp; this generally takes 3–6 weeks. At that time, full weight bearing is permitted.

b. **Prognosis and complications**

   (1) **Sciatic nerve injuries** are discussed in **IV 2.c and e.**

   (2) **Avascular necrosis of the femoral head** is the most feared delayed complication from a simple posterior dislocation of the hip. It occurs late, but various authors have noted an average time of 17–24 months from injury to time of diagnosis. Rates of approximately 6%–27% are variously reported, and figures show an incidence of 15.5% for early closed reductions, increasing to 48% if reduction is delayed. There were no good results if reduction was delayed more than 48 hours. In Epstein's classic study of 426 cases, better results were obtained with open reduction and internal fixation in patients who had associated fractures (see Selected Historical Readings). The overall rate of avascular necrosis was 13.4% with a higher rate of 18% in patients with associated fractures. For fracture-dislocations treated by open means, the avascular necrosis rate was only 5.5%. Treatment of avascular necrosis is discussed in Chap. 23, **I.I.2.**

   (3) Epstein also reported an overall rate of **traumatic osteoarthritis** of 23% following posterior hip dislocations, with a rate of 35% in dislocations treated by closed means and a rate of 17% in those treated by open means: In another series, after 14½ years of follow-up, 16% of patients had posttraumatic arthritis and arthritis developed in an additional 8% as a result of avascular necrosis (20). Similar results have been reported from other centers (2,20).

2. **Posterior dislocation with associated acetabular fracture**

   a. As previously noted, the **dislocation is reduced as soon as possible considering the patient's other injuries.** If the patient needs to undergo a lengthy trauma evaluation, then an attempt can be made in the emergency department to reduce the hip with sedation. In the patient who has been intubated for airway control, chemical paralysis totally eliminates muscle spasm. If reduction attempts fail, then the urgency for hip reduction must be transmitted to the trauma team leader so the patient can be brought to the operating room earlier in the evaluation phase. An alternative to standard closed reduction maneuvers involves inserting a 5-mm Schanz pin into the ipsilateral proximal femur at the level of the lesser trochanter. This allows more focused lateral and distal traction by a second assistant to accompany the reduction maneuver. If this maneuver fails, then open reduction is preferred via a posterior approach. A posterior wall fracture is internally fixed with lag screws and a neutralization plate after joint lavage. If a more complex acetabular fracture is present, then an experienced acetabular and pelvic surgeon should be consulted (8). If the basic posterior acetabular anatomy appears intact and the joint debridement is complete, then a CT scan should be obtained to check on the adequacy of debridement and to evaluate for associated fractures (7,9).

       b. Postoperative treatment. Historically, traction has been used postoperatively, but this is no longer recommended. With stable internal fixation, early motion is advised starting with CPM. Flexion is generally limited to 60 degrees for the first 6 weeks postoperatively for large posterior wall fractures (8). Weight bearing is limited and crutches are used for 12 weeks (10–13).

       c. Sciatic nerve injury. Direct contusion, partial laceration by bone fragments, a traction injury, or occasionally an iatrogenic injury resulting from malplacement of retractors during open reduction can cause this injury. Nerve injury should be evaluated early by a careful motor and sensory examination before reduction. If the nerve function is normal before reduction and is abnormal after reduction, then this may represent sciatic nerve entrapment in a fracture line. Emergent open reduction and nerve exploration are indicated (10–13). The peroneal portion of the sciatic nerve is most commonly injured because it lies against the bone in the sciatic notch. When the entire distal sciatic nerve function is abnormal, the tibial portion of function returns nearly 100% of the time. The peroneal portion of function is regained in 60%–70% of cases: The more dense the motor injury, the less likely is the return of good function (16). The postinjury foot drop is generally easily managed by a plastic ankle-foot orthotic. Tendon transfers at a later date remain an option.

      d. Prognosis and complications. Late traumatic arthritis and femoral head avascular necrosis can result in 20%–30% of cases (8,10–13). Of all acetabular fractures, the posterior wall injury, despite its being the simplest pattern, has the worst prognosis with regard to these complications (15,22). Total hip arthroplasty is the most acceptable reconstruction option when these complications occur: Long-term results in this situation are not as predictable as with total hip arthroplasty for arthritis (15,20). Most patients who sustain these injuries are younger than 50 years of age, so loosening of the components over the patient's lifetime is a real concern (22).

V. Fractures of the femoral head

  A. Diagnosis. Fractures of the femoral head generally occur with an associated hip dislocation. They are seen as abrasion or indentation fractures of the superior aspect of the head in association with an anterior dislocation or as shear fractures of the inferior aspect of the head in association with a posterior dislocation. Comminuted head fractures occasionally occur with severe trauma. Femoral neck or acetabular fractures may be involved. The diagnosis is established by roentgenograms and CT scan.

  B. Treatment

    1. Emergent. Early treatment must focus on reducing the hip dislocation and diagnosing the fracture pattern. Diagnosis, made by clinical examination, is confirmed by the admission anteroposterior pelvic roentgenogram. Great care should be given in evaluating the roentgenograms before reducing the hip, because nondisplaced associated femoral neck fractures may be displaced with the reduction maneuver. If these are noted, the reduction should be performed in the operating room under fluoroscopy so that, if the femoral neck fracture appears unstable with the reduction maneuver, the surgeon can proceed with an open reduction. If the closed reduction is successful, a repeat roentgenogram is obtained to confirm the reduction and a CT scan should be obtained for treatment planning.

    2. Definitive. If the femoral head fracture is an indentation fracture associated with an anterior dislocation, early CPM and mobilization with crutches (partial weight bearing) are indicated. The prognosis regarding degenerative joint disease is poor, however (1,9,18,19).

    a. If the femoral head fracture is a shear fracture associated with a posterior dislocation and is of small size **(Pipkin type I, infrafoveal),** the treatment can involve a brief period of traction for comfort followed by mobilization with a restriction of flexion to less than 60 degrees for 6 weeks. Indications for surgery include a restriction of hip motion resulting from an incarcerated fragment and multiple traumas. The fracture should be approached anteriorly for best visualization (19).

    b. If the fracture is of larger size **(Pipkin type II, suprafoveal),** the reduction should be anatomic or within 1 mm on the postreduction CT to proceed with conservative treatment as outlined earlier. If it is displaced, open reduction and internal fixation with well-recessed (countersink) screws using an anterior approach is indicated (19).

    c. If the fracture is associated with a femoral neck fracture **(Pipkin type III),** both fractures should be internally fixed via an anterior approach, and early motion with CPM should be initiated. The prognosis for this combination injury is not as favorable as with isolated femoral head fractures because of the higher incidence of posttraumatic osteonecrosis associated with the neck fracture.

    d. Femoral head fractures associated with acetabular fractures **(Pipkin type IV)** should be managed in tandem with the acetabular fracture. Generally this is accomplished operatively by an experienced pelvic surgeon (10–12).

VI. Acetabular fractures without posterior dislocation

  A. Mechanism of injury. These fractures result from a blow on the greater trochanter or with axial loading of the thigh with the limb in an abducted position.

  B. Physical examination. These patients often have multiple injuries, so the management of the patient is the same as outlined in Chap. 1. A careful examination of the sciatic nerve function must be conducted. The muscles innervated by the femoral and obturator nerves must also be examined, because they can occasionally be injured with complex anterior column fractures. The anteroposterior pelvis admission trauma film and the two 45-degree pelvic oblique views described by Judet (Fig. 22-1), as well as a CT scan of the pelvis (10–13), are used to evaluate the fracture pattern. The scan is helpful in determining the presence of intraarticular bone fragments, femoral head fractures, and displacement in the weight-bearing region of the acetabulum (17). Roof arc measurements are useful for treatment planning (Fig. 22-1.).

  C. Treatment

    1. Nonoperative. Traction was once the recommended treatment for all acetabular fractures (6). With modern techniques, nearly all significantly displaced acetabular fractures can be fixed safely and effectively, even in elderly individuals (5,8,10–13). As definitive therapy, traction is not currently generally recommended. It is generally reserved for temporary treatment of displaced transverse acetabular fractures in which the femoral head is articulating on the ridge of the fracture edge on the lateral portion of the joint. Traction prevents further cartilage injury and femoral head indentation; however, it must be heavy (35–50 lb) and with a distal femoral pin. Trochanteric pins to provide a lateral traction vector should never be used if open reduction is an option at any time in the patient's management. If nonoperative management is selected, then bed-to-chair mobilization for 6–8 weeks is the best option, followed by gradual return to weight bearing. Total hip arthroplasty is an effective salvage technique as long as the acetabular anatomy is not too distorted (15,22).

    2. Operative. In young patients, displacement of 2–3 mm in the major weight-bearing portions of the acetabulum is an indication for open reduction (10–13). Numerous surgical approaches to reduction are available, including the Kocher-Langenbach posterolateral approach, the ilioinguinal, the extended iliofemoral, and combined approaches. These procedures should be undertaken by experienced acetabular surgeons because the techniques for reduction and fixation are numerous and require much special equipment; inferior results are documented by surgeons who are inexperienced (8). Postoperatively, CPM is frequently used along with 12 weeks of "touch down" weight bearing with crutches. If posterior wall involvement is significant, then flexion is restricted to 60 degrees for the first 6 weeks: Complications include infection (1%–2%), heterotopic ossification (4%–6% functionally limiting), avascular necrosis (5%), deep venous thrombosis (10%–20%), pulmonary embolus (1% fatal), degenerative arthritis (20%–30%, generally associated with posterior wall fractures), and sciatic nerve injury (2%–5%) (4,5 ,8,14,21). Heterotopic ossification is most commonly associated with extended posterior (the extended iliofemoral) and combined approaches (4): All of these complications occur more often when surgeons are inexperienced. Effective prophylaxis includes indomethacin, 25 mg tid for 6 weeks, and low-dose irradiation (800–1,000 R) in the first week postoperatively (8,14).

VI. **Acetabular fractures in association with fractures of the femoral head, neck, or shaft.** Associated injuries of the femur are not uncommon. They should be dealt with by internal fixation, then the acetabular injury should be treated as outlined previously (10–13). Attempts at treating both injuries by traction have not been satisfactory.

VII. **Traction.** The use of traction in the lower extremity is discussed in Chap. 9, **VII.** Classic balanced traction with a half or a full ring Thomas splint is not only cumbersome but also restricts the use of the hip in the muscle rehabilitation program. A hip exerciser such as that described by Fry should be considered. These techniques must be learned because they are occasionally needed in treating problems associated with severe preexisting systemic disease or local skin problems.

VIII. **Traumatic dislocation of the hip joint in children.** This condition is fairly uncommon.
   A. **Immediate reduction is essential.** Delaying reduction for more than 24 hours increases the incidence of avascular necrosis.
   B. **Weight bearing should be prohibited for 3 months** (a spica cast is recommended for children younger than 8 years of age), at which time it usually is possible to determine the degree of avascular necrosis, although a 3-year follow-up period is necessary to assess this complication fully. Institution of prompt treatment and protected weight bearing as for Legg-Calvé-Perthes disease probably is indicated. Recurrent dislocation can occur in children who are not immobilized.
   C. When reduction is achieved rapidly with no gross associated trauma, the **results are usually satisfactory,** especially in patients younger than 6 years. The incidence of avascular necrosis, however, has been reported to be approximately 5%–10%.

HCMC Treatment Recommendations

Hip Dislocations

   Diagnosis: Anteroposterior pelvic radiograph, and physical examination. Leg is shortened and internally rotated for posterior dislocation and flexed and externally rotated for anterior dislocation. Judet views and CT scan are obtained after redcuction.

   Treatment: Reduction in emergency department with sedation and analgesia; reduction in operating room if other injuries so require

   Indications for surgery: Irreducible dislocation, intraarticular loose bodies diagnosed on postreduction radiographs or CT scan

   Recommended technique: Hip arthroscopy for small loose bodies, arthrotomy with posterior approach for irreducible dislocation

---

HCMC Treatment Recommendations
Femoral Head Fractures
  Diagnosis: Anteroposterior pelvis radiograph and physical examination—these nearly always accompany a hip dislocation, 90% of which are posterior dislocations
  Treatment: Closed reduction of hip (see previous discussion) followed by CT scan to assess size and reduction of fragment. If reduction is anatomic, limited weight bearing with crutches for 6 weeks
  Indications for surgery: Displaced large head fragment (Pipkin II, >2 mm displaced) or displaced type III or IV fracture
  Recommended technique: Open reduction with internal fixation (ORIF) via anterior approach, fixation with counter sunk lag screws

---

HCMC Treatment Recommendations
Acetabular Fractures
  Diagnosis: Anteroposterior pelvic and Judet views, CT scan, physical examination
  Treatment: ORIF of displaced (>2 mm) intraarticular components, 6–8 weeks of partial weight bearing for nondisplaced fractures
  Indications for surgery: Displaced articular component
  Recommended technique: Surgical approach of ilioinguinal, Kocher-Langenbach or extended approach based on fracture pattern and experience of surgeon. Fixation with lag screws and reconstruction plates. Limited weight bearing for 12 weeks.

References

1. DeLee JC, Evans JA, Thomas J. Anterior dislocation of the hip and associated femoral head fractures. *J Bone Joint Surg (Am)* 1980;62:960.
2. Dreinhofer KE, Schwarzkopf SR, Haas NP, et al. Isolated traumatic dislocation of the hip; long-term results in 50 patients. *J Bone Joint Surg (Br)* 1994;76:6–12.
3. Frick SL, Sims SH. Is computed tomography useful after simple posterior hip dislocation? *J Orthop Trauma* 1995;9:388–391.
4. Ghalambour N, Matta JM, Bernstein L. Heterotopic ossification following operative treatment of acetabular fracture. An analysis of risk factors. *Clin Orthop* 1994;305:96–105.
5. Helfet DL, Borrelli J, DiPasquale T, et al. Stabilization of acetabular fractures in elderly patients. *J Bone Joint Surg (Am)* 1992;74:753–764.
6. Hesp W, Goris R. Conservative treatment of fractures of the acetabulum: results after long-term follow-up. *Acta Chir Belg* 1988;88:27.
7. Hougaard K, Jaersgaard-Anderson P, Kuut E. CT scanning following traumatic dislocation of the hip. *Int J Orthop Trauma* 1994;4:68–69.
8. Kaempfte FA, Bone LB, Border JR. Open reduction and internal fixation of acetabular fractures: heterotopic ossification and other complications of treatment. *J Orthop Trauma* 1991;5:439–445.
9. Konrath GA, Hamel AI, Guemin J, et al. Biomechanical evaluation of impaction fractures of the femoral head. *J Orthop Trauma* 1999;13:407–413.
10. Matta JM, et al. Fractures of the acetabulum: A retrospective analysis. *Clin Orthop* 1986;205:230.
11. Matta JM. Fractures of the acetabulum: accuracy of reduction and clinical results in patients managed operatively within three weeks after the injury. *J Bone Joint Surg (Am)* 1996;78:1632–1645.
12. Matta JR, Mehne DK, Roffi R. Fractures of the acetabulum: early results of a prospective study. *Clin Orthop* 1986;205:241.

13. Mayo KA. Fractures of the acetabulum. *Orthop Clin North Am* 1987;18:43.
14. McLaren AC. Prophylaxis with indomethacin for heterotopic bone after open reduction of fractures of the acetabulum. *J Bone Joint Surg (Am)* 1990;72:245–247.
15. Rumness DW, Lewallen D. Total hip arthroplasty after fracture of the acetabulum. *J Bone Joint Surg (Br)* 1990;72:761–764.
16. Seddon HJ. *Surgical disorders of the peripheral nerves,* 2nd ed. New York: Churchill Livingstone, 1975.
17. St: Pierre RK, et al. Computerized tomography in the evaluation and classification of fractures of the acetabulum. *Clin Orthop* 1984;188:234.
18. Swiontkowski MF. Femoral head fractures. *Curr Orthop* 1991;5:99.
19. Swiontkowski MF, Thorpe M, Seiler JG, et al. Operative management of displaced femoral head fractures: case matched comparison of anterior versus posterior approaches for Pipkin I and Pipkin II fractures. *J Orthop Trauma* 1992;6:437.
20. Upadhyay SS, Moulton A, Srikrishnamurthy K. An analysis of the late effects of traumatic posterior dislocation of the hip without fractures. *J Bone Joint Surg (Br)* 1983;65:150.
21. Webb LX, Rush PT, Fuller SB, et al. Greenfield filter prophylaxis of pulmonary embolism in patients undergoing surgery for acetabular fracture. *J Orthop Trauma* 1992;6:139–145.
22. Weber M, Berry DJ, Harmsen WS. Total hip arthroplasty after operative treatment of an acetabular fracture. *J Bone Joint Surg (Am)* 1998;80:1295–1305.

Selected Historical Readings

Brav EA. Traumatic dislocation of the hip joint. *J Bone Joint Surg (Am)* 1962;44:1115.
Epstein HC. *Traumatic dislocations of the hip.* Baltimore: Williams & Wilkins, 1980.
Epstein HC. Posterior fracture-dislocations of the hip. *J Bone Joint Surg (Am)* 1974; 56:1103.
Epstein HC, Harvey JP. Traumatic anterior dislocations of the hip. *Orthop Rev* 1972; 1:33.
Funk FJ Jr. Traumatic dislocations of the hip in children. *J Bone Joint Surg (Am)* 1962; 44:1135.
Hunter GAP. Posterior dislocation and fracture-dislocation of the hip. *J Bone Joint Surg (Br)* 1969;51:38.
Judet R, Judet J, Letournel E. Fractures of the acetabulum: classification and surgical approaches for open reduction. *J Bone Joint Surg (Am)* 1964;46:1615.
Letournel E. *Fractures of the acetabulum.* New York: Springer-Verlag, 1981.
Moore TM. Central acetabular fracture secondary to epileptic seizure. *J Bone Joint Surg (Am)* 1970;52:1459.
Pearson DE, Mann RJ. Traumatic hip dislocation in children. *Clin Orthop* 1973;92:189.
Pipkin G. Treatment of grade IV fracture-dislocation of the hip. *J Bone Joint Surg (Am)* 1957;39:1027.
Stewart MJ, Milford LW. Fracture-dislocation of the hip. *J Bone Joint Surg (Am)* 1954; 36:315.

23. FRACTURES OF THE FEMUR

I. **Fractures of the femoral neck**
A. **Mechanism of injury.** Femoral neck fractures are uncommon in patients younger than the age of 50 years; patients in this age group account for approximately 5% of the total number of cases (55). These fractures result from high-energy trauma. They become more common with increasing age, and always involve some trauma, generally a fall onto the side of the fracture. Osteoporosis is a common finding and factors such as early menopause, alcoholism, smoking, low body weight, steroid therapy, phenytoin treatment, and lack of exercise all predispose patients to femoral neck fractures. Excessive use of sedative drugs has also been implicated (46). Typical patients are female, fair, thin, and with a history of early menopause and poor dietary habits. Individuals in whom a femoral neck fracture develops have a greater degree of osteoporosis than other individuals; some element of trauma is a factor. Efforts at preventing falls in elderly persons seem to have the most potential for controlling this phenomenon. Stress fractures that occur in highly active patients with normal bone along the superior aspect of the femoral neck are called *tension fractures*. These fractures can also occur in elderly patients who have been inactive for long periods of time and who suddenly become active. The compression stress fracture, which occurs at the base of the femoral neck, is even more common in these patients. These fractures are less likely to displace.
B. **Classification of fractures.** From the clinical standpoint, neck fractures are of **four basic types:** the stress fracture, the impacted fracture, the nondisplaced fracture, and the displaced fracture.
C. **Symptoms and signs of injury.** Patients with stress fractures, nondisplaced fractures, or impacted fractures may complain only of **pain in the groin** or sometimes pain in the ipsilateral knee (23). The patients with stress fractures have a history of a recent increase in activity, may only walk with an antalgic gait, and may believe themselves to have a muscle strain. In contrast, patients with nondisplaced or impacted fractures have some element of trauma. They generally have a higher intensity of pain, can associate the onset with an event, and are seen early for medical treatment. In all three groups of patients, there is no obvious deformity on physical examination, but there is generally pain with internal rotation. Patients with traumatic fractures have more discomfort. A high index of suspicion must be maintained to avoid delay in diagnosis. Patients with displaced femoral neck fractures complain of pain in the entire hip region and lie with the affected limb shortened and externally rotated. Roentgenograms obtained early diagnose impacted and nondisplaced fractures, but technetium bone scans or magnetic resonance imaging (MRI) studies may be required to diagnose stress fractures if symptoms are of recent onset. MRI has been shown to be the quickest, most cost-effective way of making the diagnosis. Comparing the impaired hip to the unimpaired on the anteroposterior pelvis film yields the diagnosis in most traumatic cases, but occasionally tomography is helpful. The diagnosis should simply be confirmed with roentgenograms; movement of the limb to elicit pain or crepitus is not necessary. An anteroposterior pelvis and high-quality cross-table lateral (obtained by flexing the uninjured, not the injured, hip) are necessary for planning treatment. Patients should be allowed to rest with the limbs in the most comfortable position, which is generally in slight flexion on a pillow. Traction is not necessary and may increase pain.
D. **Treatment**
1. **Stress fractures.** These fractures commonly occur in young, vigorous individuals and, if protected, heal without incident. They should be treated by relieving weight-bearing and stressful non–weight-bearing

positions (23). Crutches or a walker is adequate, but patients should be cautioned not to attempt straight-leg raising exercises and not to use the leg for leverage in rising or in changing positions, particularly getting up out of a chair. Partial weight bearing is safe within 6 weeks, with full weight bearing in 12 weeks, as long as the fracture shows roentgenographic evidence of healing, which is evidenced by sclerosis at the superior femoral neck. In unreliable patients or in elderly patients with a tension (superior neck) fracture, it is wise to carry out internal fixation with multiple pins (percutaneous), especially if the hip cannot be protected against increased stress. Compression types of fractures in elderly individuals generally do well with limiting activity as outlined above.

2. **Impacted fractures**
   a. These can be treated either **nonoperatively** or **operatively** (55). With the nonoperative method, the patient usually is kept in bed for a few days with the leg protected from rotation stresses until the muscle spasms subside. A program of protected ambulation, as outlined for stress fractures, is then initiated. Displacement rates are in the range of 10%–20%. Because the risk of posttraumatic osteonecrosis then doubles, the authors recommend internal fixation with multiple pins or screws.
   b. **Internal fixation** appears to have many advantages over nonoperative methods, especially using percutaneous technique. A union rate of 100% in operative cases has been reported, as opposed to 88% with closed management. The rate of avascular necrosis was not altered, however. The authors recommend multiple screw fixation, either percutaneous or by open technique, because it allows immediate weight bearing (58) (see **I.F**).

3. **Displaced fractures.** The treatment decision should be based on the activity level of the patient before the fracture because this is an indirect measure of bone density (55).
   a. Displaced fractures, in community ambulators, with or without slight comminution, should be **reduced, impacted,** and **internally fixed.** When surgical repair was carried out within the first 12 hours, a 25% rate of avascular necrosis was reported, increasing to 30% with surgery between 13 and 24 hours, 40% between 24 and 48 hours, and 100% after 1 week. Intracapsular tamponade from fracture hematoma has an unfavorable effect on femoral head blood flow, as does nonanatomic position, so there is a rationale for proceeding with some urgency (33,34,40,50,53,55,57). However, patients with dehydration or unstable cardiac conditions should be reducibly stabilized before surgery to minimize the risk of fatality (26). There is consensus that accurate reduction and impaction at the fracture site are essential to a good end result.
      (1) Authorities who stress an **anatomic reduction with impaction** believe that this allows the maximum opportunity for reestablishment of the vascular supply. Any stretch or kinking of the vessels of the ligamentum teres or retinaculum is avoided while stability of the fracture is optimized (40). Internal fixation with three pins or screws secures fracture stability; there is no value in using more than three implants (58). Fracture stability is determined by the bone density and quality of reduction rather than by the number of implants (58).
      (2) Authorities who stress a **valgus reduction** believe that this position allows for maximum bone-on-bone stability. In a valgus nailing, the nail or screw is near the center of the head, but the nail is rested along the calcar of the femoral neck to reduce the distance between the fulcrum of the nail or screw and the head. This positioning produces a shorter biomechanical

moment and less stress on the device. Concern that the fixation cuts out superiorly or anteriorly can be eliminated by proper impaction of the fracture and the use of multiple pins or a sliding fixation apparatus (40,58).

   b. The **authors believe that an anatomic reduction is preferable to the valgus reduction, but when faced with a choice between slight valgus and any varus, then slight valgus is chosen.**

E. Reduction techniques

   1. The authors favor a **closed reduction** on a fracture table that then allows for the insertion of internal fixation under two-plane image-intensifier control. Manipulative reduction should be gentle, and the authors have found the techniques of McElvenny and Deyerle to be the most satisfactory. Frequently, however, the fracture is reduced by the maneuver of applying traction on the limb with neutral adduction-abduction with internal rotation to bring the femoral neck parallel to the floor.

      a. In **McElvenny's technique,** both extremities are placed in traction with the hips in extension. The affected leg is lined up with the long axis of the body and is then maximally internally rotated by rotating the knee rather than the foot to reduce stress on the knee ligaments. Traction then is released on the contralateral side. After viewing follow-up roentgenograms, if more valgus is required, the traction may be reapplied to the affected leg. Just before releasing the traction on the opposite leg, an abduction force at the knee is applied along with a simultaneous pushing inward over the trochanter.

      b. The **Deyerle technique** achieves final alignment of the femoral neck and head in the lateral plane by a direct push posteriorly by two hands placed anteriorly over the greater trochanter while the pelvis on the contralateral side is supported to prevent ligament stress. This procedure is carried out after traction and internal rotation have reduced the fracture in the anteroposterior plane and before placement in slight valgus as described in **a.**

   2. **Open methods.** Open reduction through a **Watson-Jones anterolateral approach** with impaction and internal fixation under direct vision is most useful when a satisfactory closed reduction cannot be obtained in a patient in whom prosthetic replacement is contraindicated (55).

F. Operative techniques

   1. **Multiple screws.** The multiple screw method, using three pins, is the simplest method of obtaining internal fixation. This method can be a percutaneous procedure, thus reducing the risk of infection and the operative morbidity in elderly patients, extremely poor-risk patients, and bedridden patients. The alternative of prosthetic replacement in the low functional demand patient is chosen except when these criteria apply (51). When an adequate (anatomic) closed reduction is obtained, the screws can be placed through a small lateral incision, but a capsulotomy is recommended by extending the deep dissection anteriorly. When the reduction is nonanatomic, open reduction is advised (55,57).

   2. **Sliding screw plate fixation** is an alternative to multiple screw fixation. No mechanical advantage is obtained, however, because the fracture stability is most dependent on the quality of the reduction and the density of the bone in the femoral head. In a nonanatomic reduction, there is an advantage to the use of a hip screw because the fixation relies on the lateral cortex rather than opposition of the fracture surface (40,58). A sliding screw plate appears to have the advantage of firm fixation of the head, as well as allowing for impaction through sliding in a fitted barrel. The addition of a threaded pin or cancellous screw superiorly in the neck and head for improved torsional control is gaining popularity (40). Regardless of the particular type of mechanism used, it is essential to obtain maximum holding capacity in the head, which necessitates

the use of a 135-degree angle device in most individuals when anatomic reduction is obtained. When a valgus reduction is chosen, it is important to use a 150-degree nail plate device and to position the nail or screw in the deepest portion of the head.

3. **Prosthetic replacement.** A recent analysis of the literature has revealed improved functional outcomes for hemiarthroplasty when compared with internal fixation. Arthroplasty procedures carry a higher risk of deep infection, dislocation, and potential need for revision (31). Inserting the prosthesis via an anterior or lateral approach significantly decreases the risk of dislocation (31). A fixed head prosthesis is used for patients with very low functional demand, such as patients with multiple medical problems who are limited to household ambulation (55). Bipolar prosthesis, which allows for motion between the larger prosthetic head and a smaller head on the femoral stem, may result in less acetabular wear and is used in patients with higher functional demands, such as community ambulation. Total hip arthroplasty is also appropriate in this setting but carries the need for a more extensive surgical procedure to insert the prosthetic acetabulum and a higher risk (10%) of dislocation (17). This is the procedure of choice when femoral neck fractures occur in patients with rheumatoid arthritis. Such fractures are exceedingly rare in patients with degenerative arthritis of the hip, but total hip arthroplasty would also be appropriate in these cases.

4. **The authors' preference.** Multiple screw fixation or the sliding screw plate with an additional pin or screw appears to offer optimum fixation (55,57). The techniques are not easily learned or applied and are only effective with anatomic reduction and maximum fracture impaction at the time of surgery. Given the difficulties inherent with either technique, the uncertain end results if anatomic reduction is not obtained, and **the minimum of a 12% avascular necrosis rate,** the surgeon should consider femoral prosthetic replacement as an alternative in the older patient with low functional demands and poor bone quality (31).

G. **Failed primary fixation.** Loss of reduction, protrusion of the screw or pins into the acetabulum, and collapse with symptomatic avascular necrosis are also indications for prosthetic replacement. If the acetabulum has been damaged, total hip arthroplasty is recommended.

H. **Postoperative care and rehabilitation.** The aim of treatment is to return the patient to preoperative status by the quickest, safest method. Therefore, rehabilitation planning should begin at the time of admission, because most patients are elderly and do not tolerate prolonged periods away from familiar environments (26). Surgery is carried out as soon as possible, and the procedure should be one that allows immediate partial or full weight bearing, the first step in rehabilitation. Attempting to maintain a patient in non–weight-bearing status is frustrating for the surgeon, therapist, and family. The use of bedpans and the practice of straight-leg raising of the intact leg while in bed have been shown to produce considerable stress across the femoral neck. It is fallacious to attempt to protect the hip by non–weight bearing with crutches, because approximately half the body weight is transmitted across the so-called non–weight-bearing hip. If the knee and hip are fully flexed, the forces at the hip approximate total body weight. The dependent position without the normal pumping action of muscles also predisposes to edema, venostasis, and thrombophlebitis. The authors' experience indicates that, as long as stable internal fixation is achieved, gains from early weight bearing far outweigh the risks. Patients are encouraged to ambulate and to apply as much weight as is comfortable. Initially, a walker is used, and then gradual progress is made to crutches, if practical, and eventually a cane. In the case of the patient with balance problems, the walker or cane may be used indefinitely to help prevent more falls.

I. **Non-union and avascular necrosis**

1. In the past, **non-union** has been an important complication, but with proper reduction, impaction, and internal fixation, its incidence should

be reduced to less than 10% (31,55). Most fractures heal promptly and the union is well established within 4 months. Occasionally, there is some resorption at the fracture site, probably a result of insufficient impaction at surgery and therefore some fracture instability. Further impaction and eventual healing usually occur, but the incidence of avascular necrosis is significantly higher than in patients who obtain primary union.

2. **Avascular necrosis**
   a. The **roentgenographic signs** of avascular necrosis, with associated collapse, can occur at any time postoperatively. For practical purposes, however, changes with collapse are usually seen within 3 years. The incidence of avascular necrosis is variously reported to be within 12%–35%, and it must be appreciated that for displaced femoral neck fractures, the head, or at least a major portion of it, is rendered avascular at the time of injury (31,55). The lower figure of 12% is identical to that reported by most authors for impacted valgus fractures and probably represents the lowest possible incidence. When avascular changes are identified, the patient should be managed according to symptoms. In many older patients, the condition may not be severe enough to warrant any further surgery, but in patients with complete collapse of the femoral head and increasing pain, early total hip replacement is the treatment of choice.
   b. The **role of bone grafting for either prevention or treatment of avascular necrosis remains uncertain.** Currently, evidence for use of bone grafting for either of these conditions on a routine basis is lacking.

J. **Prognosis.** Anticipated complications and end results have been discussed for each fracture. Because of the advanced age of the typical patient, development of degenerative articular changes over a long period is difficult to assess, but it does not appear to be a frequent complication. The **morbidity and mortality rates (12% for the 12 months following fracture) are high, but they can be notably decreased by treating this fracture with early reduction and early ambulation.** The mortality rates return to those of age-matched control subjects after 1 year.

K. **Fractures of the neck of the femur in children** (27,54)
   1. **Treatment**
      a. **Transepiphyseal fractures** are uncommon, and there is no series of sufficient size to make any conclusions about the treatment of choice. The authors recommend reduction with capsulotomy and fixation with smooth pins (54).
      b. **Undisplaced and minimally displaced cervicotrochanteric fractures** carry a risk of avascular necrosis. The pathophysiology may involve intracapsular tamponade of the vessels supplying the femoral head (54). The authors recommend capsulotomy, reduction if necessary, and fixation with lag screws short of the femoral head epiphysis. The screws are generally sufficient because of the density of the bone. In children 8 years old and younger, postoperative spica cast immobilization is also used for 6–12 weeks. Displaced fractures are treated in the same way. These fractures must be treated emergently to minimize the complication of avascular necrosis.
   2. **Prognosis.** These fractures have nearly a 100% rate of union with optimum management.
   3. **Complications**
      a. **Coxa vara.** Although this complication is commonly reported, it is generally associated with nonoperative management.
      b. **Avascular necrosis.** This complication affects 0%–17% of patients who undergo emergent treatment. The long-term consequence is generally degenerative arthritis, which requires total hip arthroplasty in patients in their 40s to 60s.

      c. **Premature closure of the epiphysis** occurred in 7% of the patients in Lam's series (27). This complication is not a significant long-term problem except when it occurs in children younger than 8 years.

II. Intertrochanteric fractures (29)

A. Surgical anatomy

1. **The classic intertrochanteric fracture occurs in a line between the greater and lesser trochanters.** Although in theory such a fracture is totally extracapsular, the distinction between an intertrochanteric fracture and a basilar femoral neck fracture is not always clear. In peritrochanteric fractures, the internal rotators of the hip remain with the distal fragment, whereas usually at least some of the short, external rotators are still attached to the proximal head and neck fragment. This factor becomes important in reducing the fracture, because in order to align the distal fragment to the proximal one, the leg must be in some degree of external rotation. This requires a distinctly different maneuver in the operating room with the patient on the fracture table to reduce the fracture.

2. When the forces producing the fracture are increased, the greater trochanter and lesser trochanter can be separately fractured and appear as separated fragments **(four-part fracture).** Secondary comminution is not infrequent and usually involves one of the four major fragments. Anatomic restoration becomes a major undertaking but is not necessary to obtain a satisfactory result from a functional point of view. Occasionally, a subtrochanteric extension of the fracture is encountered.

B. Mechanism of injury.
The intertrochanteric fracture almost invariably occurs as a result of a fall in which both direct and indirect forces are acting. Direct forces act along the long axis of the femur or directly over the trochanter. Indirect forces include the pull of the iliopsoas muscle on the lesser trochanter and that of the abductors on the greater trochanter.

C. Classification.
A number of classifications and subclassifications have been proposed (2,28). From the standpoint of treatment and prognosis, a simple classification into stable or unstable fractures is most satisfactory.

1. A **stable intertrochanteric fracture** is one in which it is possible for the medial cortex of the femur to butt against the medial cortex of the calcar of the femoral neck fragment. Not uncommonly, the lesser trochanter is fractured off as a small secondary fragment, but this does not interfere with the basic stability of the fracture.

2. The **unstable intertrochanteric fracture** is one in which there is comminution of the posteromedial-medial cortex (along the calcar femorale). In the most common unstable pattern, a large posteromedial fragment encompasses the lesser trochanter, with or without a fracture through the greater trochanter (four-part fracture). A fracture with high obliquity may be considered unstable because of the high shearing force at the fracture site despite anatomic reduction and internal fixation.

D. Physical examination.
The fracture occurs primarily in the elderly, the average age reported being 66–76 years, which is slightly older than for femoral neck fractures. There is a predominance in women, with a ratio of occurrence in women to men of 2:1 to 8:1. The leg is shortened and lies in marked external rotation. Any movement of the extremity is painful and should not be attempted. If traction is applied with a Thomas splint for patient transport, it should be removed before roentgenograms are obtained because the ring interferes with proper assessment of the fracture. Both anteroposterior and lateral roentgenograms should be made to confirm the diagnosis and to delineate the fracture pattern. The lateral film is obtained as a cross-table view, which can be obtained by flexing the uninjured hip.

E. Treatment.
Operative treatment is the procedure of choice if a skilled anesthesiologist and surgeon are available. The more debilitated the patient, the

more emergent the indications. The goal of treatment must be to restore the patient to preoperative status as early as possible, which can be achieved best through reduction and internal fixation in a stable fashion so as to allow early ambulation. As with intracapsular fractures, if the patient is first seen with unstable medical conditions, these should be stabilized before surgery to minimize the risk of perioperative morbidity and mortality (26). If there are complicating injuries or illnesses that make it impossible to carry out operative reduction and fixation, well-leg traction is remarkably well suited to this situation. The leg must be held in some external rotation to maintain reduction of the fracture. This treatment allows movement from bed to chair and eliminates cumbersome traction apparatus for transport. Because treatment necessitates the use of crutches following the period of bed rest, weights should be used for strengthening the upper extremities. Great care must be taken to avoid secondary complications such as pressure areas over the sacrum and the heels, equinus contractures of the foot, and thromboembolic disease. Traction must be maintained until there is callus seen on roentgenograms—usually approximately 8 weeks. Following this period, mobilization may begin using non–weight bearing and parallel bars, a walker, or crutches. The hip must be protected until there is mature callus and bridging bone—an additional 4–6 weeks. The use of a cane in the opposite hand should be encouraged indefinitely to help prevent subsequent falls and injury.

1. **Operative treatment of stable intertrochanteric fractures.** Most of the current available internal fixation devices for treatment of intertrochanteric fractures can be expected to yield satisfactory results. "Fixed angle" devices that do not allow collapse of the fracture produce inferior results (2). If the fracture is displaced, it must be reduced to a stable position; that is, the medial cortices must abut each other anatomically. What is potentially a stable fracture can be converted into an unstable situation by inadequate reduction of the medial cortices. The reduction is accomplished on a fracture table by direct traction, slight abduction, and external rotation. If these maneuvers do not produce an anatomic reduction, the fracture site should be opened to ensure stability of the reduction. Not infrequently, there is some posterior displacement at the fracture site that requires the femur shaft to be lifted anteriorly to secure an anatomic reduction at the time of fixation. Regardless of the internal fixation used, in the elderly osteoporotic patient, the neck itself might be little more than a hollow tube; to gain purchase, it is essential to insert the nail or screw well into the head. The authors recommend insertion to within 0.5 inch of the subchondral bone. The position should be in the center of the femoral head on both views (3,4). Baumgaertner has popularized the "tip-apex distance" as a way to emphasize the center/center position within the femoral head. The plate should be securely fixed across both femoral cortices by four screws. **The authors believe that a properly inserted sliding screw plate with the wide, threaded, blunt-nosed screw offers the best mechanical fixation for intertrochanteric fractures** (Fig. 23-1). Although intramedullary devices such as the Gamma nail have been advocated to minimize blood loss and allow early full weight bearing, they have not proved superior to sliding anteroposterior screws and may carry a higher complication rate (20,21,44).

2. **Operative treatment of unstable intertrochanteric fractures.** The following procedures, which are all designed to enhance medial contact of the major fragments, are mechanisms to obtain a stable reduction of an unstable fracture.

   a. **Secure the lesser trochanteric fragment** to the femoral shaft, if possible, to provide a stable buttress for reduction of the neck portion by the use of lag screws or cerclage with wire or bands. This technique has been successful in the hands of those who have become

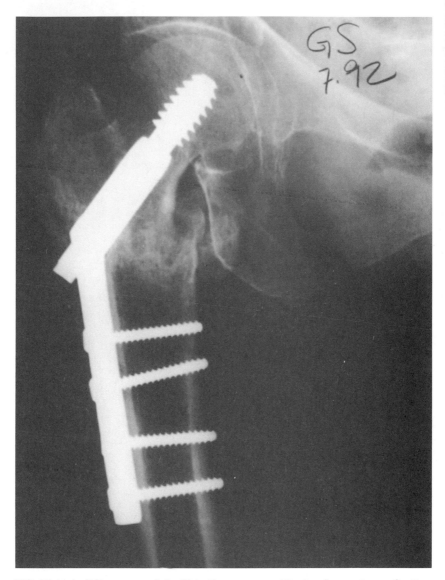

FIG. 23-1. A sliding screw plate. Note the proper positioning for maximum fixation with the screw centrally seated in the head within 1 cm of the subchondral bone. Four screws are used to insert the slide plate onto the femur.

skilled in its use but cannot be expected to work in all instances, particularly if there is significant comminution.

   b. **A sliding screw or nail plate device** can be inserted that allows the fracture fragments to impact and thus seek their own stability. With unstable fractures, shortening and medial displacements almost invariably occur, but the fractures progress to prompt union (6). Dramatic collapse during healing does result in poor function (6). If a stable reduction is not obtained at the time of insertion, the sliding apparatus is forgiving and allows for subsequent displacement to achieve stability. **The authors believe that the sliding screw plate is most satisfactory for treating this type of fracture,** and the postoperative treatment outlines are based on its use. Improving the medial contact as noted in **a.** minimizes the amount of shortening that occurs.

   c. Elective medial displacement of the femoral shaft has been used by Dimon and Hughston to achieve stability, followed by internal fixation with a shortened nail plate device. The same authors and Sarmiento and Williams have advocated an **osteotomy** to position the head and neck fragments in more valgus, thus securing better medial stability than can be achieved by simple medial displacement. They then recommend fixation by a fixed nail plate device. These osteotomies have not proven to be necessary with sliding screw devices (15).

   d. In **osteoporotic patients** with highly comminuted fractures, prosthetic replacement may rarely be indicated (19).

F. Postoperative treatment. There is little agreement in the literature as to what constitutes the best postoperative management of intertrochanteric fractures. Our recommendation for rehabilitation is that patients be moved to at least a sitting position on the first postoperative day. In 2–3 days, they should be taken to the physical therapy department where ambulation can be started using the parallel bars. Patients may be allowed to place as much weight on the fractured extremity as they wish. They are not forced to go beyond what is comfortable for them but are reassured that some weight bearing is desirable and not to be feared. As soon as they feel secure using the parallel bars, patients should be transferred to a walker or crutches, depending on their abilities based on their prefracture status. With this program, it is rare that individuals who were able to walk without support before fracture cannot be returned to a self-sufficient state within 10–14 days using either a walker or crutches. Patients may disregard the walker or crutches at any time they feel secure. The long-term use of a cane is encouraged as a preventive measure in elderly patients to avoid falls and injury.

G. Prognosis and complications. Because of the age of patients (many suffer from other debilitating conditions at the time of injury), **mortality and morbidity rates will always be significant.** With an aggressive treatment program, mortality rate should be 10%–15% for the first year after the fracture; subsequently, the mortality rate returns to that of age-matched controls. Mechanical failure and non-union can be reduced to 1% or less. Avascular necrosis is rare but has been reported (32). Infection is still a problem, with most series reporting an incidence of 1%–5% deep infections. This rate can be significantly decreased by careful soft tissue technique (9,33) and the use of prophylactic antibiotics for 24 hours. With prompt internal fixation and an aggressive postoperative rehabilitation program stressing early weight bearing, complications from thromboembolic disease can be sharply reduced. The authors recommend the use of sequential compression devices and aspirin for all patients with the use of a low-dose warfarin or enoxaparin regimen. **Even with optimum treatment, it is scarcely possible to return more than 40% of the patients to their true prefracture status, but one can obtain satisfactory results from treatment in approximately 80% of patients.** Prophylactic antibiotics are recommended as discussed in Chaps. 8 **(IV.D)** and 10 **(I.B.2).**

III. Trochanteric fractures

  A. Isolated avulsion or comminuted fractures of the greater trochanter occasionally are seen. **Unless displacement of the fragment is greater than 1 cm,** the fracture is treated as a soft-tissue injury with protected weight bearing until the patient is asymptomatic. Several days of bed rest are usually required, followed by walker or crutch ambulation for 3–4 weeks. **In elderly patients, even with separation greater than 1 cm, operative treatment with internal fixation rarely is indicated.**

  B. In the younger patient, **when displacement is greater than 1 cm,** it is advisable to fix the fracture fragment internally with either two cancellous screws or a wire loop to secure fragments. This maneuver reconstitutes the abductor mechanism. Postoperatively, the extremity is protected until soft-tissue healing is secured. Then the patient is allowed to ambulate without weight bearing for 3–4 weeks, followed by partial weight bearing for another 3–4 weeks until limp-free walking can be achieved.

IV. Isolated avulsion fractures of the lesser trochanter

  A. These fractures are seen mainly in children and athletic young adults. **Unless displacement is greater than 2 cm,** operative fixation is not indicated and the end result is excellent.

  B. With displacement greater than 2 cm, it is advisable to replace the avulsed fragment with a cancellous screw or a cortical screw, securing it to the opposite cortex. This procedure is most readily accomplished through a medial approach to the hip. Complications are minimal, and the end result is most satisfactory. In patients older than 50 years of age, this fracture may be the first sign of metastatic disease and a full evaluation is indicated.

V. Subtrochanteric fractures

  A. Subtrochanteric fractures occur as extensions of intertrochanteric fractures or as independent entities (33). The mechanism is direct trauma, and significant forces usually are required. This type of fracture is ordinarily seen in younger individuals as compared with the intertrochanteric or femoral neck fracture. Subtrochanteric fractures, which are extensions of intertrochanteric fractures, are seen in elderly patients. Thus, these fractures have a bimodal distribution.

  B. Classification. Fielding classified subtrochanteric fractures as occurring in three zones: zone I, those at the level of the lesser trochanter; zone II, those 1–2 inches below the upper border of the lesser trochanter; zone III, those 2–3 inches below the upper border of the lesser trochanter. Although we do not wish to propose a new classification, for the purposes of this discussion, the concept of unstable and stable fractures is used, with stability being determined by the ability to establish bone-on-bone contact of the medial cortex. Seinsheimer's classification and results have emphasized the importance of the posteromedial fragment. Internal fixation then acts as a tension band on the outer (distracting) cortex and allows for impaction and weight bearing directly through the medial cortex. If this internal fixation is not possible, the fracture pattern is unstable.

  C. Physical examination. Because the forces required to produce the fracture are substantial, other injuries in the same extremity and elsewhere in the body often occur. Emergency splinting in a Thomas splint generally is required. Hemorrhage in the thigh may be significant, so the patient should be monitored for hypovolemic shock, and blood replacement may be necessary. Good anteroposterior and lateral roentgenograms are necessary to assess clearly the extent of the fracture.

  D. Treatment. Operative stabilization to allow early rehabilitation is the treatment of choice. Traction may rarely be necessary for the severely comminuted fracture, but the healing time is longer than for an intertrochanteric fracture, and delayed unions and malunions frequently are encountered. Skeletal traction should be used and applied in such a way as to align the distal fragment to the proximal fragment. If the lesser trochanteric fragment with its attached iliopsoas muscle remains intact on the head and neck fragment, it is necessary to flex and externally rotate the distal fragment to obtain reduction. The strong adductors attached to the femoral shaft tend to cause varus angulation, and attempts to correct this by abduction of the hip often exert pull on the adductors and cause bowing at the fracture site or medial displacement of the shaft fragment. In this event, it is best for the patient to undergo treatment in a neutral position with reference to abduction-adduction and to increase the traction. When the fracture is comminuted and the lesser trochanter is off as a separate piece, treatment is the same as for intertrochanteric fractures. If traction treatment is used, it should be maintained until there is roentgenographic evidence of union. The patient is then placed in a single spica cast for protected weight bearing until the callus matures.

E. **Operative treatment**
  1. **Stable fractures at the level of the lesser trochanter** (Fielding zone I). Fractures in this region may be treated like intertrochanteric fractures. When there is a single fracture line through the medial cortex, anatomic reduction should be obtained. Internal fixation that is sufficiently strong to provide a tension band effect laterally and to maintain a reduction is the treatment of choice. If the fracture is transverse, an angled blade plate can achieve this effect (33). A Zickel nail will also meet these requirements but is very stiff and does not allow distal interlocking (7). Reconstruction type intramedullary nails that use two screws in the head and neck fragment are generally thought to be the most satisfactory implant. They can be inserted with relative ease only when the piriformis fossa of the proximal femur remains intact.
  2. **Stable fractures below the lesser trochanter** (Fielding zones II and III). The same principles apply as outlined in **1,** except that with these fractures it is not possible to insert a fixed or sliding nail plate device across the fracture site and allow for medial displacement. If there is a secure ring of diaphyseal bone for approximately 2 cm below the lesser trochanter, the authors favor intramedullary nailing with a standard interlocking nail (64,65). Compression plating is equally satisfactory in the hands of persons familiar with its application, but it is not used routinely because of the large surgical dissection required.
  3. **Unstable fractures at or above the lesser trochanter** when the greater trochanter head and neck are not in a single piece. These should be managed as unstable, intertrochanteric fractures, using a technique of either a sliding screw or condylar plate inserted into the head and neck fragment at the fracture site to gain stability by medial displacement and impaction (33). Although osteotomy and medial displacement may be used to gain stability before internal fixation, they are not routinely recommended. If the proximal fragment is a single piece, a reconstruction nail can be used, but this requires skill and experience.
  4. **Unstable fractures extending distal to the lesser trochanter.** Occasionally, the subtrochanteric fracture is unstable because of a single, large displaced medial fragment. In these circumstances, stability can be obtained by reducing the fragment and holding it with two lag screws or cerclage and one of the sliding screw plate devices or a condylar plate to maintain the fracture reduction. This is a satisfactory solution when care is taken to ascertain that the medial fragment is truly secure, thus allowing direct weight to be borne through the medial cortex with the fixation device acting as a tension band laterally. Frequently, the medial cortex is comminuted or fractured in such a way that stability cannot be achieved. In this event, far too much tension is placed on any of the fixation devices, with the result that mechanical failure is frequent; delayed unions, malunions, and non-unions are common. In such cases, the standard sliding screw or blade plate fixation should be supplemented by bone grafting at the fracture site or by maintaining the patient in traction or a spica cast for additional protection until union is achieved. Indirect

reduction techniques may eliminate the need for bone grafting (33). A
Gamma or reconstruction type nail can be successfully used in this setting by a surgeon experienced in the application of these devices.

F. **Postoperative management.** Stable subtrochanteric fractures or those
that can be rendered stable by operative treatment can be managed much
as intertrochanteric fractures. The unstable subtrochanteric fracture must
be supported and protected from weight bearing until the union is secure.

G. **Complications.** In the event of a frank non-union or a delay in union of an
intertrochanteric or subtrochanteric fracture, a careful assessment of the
cause of this failure should be made. Too often it is caused by less-than-strict
adherence to the treatment principles outlined. If the fixation is secure and
the reduction adequate, bone grafting may suffice. As soon as problems with
union are recognized, optimal position of the fracture should be obtained
and standard internal fixation combined with fresh autogenous cancellous
grafting carried out. Osteotomy may be required. Once this process is completed, the management is the same as for a fresh fracture, except that it
may be necessary to delay patient activity until discomfort from the graft
donor site has subsided.

VI. **Intertrochanteric and subtrochanteric fractures in children.** These fractures may be treated in **balanced skeletal traction,** aligning the distal fragment to the proximal one. Traction is maintained until the fracture is stable
(4–6 weeks), at which time the extremity is placed in a single spica cast for immobilization until union is solid (approximately 12 weeks). Increasingly, percutaneous pin or screw fixation with supplemental spica casting is used. The
authors favor reduction and percutaneous Steinmann pin fixation followed by
supplemental spica casting.

VII. **Femoral diaphyseal fractures in adults** (10,24,63,65)

A. Diaphyseal fractures are the result of significant trauma and usually are associated with considerable **soft-tissue damage.** Blood loss of 2–3 units is
common. In addition, these fractures have a high incidence of associated injury in the same extremity (61,62), including fractures of the femoral neck
(41), posterior fracture-dislocations of the hip, tears of the collateral ligaments of the knee (62), and osteochondral fractures involving the distal
femur or patella and fractures of the tibia (61).

B. **Examination.** Diagnosis usually does not present any clinical problem if
care is taken to rule out the other associated injuries by physical examination and radiographs.

C. **Roentgenograms.** Films are obtained primarily to confirm the diagnosis
and for preoperative planning. It is **essential** to view the joint above and
the joint below the fracture. Films of the uninjured femur are helpful for se-
lecting the appropriate internal fixation device. An anteroposterior and lateral roentgenogram of the injured femur should be supplemented by the
anteroposterior pelvis to obtain optimum views of the femoral neck (56).

D. **Treatment**

1. Emergency treatment consists of the immediate application of a
Thomas splint before roentgenograms are obtained. Unless there is
gross comminution or the patient is not a surgical candidate, fractures
of the shaft of the femur from 2 cm below the lesser trochanter to approximately 10 cm above the knee joint should be treated by **closed
interlocking nailing** (see Fig 25-3), with reaming of the canal using
flexible reamers and prebent nails (63,65). Once associated body cavity and other extremity injury is ruled out, the patient should receive
urgent operative stabilization. The more severely injured the patient,
the more critical is solid fixation of the femur fracture. Early fixation
has been shown to be associated with decreased narcotic use, reduced
pulmonary complications (e.g., adult respiratory distress syndrome),
and decreased mortality rate (10). Even patients with isolated femoral
shaft fractures, including elderly patients, benefit from urgent (within
24 hours of admission) stabilization of the femur with an interlocking

nail (10,14,38). These procedures are carried out on a fracture table in the operating room under fluoroscopic control. Although many authors recommend routine supine positioning because of the ease of placement of locking bolts, we favor the lateral position on the fracture table when the patient does not have chest, abdominal, or pelvic injuries. This allows greater ease of access to the greater trochanter and use of smaller incisions in large patients. When the patient is severely traumatized, fracture stability can be achieved with external fixation or plates much more rapidly on a standard table. The fixator is generally exchanged for an interlocking nail within the first 5–7 days when the patient's condition has stabilized. Primary interlocking nailing after debridement is the procedure of choice for most open femoral shaft fractures. Intramedullary nailing can be performed with the patient supine on a radiolucent table (25). Recently, there has been an interest in using small diameter locked nails without reaming; this has been associated with longer healing time and implant failure (8,36,60).

2. Recently, implants for retrograde locked nailing have been developed (16,42). Indications for further use include bilateral fractures and ipsilateral patella (or femoral neck fracture) (35,45).

3. Balanced suspension skeletal traction may be used until a cast-brace can be applied only when the equipment or expertise necessary for locked nailing is unavailable and when the patient cannot be transported (24).

E. **Complications**
1. **Associated vascular and nerve damage,** especially a transient peroneal or pudendal nerve palsy, is not uncommon. These problems are generally associated with excess traction.
2. **Shortening and malrotation** of the extremity frequently occur, especially when intramedullary nailing is not performed. Slight shortening is associated with earlier fracture union, and shortening up to 0.5 inch should be accepted without hesitation.
3. **Skin breakdown** over bony prominences and pin traction infections are complications of traction.
4. **Infection is extremely rare with the closed nailing technique** (49).
5. **Non-union** occurs in approximately 1% of fractures treated with nailing. This problem is easily managed with nail removal, reaming, and renailing.
6. Rotational malunion occurs in 10%–20% of patients; the deformity is generally external rotation (11).
7. Weakness of the abductor muscles and hip pain can occur in one third of patients (1,5).
8. Knee injuries are common after femoral shaft fractures (37).

VIII. **Diaphyseal fractures in children**
A. **For children younger than 6–8 years** with an uncomplicated, isolated femoral shaft fracture, a spica cast can be used for primary treatment. The technique is as follows (52):
1. When the patient's general condition has stabilized, usually after at least 24 hours of observation in 2–3 lb of Buck's traction, the patient is placed under general anesthesia on a fracture table. The feet are placed in stirrups, and traction is applied. The fractured thigh may be supported by a sling to an overhead bar if necessary to restore the normal anterior bow of the femur. For a child younger than 2 years, it may be desirable to flex the hip and knee to 90 degrees. For the older child, the hip is flexed approximately 20–30 degrees, abducted 20 degrees, and externally rotated to best align the distal fragment to the proximal fragment. The knees are kept extended. Roentgenograms are made to verify the reduction. The object of manipulation is to provide approximately 1 cm of overriding of the fragments (bayonet apposition in good alignment in both planes). When this position has been achieved, the

skin between the knees and ankles is then sprayed with medical adhesive B. A single layer of bias-cut stockinet is wrapped over the entire area as described for extremity casting (see Chap. 7). Quarter-inch felt, sponge rubber, or several additional turns of Webril may be used over bony prominences except between the knee and ankle. A **double hip spica cast** is then applied, molded carefully around the pelvis, and extended to embrace the rib margin. When the cast has hardened, the foot pieces of the fracture table are removed, and if roentgenograms confirm the proper position, the cast is extended to include both feet and ankles, which are well padded, in a neutral position. A crossbar is added to the cast.

2. **Postcasting treatment.** Follow-up roentgenograms are made at 1, 2, and 3 weeks to be certain of the maintenance of position. The cast is worn for 6–12 weeks, depending on the age of the patient and the type of fracture. The family must be instructed in cast care and told to alert the physician if there is any evidence of pain, fever, or loss of extension of the great toe.

B. **Children older than 8 years** or patients for whom this method of treatment is not considered practical should undergo treatment with fixed or balanced suspension skeletal traction followed by a spica cast or external fixation. For transverse, length stable fractures, retrograde flexible nailing has gained increase acceptance. When the child is 12–13 years or older, intramedullary nailing should be considered for fractures of the diaphysis of the femur. The starting point for the nail should be moved slightly lateral to decrease the risk of avascular necrosis.

C. **Children with head injuries** or multiple trauma should be managed with operative stabilization. In patients younger than 12 years, this should involve plates, retrograde flexible nails, or external fixators. Children older than 12 years may undergo treatment with intramedullary nails.

IX. **Unicondyler, supracondylar, and intracondylar fractures** (49)
A. **Mechanism of injury.** In older individuals, these fractures are sustained with minimal trauma. In young people, these fractures generally are caused by massive trauma and often are associated with vascular and other soft-tissue injuries. This fracture has a bimodel age distribution as well.

B. **Examination.** A careful assessment of nerve and vascular status distal to the fracture is critical here as with any fracture. Care must be taken to ascertain any injuries to the soft tissues about the knee and whether the fracture extends into the joint.

C. **Roentgenograms.** Anteroposterior, lateral, and, occasionally, oblique views are necessary.

D. **Treatment**
1. Displaced unicondylar fractures should be treated by open reduction and internal fixation (ORIF) with lag screws; good results can be anticipated (4).

2. Undisplaced supracondylar fractures or fractures displaced less than 1 mm involving the joint surface may be treated by percutaneous screw fixation, generally with cannulated screw systems. Alternatively, a hinged knee brace or cast-brace may be used, but frequent roentgenograms must be obtained. In either case, early motion must be initiated to optimize results. Inferior results with nonoperative management for these fractures has been documented (13).

3. Extraarticular distal femur fractures or those occurring above total knee replacements can be nicely managed with retrograde supracondylar nails (12,22) or standard antegrade nails (30).

4. **Displaced intraarticular or supracondylar fractures** are managed by internal fixation (9,35,43,47). The fracture requires open reduction of the joint surface via a lateral approach to ensure that it is anatomically reduced. Minimal stripping of the soft-tissue attachments to the extraarticular fragments must be completed (9). This speeds

union and decreases the need for bone grafting while minimizing infection. A 95-degree condylar blade plate or dynamic condylar screw is the optimum device for fixing these fractures, but they require 1.5–2 cm of intact bone proximal to the compression screw or blade (35,47). With extremely comminuted fractures, a condylar buttress plate is required, which allows for more screws into the distal fragment. Rarely, a second medial approach with a second plate is required to gain the stability necessary for early motion (48). Minor malunion is common with the use of fixed angle devices (66). If the expertise or equipment to perform these procedures does not exist and the patient cannot be transported to a facility where they are available, skeletal traction can be used. A tibial pin is inserted with the knee flexed 20 degrees, and balanced suspension is used. Early active quadriceps exercises are necessary to prevent joint fibrosis. Because of the pull of the gastrocnemius, which extends the fracture, the flexed position should be maintained for the first several weeks. The distal fragment must be aligned to the proximal fragment, which is usually in external rotation.

E. **Postoperative care.** Continuous passive motion is used while the patient is in the hospital and may be extended to the early posthospitalization period (first 3 weeks) in most cases in which stable internal fixation has been achieved. A hinged-knee brace is generally used for 6 weeks. The goal of full extension and 120 degrees of flexion by 6 weeks postoperatively is standard. Full weight bearing is delayed for 10–12 weeks. Strengthening exercises can then be initiated. Patients in traction require aggressive physical therapy to regain full extension and 90 degrees of flexion. Active and gentle passive motion protocols are initiated once the fracture is clinically and radiographically healed at about 8 weeks after injury. Some permanent loss of motion is expected for fractures treated this way as well as for severe intraarticular fractures managed operatively (48).

HCMC Treatment Recommendations
Femoral Neck Fractures
Diagnosis: Anteroposterior pelvis and lateral radiographs, physical examination. Patient's leg will be shortened and externally rotated.
Treatment: ORIF of fracture with multiple pins/screws for all impacted and nondisplaced fractures and for displaced fractures in active patients with good bone density. Patients with preexisting arthritis or significant osteoporosis should receive a prosthetic replacement (hemiarthroplasty or total hip replacement).
Indications for surgery: Femoral neck fracture
Recommended technique: Hemiarthroplasty done through an anterior or posterior approach to the hip—rehabilitation is easier with the anterior approach but access to the proximal femur is slightly more difficult.

HCMC Treatment Recommendations
Intertrochanteric Hip Fractures
Diagnosis: Anteroposterior pelvis and lateral hip radiographs, clinical examination. Patient's leg will be shortened and externally rotated.
Treatment: ORIF of fracture with sliding hip screw. Rarely, extremely comminuted fractures in extremely osteoporotic individuals are treated with prosthetic replacement.
Indications for surgery: Any intertrochanteric fracture, displaced or nondisplaced
Recommended technique: Sliding hip screw applied with patient on the fracture table with C-arm control.

HCMC Treatment Recommendations

Subtrochanteric Femur Fractures

Diagnosis: Anteroposterior pelvis and lateral proximal femur radiographs, clinical examination. Again, patient's leg will be shortened and externally rotated.

Treatment: Depends on involvement of the piriformis fossa. Fractures below the piriformis fossa are treated by closed reduction and interlocking nail placement. Open reduction may be required in certain fracture patterns to ensure proper placement of the implant. If the lesser trochanter is not attached to the proximal fragment, a "second generation" interlocking nail where the proximal interlocking screws are directed into the femoral head and neck are required. Fractures above the piriformis fossa may be treated by a sliding hip screw, 95-degree condylar screw, blade plate, or proximal femoral nail.

Indications for surgery: All subtrochanteric femur fractures

Recommended technique: For isolated fractures, the implant is inserted with the patient on the fracture table in the lateral decubitus position. Nailing of fractures as described is preferred; rarely a 95-degrees device such as a condylar screw or blade plate is preferred based on fracture pattern considerations.

HCMC Treatment Recommendations

Femoral Shaft Fractures

Diagnosis: Anteroposterior and lateral radiographs of the femur, clinical examination

Treatment: Closed reduction and insertion of reamed interlocking nail

Indications for surgery: All femoral shaft fractures in adult patients

Recommended technique: For isolated fractures, closed interlocking nail placement on the fracture table with the patient in the lateral decubitus position. For patients with multisystem trauma, the nailing can be done with the patient supine on a radiolucent table with a C-arm. Rarely, a plate or the temporary use of an external fixator followed by conversion to an interlocking nail is indicated within the first 2 weeks after injury.

HCMC Treatment Recommendations

Distal Femur Fractures

Diagnosis: Anteroposterior and lateral radiographs of the distal femur, including the knee joint, clinical examination

Treatment: Internal fixation to allow range of motion of the knee joint

Indications for surgery: All displaced supracondylar fractures of the femur with or without joint extension

Recommended technique: ORIF with plate and screws for most younger patients with articular extension. Retrograde nailing with or without lag screws for patients who are obese, osteoporotic, have a fracture above a knee prosthesis. AROM and limited weight bearing for 12 weeks.

References
1. Bain GI, Zacest AC, Paterson DC, et al. Abduction strength following intermedullary nailing. *J Orthop Trauma* 1997;11:93–97.
2. Bannister GC, Gibson GF, Ackrund CE, et al. The fixation and prognosis of trochanteric fractures. A randomized, prospective controlled trial. *Clin Orthop* 1990;254:242–246.

3. Baumgaertner MR, Curtin SL, Lindskog DM, et al. The value of the tip-apex distance in predicting failure of fixation of peritrochanteric fractures of the hip. *J Bone Joint Surg (Am)* 1995;77:1058–1064.

4. Baumgaertner MR, Solberg BD. Awareness of tip-apex distance reduces failure of fixation of trochanteric fractures of the hip. *J Bone Joint Surg (Br)* 1992;79:969–971.

5. Benirschke SK, Melder I, Henley MB, et al. Closed interlocking nailing of femoral shaft fractures: assessment of technical complications and functional outcomes by comparison of a prospective database with retrospective review. *J Orthop Trauma* 1993;7:118–122.

6. Bendo JA, Weiner LS, Strauss E, et al. Collapse of intertrochanteric hip fractures with sliding screws. *Orthop Rev* 1994;Suppl:30–37.

7. Bergman GD, et al. Subtrochanteric fractures of the femur: fixation using the Zickel nail. *J Bone Joint Surg (Am)* 1987;69:1032.

8. Bhandari M, Guyatt GH, Tong D, et al. Reamed versus nonreamed intramedullary nailing of lower extremity long bone fracture: a systematic overview and meta-analysis. *J Orthop Trauma* 2000;14:2–9.

9. Bolhofner BR, Carmen B, Clifford P. The results of open reduction and internal fixation of distal femur fractures using a biologic (indirect) reduction technique. *J Orthop Trauma* 1996;6:372–377.

10. Bone LB, et al. Early versus delayed stabilization of femoral fractures: a prospective randomized study. *J Bone Joint Surg (Am)* 1989;71:336.

11. Braten M, Terjesen T, Rossvoll I. Torsional deformity after intramedullary nailing of femoral shaft fractures. *J Bone Joint Surg (Br)* 1993;75:799–803.

12. Brumback RJ, Toal TR, Murphy-Zane MS, et al. Immediate weight-bearing after treatment of a comminuted fracture of the femoral shaft with a statically locked intramedullary nail. *J Bone Joint Surg (Am)* 1999;81:1538–1544.

13. Butt MS, Krikler SJ, Ali MS. Displaced fractures of the distal femur in elderly patients; operative vs. non-operative treatment. *J Bone Joint Surg (Br)* 1995;77: 110–114.

14. Cameron CD, Meek RN, Blachut PA, et al. Intramedullary nailing of the femoral shaft: a prospective, randomized study. *J Orthop Trauma* 1992;6:448–451.

15. Chang WS, et al. Biomechanical evaluation of anatomic reduction versus medial displacement osteotomy in unstable intertrochanteric fractures. *Clin Orthop* 1987;225:141.

16. Cole JD, Huff WA, Blum DA. Retrograde femoral nailing of supracondylar, intracondylar and distal fractures of the femur. *Orthopedics* 1996;[Suppl 1]:22–30.

17. Delamarter R, Moreland JR. Treatment of acute femoral neck fractures with total hip arthroplasty. *Clin Orthop* 1987;218:68.

18. Dodenhoff RM, Dainton JN, Hutchins PM. Proximal thigh pain after nailing—causes and treatment. *J Bone Joint Surg (Br)* 1997;79:738–741.

19. Green S, Moore T, Proano F. Prosthetic replacement for the management of unstable intertrochanteric hip fractures in the elderly. *Clin Orthop* 1987;224:169.

20. Handy DCR, Descamps PY, Krallis P, et al. Use of an intramedullary hip-screw compared with a compression hip-screw with a plate for intertrochanteric femoral fractures: a prospective, randomized study of one hundred patients. *J Bone Joint Surgery (Am)* 1998;80:618–630.

21. Herscovici D, Ricci WM, McAndrews P, et al. Treatment of femoral shaft trauma. *J Orthop Trauma* 2000;14:10–14.

22. Henry SL. Management of supracondylar fractures proximal to total knee arthroplasty with the GSH supracondylar nail. *Contemp Orthop* 1995;31:231–238.

23. Jensen J, Hugh J. Fractures of the femoral neck: a follow-up study of nonoperative treatment of Garden's stage 1 and 2 fractures. *Injury* 1982;14:339.

24. Johnson KD, Johnston DWC, Parker B. Comminuted femoral-shaft fractures: treatment by roller traction, cerclage wires, and an intramedullary nail, or an interlocking intramedullary nail. *J Bone Joint Surg (Am)* 1984;66:1222.

25. Karpos PAG, McFerran MA, Johnson KD. Intramedullary nailing of acute femoral shaft fractures using manual traction without a fracture table. *J Orthop Trauma* 1995;9:57–62.

26. Kenzora JE, et al. Hip fracture mortality: relation to age, treatment, preoperative illness, time of surgery, and complications. *Clin Orthop* 1984;186:45.

27. Lam SF. Fractures of the neck of the femur in children. *J Bone Joint Surg (Am)* 1971;53:1165.
28. Larsson S, Friberg S, Hansson LI. Trochanteric fractures; influence of reduction and implant position in impaction and complications. *Clin Orthop* 1990;259:130–138.
29. Laskin RS, Gruber MA, Zimmerman AJ. Intertrochanteric fractures of the hip in the elderly. *Clin Orthop* 1979;141:188.
30. Leung KS, Shen WY, So WS, et al. Interlocking intramedullary nailing for supracondylar and intracondylar fractures of the distal part of the femur. *J Bone Joint Surg (Am)* 1991;73:333–340.
31. Lu-Yoo GL, Keller RB, Littenberg B, et al. Outcomes after displaced fractures of the femoral neck: a meta-analysis of one hundred and six published reports. *J Bone Joint Surg (Am)* 1994;76:15–25.
32. Mann RS. Avascular necrosis of the femoral head following intertrochanteric fractures. *Clin Orthop* 1973;92.108.
33. Mast J, Jakob R, Ganz R. *Planning and reduction techniques in fracture surgery.* New York: Springer-Verlag, 1989.
34. Melberg PE, Korner L, Lansinger O. Hip joint pressure after femoral neck fracture. *Acta Orthop Scand* 1986;57:501.
35. Mize RD, Bucholz RW, Grogan DP. Surgical treatment of displaced, comminuted fractures of the distal end of the femur. *J Bone Joint Surg (Am)* 1982;64:871.
36. Moed BR, Watson JT, Cramer KE, et al. Unreamed retrograde intramedullary nailing of fractures of the femoral shaft. *J Orthop Trauma* 1998;12:334–342.
37. Moore TJ, Campbell J, Wheeter K, et al. Knee function after complex femoral fractures treated with interlocking nails. *Clin Orthop* 1990;261:238–241.
38. Morgan CG, Gibson MJ, Cross AE. Intramedullary locking nails for femoral shaft fractures in elderly patients. *J Bone Joint Surg (Br)* 1989;72:19–22.
39. O'Brien PJ, Meek RN, Powell JN, et al. Primary intramedullary nailing of open femoral shaft fractures. *J Trauma* 1991;31:113–116.
40. Ort PJ, Lamont T. Treatment of femoral neck fractures with a sliding hip screw and the Knowles pins. *Clin Orthop* 1984;190:158.
41. Ostermann PAW, Neumann K, Ekkernkamp A, et al. Long-term results of unicondylar fractures of the femur. *J Orthop Trauma* 1994;8:142–146.
42. Ostrum RF, DiCiccio J, Lakatis R, et al. Retrograde intramedullary nailing of femoral diaphyseal fractures. *J Orthop Trauma* 1998;12:464–468.
43. Ostrum RF, Geel C. Indirect reduction and internal fixation of supracondylar femur fractures without bone graft. *J Orthop Trauma* 1995;9:278–284.
44. Parker MJ, Pryor GA. Gamma versus DHS nailing for extracapsular femoral fractures; metanalysis of 10 randomized trials. *Int Orthop* 1996;20:163–168.
45. Patterson BM, Routt ML Jr, Benirschke SK, et al. Retrograde nailing of femoral shaft fractures. *J Trauma* 1995;38:38–43.
46. Ray WA, Griffin MR, Downey W. Benzodiazepines of long and short elimination half-life and the risk of hip fracture. *JAMA* 1989;262:3303.
47. Sanders R, Regazzoni P, Reudi T. Treatment of supracondylar-intraarticular fractures of the femur using the dynamic condylar screw. *J Orthop Trauma* 1989;3:214.
48. Sanders R, et al. Complex fractures and malunions of the distal femur: results of treatment with double plates. *J Bone Joint Surg (Am)* 1991;73:341.
49. Schatzker J, Lambert DC. Supracondylar fractures of the femur. *Clin Orthop* 1979;138:77.
50. Sevitt S, Thompson RG. The distribution and anastomosis of arteries supplying the head and neck of the femur. *J Bone Joint Surg (Br)* 1965;47:560.
51. Sikorski JM, Barrington R. Internal fixation vs. hemiarthroplasty for the displaced subcapital fracture of the femur: a prospective randomized study. *J Bone Joint Surg (Br)* 1981;63:357.
52. Staheli LT, Sheridan GW. Early spica cast management of femoral shaft fractures in young children. *Clin Orthop* 1977;126:162.
53. Stromqvist B. Femoral head vitality after intracapsular hip fracture: 490 cases studied by intravital tetracycline labeling and TC-MDP radionuclide imagery. *Acta Orthop Scand* 1983;54[Suppl 200]:5.
54. Swiontkowski MF, Winquist RA. Displaced hip fractures in children and adolescents. *J Trauma* 1986;26:384.

55. Swiontkowski MF. Femoral neck fractures: current concept review. *J Bone Joint Surg (Am)* 1994;76:129–138.
56. Swiontkowski MF, Hansen ST, Kellam J. Ipsilateral fractures of the femoral neck and shaft. *J Bone Joint Surg (Am)* 1984;66:260.
57. Swiontkowski MF, Winquist RA, Hansen ST. Fractures of the femoral neck in patients between the ages of twelve and forty-nine years. *J Bone Joint Surg (Am)* 1984;66:837.
58. Swiontkowski MF, et al. Torsion and bending analyses of internal fixation techniques for femoral neck fractures: the role of implant design and bone density. *J Orthop Res* 1987;5:433.
59. Torentta P, Ritz G, Kanton A. Femoral torsion after interlocking nailing of unstable femoral fractures. *J Trauma* 1995;38:213–219.
60. Tornetta P, Tiburzzi D. Reamed versus nonreamed antegrade femoral nailing. *J Orthop Trauma* 2000;14:15–19.
61. Veith RG, Winquist RA, Hansen ST. Ipsilateral fractures of the femur and tibia. *J Bone Joint Surg (Am)* 1984;66:991.
62. Walling AK, Seradge H, Spiegel PG. Injuries to the knee ligaments with fractures of the femur. *J Bone Joint Surg (Am)* 1982;64:1324.
63. Winquist RA, Hansen ST, Clawson DK. Closed intramedullary nailing of femoral fractures. *J Bone Joint Surg (Am)* 1984;66:529.
64. Wiss D, et al. Comminuted and rotationally unstable fractures of the femur treated with an interlocking nail. *Clin Orthop* 1986;212:35.
65. Wolinsky PR, Ritz G, Kanton A. Femoral torsion after interlocking nailing of unstable femoral fractures. *J Trauma* 1995;38:213–219.
66. Zehntner MK, Marohesi DG, Burch H, et al. Alignment of supracondylar/intracondylar fractures of the femur after internal fixation by AO/ASIF technique. *J Orthop Trauma* 1992;6:318–326.

Selected Historical Readings

Arnold WD. The effect of early weight bearing on the stability of femoral neck fractures treated with Knowles pins. *J Bone Joint Surg (Am)* 1984;66:847.
Barnes JT, et al. Subcapital fractures of the femur: a prospective review. *J Bone Joint Surg (Br)* 1976;58:2.
Blickenstaff LD, Morris JM. Fatigue fracture of the femoral neck. *J Bone Joint Surg (Am)* 1966;48:1031.
Casey MJ, Chapman MW. Ipsilateral concomitant fractures of the hip and femoral shaft. *J Bone Joint Surg (Am)* 1979;61:503.
Childress HM. Well leg traction? An efficient but neglected procedure. *Clin Orthop* 1967;51:127.
Clawson DK. Intracapsular fractures of the femur treated by the sliding screw plate fixation method. *J Trauma* 1964;4:53.
Clawson DK. Trochanteric fractures treated by the sliding screw plate fixation method. *J Trauma* 1964;4:737.
Clawson DK, Smith RF, Hansen ST Jr. Closed intramedullary nailing of the femur. *J Bone Joint Surg (Am)* 1971;53:681.
Devas MB. Stress fractures of the femoral neck. *J Bone Joint Surg (Br)* 1965;47:1614.
Dimon JH, Hughston JC. Unstable intertrochanteric fractures of the hip. *J Bone Joint Surg (Am)* 1967;49:440.
Ernst J. Stress fractures of the neck of the femur. *J Trauma* 1964;4:71.
Fielding JW. Subtrochanteric fractures. *Clin Orthop* 1973;92:86.
Garden RS. Malreduction and avascular necrosis in subcapital fractures of the femur. *J Bone Joint Surg (Br)* 1971;53:183.
Hinchey JJ, Day PL. Primary prosthetic replacement in fresh femoral neck fractures. *J Bone Joint Surg (Am)* 1964;46:223.
Kempf I, Grosse A, Beck G. Closed locked intramedullary nailing: its application to comminuted fractures of the femur. *J Bone Joint Surg (Am)* 1985;67:709.
Kyle RF, Gustilo RB, Premer RF. Analysis of 622 intertrochanteric hip fractures. *J Bone Joint Surg (Am)* 1979;61:216.
Lesin BE, Mooney V, Ashby ME. Cast-bracing for fractures of the femur. *J Bone Joint Surg (Am)* 1977;59:917.

Lunceford EM. Use of the Moore self-locking vitallium prosthesis in acute fractures of the femoral neck. *J Bone Joint Surg (Am)* 1965;47:832.

Massie WK. Treatment of femoral neck fractures emphasizing long-term follow-up observations on aseptic necrosis. *Clin Orthop* 1973;92:16.

McElvenny RT. The importance of the lateral x-ray film in treating intracapsular fractures of the neck of the femur. *Am J Orthop* 1962;4:212.

Neer LS, Grantham SA, Shelton ML. Supracondylar fractures of the adult femur. *J Bone Joint Surg (Am)* 1967;49:591.

Olerud S. Operative treatment of supracondylar-condylar fractures of the femur. *J Bone Joint Surg (Am)* 1972;54:1015.

Seinsheimer F. Subtrochanteric fractures of the femur. *J Bone Joint Surg (Am)* 1978;60:300.

Singh M, Nagrath AR, Main PS. Changes in trabecular patterns of the upper end of the femur as an index of osteoporosis. *J Bone Joint Surg (Am)* 1970;52:457.

Stewart MN, Sick TO, Wallace SL. Fractures of the distal third of the femur. *J Bone Joint Surg (Am)* 1966;48:784.

Zickel RE. A new fixation device for subtrochanteric fractures of the femur. A preliminary report. *Clin Orthop* 1967;54:115.

24. KNEE INJURIES: ACUTE AND OVERUSE

I. **Foundation of injury diagnosis.** Knee injuries are common in active individuals. Both acute and overuse injuries occur, and they require different investigative processes to diagnose and treat them properly.
   A. **Subdivision** of clinical categories
      1. **Acute injury** is an injury that occurs when a single application of force creates musculoskeletal damage, for example, in athletics, motor vehicle trauma, and falls from a height.
      2. **Acute on chronic injury** is an injury that results in a disabled state that can be quiescent over time and results in a new injury episode at a later time. This new injury represents an acute injury. However, the new injury does not depend on abnormal forces to create the injury, rather there must be preexisting damage to the musculoskeletal tissue. Common examples include recurrent patella instability and recurrent shoulder subluxation.
      3. **Overuse injury** is an injury characterized by the absence of an acute injury or at least no injury significant enough to explain the current clinical situation. This kind of injury results from repetitive submaximal or subclinical trauma that results in macroscopic or microscopic damage to a structural unit or its blood supply. This overuse pattern can be seen in all musculoskeletal tissue, but is most common in bone (overuse pattern resulting in stress fracture), bursal tissues (overuse pattern resulting in bursitis), tendon (overuse pattern resulting in tendinitis).
   B. **Clinical correlation:** The clinical approach to a knee injury (acute or chronic) depends on four cornerstones:
      1. History
      2. Physical examination
      3. Tests and their interpretations
      4. Treatment
II. **Approach to the acutely injured knee**
   A. **History**
      1. **Mechanism of injury** helps to identify potential structures that may have been damaged by the application of force, either direct (contact) or indirect (twisting mechanism). If the injury was a contact injury, one should look for external signs at the point of force application and what structures might have been injured as that force continues. For instance, a blow to the anterior tibia might create upper tibial bruising. This force creates a posterior displacement of the tibia on the femur, potentially injuring the posterior cruciate ligament. Noncontact injuries frequently involve rotatory twisting; the lower limb remains fixed as the upper body twists around the knee.
      2. **Was a pop heard or felt?** A pop is frequently associated with tearing of a ligament, most commonly the anterior cruciate ligament.
      3. **Return to play.** The degree of pain or disability cannot be used as a reliable indicator of the seriousness of an injury. However, continued play with little or no impairment in performance diminishes the likelihood of a serious knee injury.
      4. **Has the joint been previously injured?** Frequently this question uncovers an acute on chronic injury.
      5. **Knee joint swelling** within 12 hours after an injury is, by definition, hemorrhage into the joint. An effusion that occurs after 12 hours suggests synovial fluid accumulation caused by reactive synovitis.
      6. The **differential diagnosis** of an acute knee hemarthrosis (what inside the knee can bleed?) is as follows (2):
         a. **Ligament injury.** The anterior cruciate ligament (ACL) and posterior cruciate ligament (PCL) are intraarticular/extrasynovial

structures. The superficial medial collateral ligament (MCL) is an extraarticular structure. However, the deep MCL is a thickening of the joint capsule and is intraarticular. In a complete tearing of the MCL, both structures are torn. The lateral collateral ligament (LCL) is an extraarticular structure. It is rare that this ligament is torn in isolation. The most common ligament torn in acute hemarthrosis is the ACL (approximately 70%) (7).

    b. Peripheral meniscus tear. The outer, or peripheral, one third of the meniscus is vascular, and a tear in this region results in a hemarthrosis. Meniscus tears in this zone have the potential for healing and are repairable. Tears in the inner two thirds of the meniscus are more often associated with synovial irritation, leading to a serous effusion.

    c. Fractures. Any fracture that involves the joint surface results in a joint hemarthrosis. In addition to obvious condylar/patellar fractures, occult osteochondral fractures can be a source of hemarthrosis. These can include avulsion fractures of the PCL and ACL (more common in developing adolescents), and fractures resulting from patella dislocation.

    d. Synovial and capsular tears. Patella dislocations, even in the absence of fractures, are a source of hemarthrosis because the medial patellofemoral ligament and medial retinacular restraints are torn.

B. Physical examination

  1. Inspection

    a. Swelling. The absence of notable intraarticular swelling does not signify a less severe injury. Severe ligament disruptions are associated with large capsular disruptions and fluid typically escapes into the surrounding tissue. The absence of knee swelling may indicate an extraarticular source of pain.

    b. Localized bruises and abrasions. These can be useful to identify the point of application of force in a contact injury. These can indicate the direction of the force, which helps to indicate what structures may be injured.

  2. Palpation

    a. Direct palpation of the injured area corresponds to the anatomic structure underneath that area. This is most useful in meniscal, patellofemoral, and collateral ligament injuries. The cruciate ligaments do not have a palpable attachment to the capsule, and, therefore, direct palpation is not possible. However, injury to the ACL is associated with anterolateral subluxation of the tibia on the femur, making anterolateral joint line tenderness common.

    b. Patella subluxation/dislocation is associated with medial tenderness along the patella retinaculum, especially at the medial epicondyle where the medial patellofemoral ligament (MPFL) inserts or along the superior medial portion of the patella.

  3. Range of motion

    a. A **locked knee** is defined as the inability to obtain full passive motion of the joint as a result of a mechanical block. This does not mean that the knee is in one position, but rather that there is an inability to obtain full motion. Common causes are a displaced meniscus tear or loose body.

    b. Pseudo locked knee is the inability to obtain full range of motion because of pain (resulting in hamstring spasm) or intraarticular knee swelling.

    c. Active range of motion assesses the integrity of the motor units surrounding a joint. Even in a severely injured knee, the patient typically retains the ability to lift the leg. Therefore, active straight-leg raising and range of motion should be assessed. Frequently missed acute knee injuries are disruptions of the extensor mechanism, which include quadriceps tendon and patella tendon injuries.

4. **Stability testing.** The *sine qua non* of a ligament disruption is the presence of pathologic joint motion.

   a. **Straight plane instabilities** are the easiest instabilities to test on a knee. This represents the ability to move the tibia away from the femur in four known planes.

      (1) **Medial instability** is associated with injury to medial or tibial collateral ligament (MCL).

      (2) **Lateral instability** is associated with injury to lateral or fibular collateral ligament (LCL).

      (3) **Anterior instability** is associated with injury to anterior cruciate ligament (ACL).

      (4) **Posterior instability** is associated with injury to posterior cruciate ligament (PCL).

   b. **Rotatory instabilities** refers to the rotation of the tibia around its vertical or longitudinal axis (Fig. 24-1).

      (1) **Anterior lateral instability** is associated with ACL injury.

      (2) **Posterior lateral instability** is associated with structures of the posterolateral corner of the knee (iliotibial band [ITB], arcuate complex, and popliteal tendon). These are frequently associated with PCL and LCL injuries.

      (3) **Posterior medial injuries** are rare and are commonly associated with PCL injury with or without MCL injury.

      (4) **Anterior medial injuries** are associated with ACL and MCL injuries.

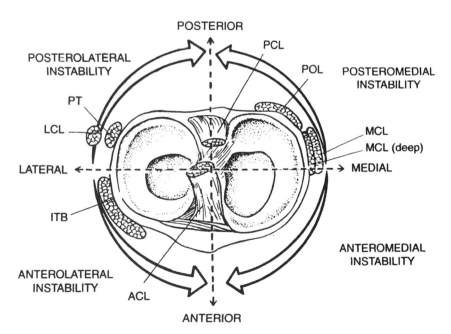

FIG. 24-1. Rotatory instability of the knee. PCL, posterior cruciate ligament; POL, posterior oblique ligament; MCL, medial collateral ligament; ACL, anterior cruciate ligament; ITB, iliotibial band; LCL, lateral collateral ligament; PT, popliteal tendon. (From Arendt EA. Assessment of the athlete with a painful knee. In: Griffin LY, ed. *Rehabilitation of the injured knee,* 2nd ed. St. Louis: Mosby, 1990, with permission.)

c. Extensor mechanism instability

    (1) Apprehension sign. Passive lateral movement of the patella causing pain or quadriceps contraction is suggestive of patellofemoral subluxation or dislocation.

    (2) Straight-leg raising against gravity confirms the integrity of the extensor mechanism, including quadriceps tendon, patella, and patella tendon. A "lag" sign represents the difference between passive and active extension of the knee. A lag signifies disruption or weakness of the extensor mechanism.

    (3) Medial and lateral patella restraints. Stability testing of the patellofemoral joint involves assessing the degree of passive patella motion in a medial and lateral direction of the patella. This is typically measured against an imaginary midline of the patella in the resting position (Fig. 24-2). This maneuver tests the static restraints of the medial and lateral extensor retinaculum complex. Any change from the patient's "normal" measured against their normal contralateral knee is suggestive of extensor mechanism disruption. Most particularly, an increase in lateral patella motion represents laxity or incompetence of the MPFL and medial retinacular structures associated with past or present patella dislocation.

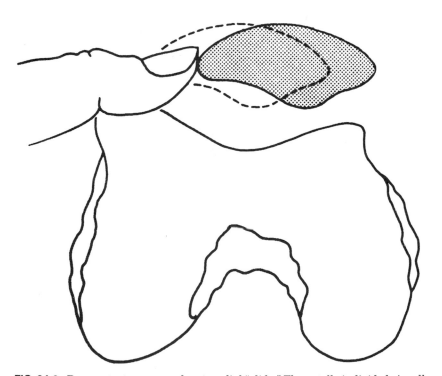

FIG. 24-2. Demonstrates one quadrant medial "glide." The patella is divided visually into four quadrants. Holding the patella between the examiner's thumb and index finger, the limits of medial and lateral motion are assessed and recorded as "quadrants" of motion. (From Halbrecht JL, Jackson DW. Acute dislocation of the patella. In: Fox JM, Pizzo WD, eds. *The patellofemoral joint.* New York: McGraw-Hill, 1993, with permission.)

C. **Tests** and their interpretation
  1. **Plain radiographs**
     a. **Anteroposterior view.** The primary utility of this view is to rule out diagnoses and assess overall tibiofemoral alignment. Standing views are preferred, but if pain and swelling limit full extension or full weight bearing, supine views are obtained.
     b. **Lateral view** evaluates the caudad/cephalad position of the kneecap. Patella alta, or increase in the cephalad position of the kneecap, suggests a patella tendon injury, especially when the kneecap on the injured side is higher than on the opposite side. Avulsion fractures, especially that of the PCL, are typically visualized along the posterior aspect of the tibia in this view.
     c. **Axial view** evaluates the position of the patella in its relationship to the trochlear groove. Oftentimes, osteochondral fragmentation following a patella dislocation can be visualized on this view. Typically, one would see fragmentation of the medial patella facet or lateral femoral condyle in an acute patella dislocation (Fig. 24-3). Different views have been established (Laurin's, Merchant's) (5). The clinician should become familiar with one technique. Axial views are necessary for complete evaluation of all acute knee injuries.
     d. **Notch or tunnel view** is most useful for evaluation of avulsion fractures of the tibia, osteochondritis dissecans (OCD), and loose bodies. This view is not standard for an acute knee injury.
  2. **Stress radiographs** can be used to document ligamentous disruption of the knee, but are infrequently performed. Stress radiographs, however, are most useful to rule out unstable epiphyseal growth plate injuries.
  3. **Bone scans** are most useful in occult infections and to rule out stress fractures. Their usefulness in diagnosing reflex sympathetic dystrophy is variable. This is not a common diagnostic test ordered for acute knee injuries.
  4. **Computed tomography** has few specific applications for routine imaging of acute knee injuries. It continues to have utility for evaluating complex fractures around the knee, especially those involving articular surfaces. When used with contrast, it can be useful to evaluate the cartilage integrity of osteochondral defects such as OCD.
  5. **Magnetic resonance imaging (MRI)** for the knee has its largest application in evaluating meniscus and cruciate ligament injury. The overall accuracy is greater than 90% (26). An MRI scan is typically an adjunct in the evaluation of an acutely injured knee. It should be performed only if it will alter the treatment protocol and is typically ordered by the

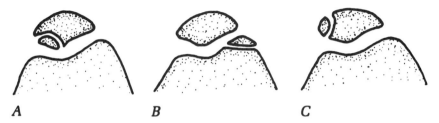

A   **B**   **C**

FIG. 24-3. Three type of fractures associated with patella dislocation. **A:** Osteochondral fracture of the medial patella facet. **B:** Osteochondral fracture of the lateral femoral condylar. **C:** Avulsion fragment of medial patella femoral ligament off medial epicondyle (osseous-nonarticular). (From Halbrecht JL, Jackson DW. Acute dislocation of the patella. In: Fox JM, Pizzo WD, eds. *The patellofemoral joint.* New York: McGraw-Hill, 1993.)

physician who will be giving definitive treatment. It should never be used in the absence of a thorough and knowledgeable history and physical examination. Posterior lateral knee structures are not well visualized in the standard knee MRI views.

D. General treatment

1. **Joint aspiration** is not advised as a necessary part of the evaluation of knee injury. However, aspiration that contains fat droplets may be helpful in diagnosing a fracture. At times, aspiration can be therapeutic, as in the case of a tense effusion.

2. **Immobilization and crutches** are the safest way to protect an injured knee until a repeat examination or definitive treatment can be performed by the same or a referral physician. When feasible, however, removal of the brace to perform gentle range-of-motion exercise is useful to help resolve an effusion. Partial weight bearing, depending on the patient's comfort level and the working diagnosis, can also be therapeutic and is encouraged. Strategies to reduce swelling should be included in the initial treatment recommendation. These include ice, gentle passive or active assisted range of motion, elevation, and compression.

3. **Repeat examination** is helpful in establishing a more firm diagnosis, especially when pain, swelling, or apprehension limits the initial examination.

4. **Antiinflammatory medication** is commonly used to control pain. The efficacy in the reduction of an acute effusion or inflammation of injured tissues is debated. Antiinflammatory medications also change the role of platelet function and can increase bleeding of an injured site.

III. Specific acute knee injuries

A. Fractures of the patella

1. **Anatomic considerations.** The patella is a sesamoid bone that is contained within the extensor mechanism. Its main function is to provide a lever arm for superior mechanical functioning of the extensor mechanism. The strong quadriceps muscle complex is attached to its superior pole.

2. Common types of **fractures**

   a. **Transverse fractures,** with or without comminution, can be caused by direct or indirect violence. They frequently are associated with disruption of the extensor mechanism and need to be surgically stabilized to regain the mechanical function of the extensor mechanism.

   b. **Vertical fractures** of the patella frequently are due to a direct injury; infrequently they represent an overuse injury of the patella. When they are associated with no or minimal displacement, they do not constitute a disruption of the extensor mechanism and can be treated conservatively.

   c. **Chip fractures** of the medial border are commonly seen with a patella dislocation; infrequently they can be associated with direct trauma (see **B**).

3. **Treatment**

   a. **Extraarticular fractures** and **undisplaced fractures** may be treated symptomatically without surgery. However, they must be protected from further damage. Immobilization in a knee immobilizer for 2–4 weeks is sufficient, with weight bearing as tolerated. Quadriceps isometric exercises can be performed during this time. Gentle, passive range of motion as per the patient's comfort level is recommended.

   b. For **displaced fractures** involving the articular surface, an anatomic reduction is essential. Open reduction and internal fixation of the fragments with a tension band wire or lag screw is the treatment of choice (25) (Fig. 24-4).

   c. **Comminuted fractures** require surgical treatment. A patellectomy is necessary if the entire patella cannot be internally fixed to

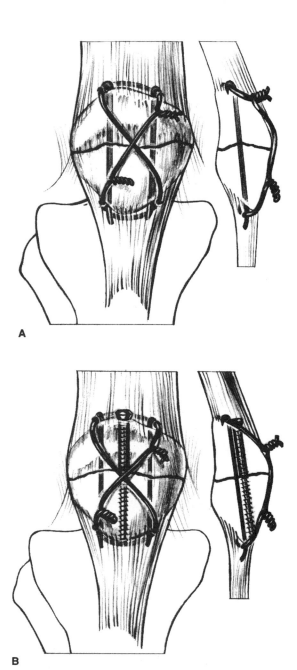

FIG. 24-4. A: Internal fixation of a transverse patellar fracture using standard tension-band wiring technique. **B:** Internal fixation of a transverse patellar fracture using an additional 3.5-mm lag screw. The superior fragment is overdrilled to 3.5 mm. (Modified fronm Hansen ST, Swiontkowski MF. *Orthopaedic trauma protocols.* New York: Raven, 1993:309, with permission.)

gain stability (33). If more than half of the patella remains intact, then the comminuted pieces may be excised and the tendon sutured just above the subchondral bone into the remaining pole of the patella. Occasionally, fragments are large enough to fix with tension band wiring or 2.7-mm cortical lag screws (25).

d. If an **osteochondral fracture** is suspected, an arthroscopy to inspect the joint and remove small fragments of bone and cartilage should be performed. This is often the result of a patella dislocation (see **B**). At times, typically the result of direct trauma, a large osteochondral fragment can be present and if the chondral fragment has an osseous layer backing it, fixation should be attempted. This might be most readily accomplished by using bioabsorbable implants. Cartilage injuries are ominous for the future health of the joint (19,23).

e. **Postoperative treatment** must be individualized according to the type of fracture and the security of the repair. Most knees are initially placed in a compressive dressing with a posterior splint or knee immobilizer. If rigid internal fixation is achieved and the patient is trustworthy, early protective passive range of motion is initiated, progressing to active motion. Typically, 6 weeks of some form of immobilization is necessary for healing of the fractures. Quadriceps muscle strength within the limits of the allowed knee motion should be encouraged throughout this time.

f. The **prognosis** of patella fractures depends on the degree of articular damage and the ability to reestablish quadriceps strength. Both are necessary for full recovery of the extensor mechanism complex. If articular damage is minimal and good extensor mechanism strength can be restored, the prognosis of patella fractures is excellent.

B. **Patella dislocations**

1. **Mechanism of injury.** This injury can result from a direct blow, but it is more commonly associated with a noncontact twisting injury involving an externally rotated tibia combined with a forceful quadriceps contraction. The patella is dislocated laterally, which disrupts the medial retinaculum. Frequently, spontaneous reduction occurs. When the patella relocates, osteochondral fragments can occur, because the medial patella facet hits the lateral femoral condyle. These two areas, in particular, should be scrutinized for osteochondral damage (Fig. 24-3). **Medial** patellar dislocations are rare in knees that have not had previous surgery. It is most often associated with iatrogenic causes, in particular a lateral retinacular release (11).

2. **Physical examination.** The patient will invariably have medial retinacular tenderness, especially at the medial femoral condylar region. If an attempt is made to displace the patella laterally, the patient resists this (patella apprehension test). A straight leg raising effort should be requested. The patient should be able to lift the leg, although he/she will report pain with this maneuver. This is frequently associated with minimal extension lag (the difference between passive and active extension).

3. **Roentgenograms.** An axial view is necessary for a complete evaluation of patellofemoral or extensor mechanism injury. If the patient is seen before spontaneous reduction of the patella, axial views will reveal the dislocated patella. Once the injury is reduced, the axial view reveals any residual tilt or subluxation as well as the presence of osteochondral fragmentation. Axial views obtained in lower degrees of flexion (Laurin's 20-degree views or Merchant's 30-degree views) are more likely to show minor degrees of continued subluxation (16,17,21).

a. If the patella **remains dislocated,** then a reduction should be performed without delay to relieve pain. Intravenous analgesia with morphine sulfate and a hypnotic should be obtained before reduction is attempted. Once the patient's muscles are relaxed, the knee is placed in full extension and the patella is reduced into place by a gentle, medially directed pressure. Slight elevation of the medial border of the patella during this maneuver is ideal. General or regional block anesthetic is rarely required.

b. If a large associated **hermathrosis** is present, aspiration is suggested because this can be therapeutic in relieving pain.

c. There is no consensus in **surgical treatment** for patella dislocations. There is universal agreement that, if it is associated with osteochondral fragmentation, then an arthroscopy with irrigation and debridement is necessary. Whether surgical repair of the injured structures is necessary or whether it produces superior functional outcome is unclear (8).

d. When **acute surgical repair** is performed, it is directed at the medial retinacular structures, in particular the MPFL (8). This may also involve a lateral retinacular release or a medial transfer of the tibial tubercle (9).

e. If there is no evidence of a fracture or continued radiographic subluxation or tilt, **nonoperative treatment** can be elected. Nonsurgical treatment is directed at providing an environment in which the patella does not dislocate. Typically, the injury should be treated initially with crutches and a knee sleeve, encouraging gentle motion. In the presence of a significant hemarthrosis, a compression dressing and immobilization in extension is appropriate until early motion is comfortable. The knee sleeve is used for 4 -6 weeks while an aggressive quadriceps rehabilitation program is pursued. Typically, 6 weeks of monitored activities, keeping the knee out of pivoting and twisting activities, is recommended. The most important thing to accomplish in the first 6 weeks postoperatively is return of normal quadriceps strength. Return to full functional activities should be based on functional strength rather than a specific time period from the original injury.

5. **Complications**

a. **Recurrent dislocation.** The main physical examination feature associated with recurrent dislocation is continued quadriceps weakness. Recurrent dislocations that have successfully gained strength comparable to their other side will likely need surgical reconstruction to stabilize the patella. Recurrent patella dislocations are frequently associated with recurrent effusions at the time that the dislocation occurs; a history that "my knee gives out" following an initial patella dislocation may represent quad weakness and not necessarily another dislocation.

b. **Degenerative joint changes** of the patellofemoral joint may occur when significant cartilage trauma is present from the initial or recurrent patella subluxations.

C. **Meniscus injuries** about the knee

1. **Anatomic concerns.** Menisci are two C-shaped structures that rest on the medial and lateral sides of the tibial plateau; their main function is shock absorbency of the knee joint. Because their outer perimeter is thicker than their inner rim, some stability is afforded by their anatomic construct as well.

2. **Mechanism of injury.** Most isolated injuries of the meniscus (not associated with ligamentous injuries) occur with a rotatory stress on a weight-bearing knee. Isolated meniscal injuries occur from trapping of the meniscus between the femoral condyle and the tibia while the knee is weight bearing, typically in flexion. A history of locking or clicking is helpful, but it is frequently misleading. In a young patient (typically younger than age 30 years), significant trauma is necessary to injure a meniscus. However, in the older knee, a degenerative tear can occur simply from normal activity.

3. **Physical examination**
   a. **Joint line tenderness** is typically present along the medial (medial meniscus tear) or lateral (lateral meniscus tear) joint lines. This joint line pain increases with attempts at full extension or full flexion.
   b. The **McMurray test.** An audible, palpable, and often painful clunk is produced when the knee is extended from the full flexed position while the tibial is forcefully internally rotated (medial meniscus) or externally rotated (lateral meniscus). This sign is associated with a torn meniscus. Crepitus or pain along the joint line when this maneuver is performed, even in the absence of an audible clunk, is also suggestive of a medial/lateral meniscus tear.
   c. The presence of an **effusion** is frequent in a meniscus tear. Typically, the normal knee has less than 10 mL of fluid and is not detectable on physical examination. As much as 10–30 mL can be detected by "milking" the suprapatellar pouch and looking for a fluid wave as one tries to push the fluid from the lateral side of the knee to the medial side of the knee. This maneuver is the best way to detect small amounts of swelling. The presence of an effusion limits complete extension of the joint and may be a cause of "locking" or lack of full extension.

4. **Roentgenograms**
   a. A meniscus tear is not seen on **plain roentgenographs.** However, in an older patient, medial or lateral joint space narrowing may give some indication as to the likelihood of a degenerative meniscus tear.
   b. An **MRI** scan is frequently requested to confirm the presence of a meniscus tear. The MRI study has high accuracy in diagnosing a meniscus tear (greater than 93%) (6,29).

5. **Treatment**
   a. An **isolated meniscus tear** in the repairable zone in a young person should be repaired. The re-tear rate of a meniscus repair in a stable knee (not associated with a ligamentous tear) has a higher re-tear rate than those meniscus tears associated with ligamentous instability when both meniscus and ligament injuries are surgically treated (4). Nonetheless, an attempt to save young meniscus when possible is recommended.
   b. A **symptomatic meniscus tear in the nonrepairable zone** or a complex meniscus tear should be arthroscopically debrided. This is advised in any age group if symptoms, such as pain, continued swelling, or instability, persist.
   c. In the **older age group** in whom one suspects a degenerative meniscus tear, the meniscus tear is a reflection of generalized early arthritis of the knee joint. This "tear" should be treated symptomatically according to the patient and physician's discussion. The presence of a degenerative meniscus tear on MRI scan is not an indication to treat. If the symptoms associated with a degenerative meniscus tear can be quieted down with rest, relative rest, or antiinflammatory, then surgical treatment may not be necessary.

D. **Ligamentous injuries** of the knee
   1. **Anatomic considerations.** The cruciate ligaments are intraarticular, extrasynovial structures. When the cruciate ligaments are torn, they can create a hemarthrosis or bleed into the joint. The LCL and superficial MCL are extraarticular structures. The deep MCL is a thickening of the joint capsule and thus is intraarticular.
   2. **Mechanism** of injury
      a. **Ligamentous injuries** can be the result of a direct or indirect trauma. Indirect trauma frequently occurs when the body rotates around a relatively fixed foot or leg. Direct injuries are a consequence of force directed to the knee or limb. Typically, the ligament opposite the area of contact is the ligament that is the most vulner-

able. For instance, a blow to the lateral side of the knee places the MCL most under stress for injury. Straight plain instabilities (anterior, posterior, medial, lateral) are most readily assessable by direct physical examination. Rotatory instability of the knee (anterolateral and posterolateral) require more sophisticated physical examination skills.

  b. In an **isolated tear of the MCL,** palpable discomfort can be detected anywhere along the ligament from its origin on the medial femoral condyle to its insertion on the tibia (approximately three finger breadths below the joint line). The deep capsular ligament is a thickening at the joint line. Medial joint line tenderness is also associated with MCL injuries. However, different from a meniscal injury, an MCL injury would create pain to stressing the knee in a valgus direction as well as to externally rotating the leg with the knee flexed.

  c. **Isolated injuries of the LCL** are rare. Frequently accompanying complete tears of the LCL are tears of the posterior lateral complex with or without cruciate involvement. If one suspects a lateral/posterior lateral injury, physical examination must include close inspection of peroneal nerve function distally in the leg and foot region.

  d. **Isolated tears of the PCL** are frequently associated with a hyperextension injury (indirect injury) or a blunt contusion to the front of the tibia (direct injury).

  e. **Isolated ACL injuries** can be sustained through a number of mechanisms, most commonly a deceleration injury or an external rotation valgus injury of the knee.

3. **Physical examination.** The amount of joint line opening or motion between the tibia and femur that occurs with manual testing is graded according to American Medical Association (AMA) guidelines: grade 1 injuries, less than 5 mm of joint line opening; grade 2 injuries, 5–10 mm; grade 3 injuries, complete tear is more than 10 mm of opening (1).

  a. The main **clinical motion test** for providing an analysis of the severity of MCL complex injuries is a valgus stress test with the knee flexed at 30 degrees. The leg is put over the side of the examining table, the fingers are placed over the medial joint line to assess the amount of joint line opening and rotation, and a valgus stress is applied to the knee by moving the leg to the outside. The reverse of this, placing a varus stress on the knee, is the main clinical motion test to analyze LCL instability.

  b. Typically, injuries to the LCL also involve injury to the **posterior lateral complex.** Motion tests to determine the amount of injury to the posterior lateral complex of the knee are the most complex of all knee examinations (15).

  c. The main clinical motion test for an analysis of ACL injuries is the **Lachman test** (32). This is performed with the knee in approximately 30 degrees of flexion with the leg in neutral rotation. The examiner holds firmly the distal femur in one hand and the proximal tibia in the other hand, then places an anterior directed force on the proximal tibia. Grading of displacement of the tibia on the femur is along the AMA guidelines. ACL injuries are also with anterior lateral rotatory tibial subluxation that is best evaluated through the pivot shift maneuver or Losee maneuver (18).

  d. The main clinical motion test to detect injuries of the PCL is the **posterior drawer test,** which is performed by placing the knee at 70–90 degrees of flexion. A posterior force is applied to the tibia and the extent of translation and the quality of the endpoint is recorded. Again, AMA guidelines are used to assess the degree of translation. The key to this test is accurately assessing the starting point of the tibia (22).

e. An acute knee examination should include **all major ligamentous structures** within the knee. Significant anteroposterior translation (greater than 10 mm) with the drawer or Lachman's test may suggest an injury to both the ACL and the PCL. Varus and valgus stress testing should be performed both at 0 and 30 degrees of knee flexion. Varus or valgus asymmetry laxity that exists at 0 degree of knee extension suggests a cruciate as well as collateral ligament injury. Varus or valgus asymmetry laxity existing at 30 degrees of flexion but not at 0 degree is most indicative of an isolated collateral ligament injury.

4. **Treatment**
   a. **Isolated tears** of ligamentous injuries
      (1) Complete isolated tears of the **MCL** can be treated conservatively (12,14). The most rigorous form of treatment is progressive weight bearing on crutches, in a brace, limiting valgus stress for 4–6 weeks. In the absence of a complete tear of the MCL, one can bear weight as pain and motion permit. Complete recovery after isolated MCL injuries is the norm.
      (2) **Isolated tears of the PCL** are frequently treated nonoperatively. In the rehabilitation process, special emphasis on quadriceps strength is important to maintain a muscular support to limit posterior displacement of the tibia.
      (3) **Isolated tears of the ACL** are prone to subluxation events when jumping and pivoting activities are performed. In young active patients, or in middle-aged patients with high-demand jobs or recreational aspirations, ACL reconstruction is typically advised.
      (4) **Multiligamentous knee injuries** most commonly involve the ACL and MCL or PCL with posterior lateral injuries. Operative treatments yields the best functional results in two-ligament knee injuries.

E. **Knee dislocations**
   1. **Evaluation and treatment.** This relatively rare dislocation requires immediate reduction and evaluation for joint stability. Reduction under anesthesia is frequently necessary (24,30). Immediate and continuous evaluation of vascular status of the leg reduction is important. If there is any question of the vascular supply, an arteriogram and surgical vascular repair must be performed immediately (10). Prophylactic fasciotomy should be considered to prevent a compartment syndrome following vascular repair. If a vascular repair is present combined with severe knee instability, an external fixator is typically applied to protect the vascular construct until definitive surgical treatment of the torn ligament ensues.
   2. **Early repair** of torn ligaments offers the best outcome (30). If the injury is associated with a vascular repair or significant disruption to the skin, a subacute reconstruction is indicated (0–3 weeks). Late surgical approach (>4 weeks) is more difficult because of soft-tissue scarring, particularly if it involves a posterior lateral corner, in which individual structures can become more difficult to dissect. In dislocated knees that are approached late (>6 weeks), reconstructive efforts aimed at collateral ligament injuries are frequently necessary (in deference to a primary repair if done early). The cruciate ligament injuries are frequently reconstructed in acute and late surgeries in deference to a repair. Because of the typically severe nature of these injuries, allograft tissue in deference to autograft tissue from the same or contralateral knee is the norm. If the original injury has no injury to the joint surface and a functioning vascular system, then, typically, functional use of the leg will parallel the ability to get back satisfactory strength and motion. Satisfactory function for day-to-day activities is common following these injuries. However, high-level activities following knee dislocations are rare.

F. Extensor mechanism disruptions
  1. **Anatomic considerations.** The extensor mechanism consists of the quadriceps muscle complex, quadriceps tendon, patella, patella tendon, and patella tendon insertion into the tibial tubercle. Disruption of the extensor mechanism along any one of its parts can result in failure of the patient to perform a straight-leg raising effort. A partial tear frequently results in the patient's ability to lift the leg, but with a considerable lag (difference between passive and active extension of the leg).
  2. **Clinical considerations.** A quadriceps tendon disruption is difficult to assess on physical examination unless one requests a straight-leg raising effort by the patient. **Quadriceps tendon ruptures** are a frequently missed cause of acute knee injuries. **Patella tendon disruptions** are often associated with an indirect trauma consisting of a forceful quadriceps contraction against a relatively fixed lower limb. These can be subtle injuries. If the rupture is below the inferior border of the patella (i.e., in the patella tendon or at the tibial tubercle), then patella alta would be present, which is best seen on lateral knee roentgenographic studies. Extensor mechanism disruptions commonly occur in patients with systemic illness such as diabetes or renal failure.
IV. Special concerns in the growing adolescent
  A. Physeal injuries are one cause of an acute knee injury in a growing adolescent.
    1. A **distal femur physeal injury,** particularly if it is a nondisplaced injury, can be confused with a collateral ligament injury. Pain is present, not only at the origin of the collateral ligaments but also across the anterior aspect of the femur or tibia, which is readily palpable in most children. Roentgenographs can show some widening and, at times, displacement of the physis. Stress roentgenographs can confirm the diagnosis and assess the stability of the fracture construct. Surgical reduction and stabilization for any displaced physeal fracture is imperative. Stable injuries can be treated nonoperatively (3).
    2. The **tibial apophysis** can avulse in the adolescent with closing growth plates. The tibial growth plate fuses from posterior to anterior, and an avulsion of the tibial tubercle frequently involves an interarticular fracture into the joint. By history this is associated with a strong quadriceps contraction, and radiographically this is associated with patella alta. Surgical reduction and fixation is advisable for the best outcome.
  B. Ligament avulsion. Cruciate ligament avulsions, particularly the attachments of the ACL and PCL onto the tibia, occur in the growing adolescent. When these are associated with a large bony fragment, surgical reduction and fixation is advised. The rehabilitation follows the course of a bone healing rather than that of a ligament reconstruction/revascularization.
  C. Osteochondritis dissecans (OCD)
    1. **Definition.** OCD is defined as an area of avascular bone commonly presenting in the medial femoral condyle of a skeletally immature child. The etiology of this area of avascularity is unknown. Most commonly accepted theories are trauma, abnormal ossification within the epiphysis, ischemia, or some combination of these. Approximately 40% of patients with OCD have a history of prior knee trauma to a mild or moderate degree (19). The medial condyle is involved 85% of the time versus 15% of the lateral condyle. Fifty percent of loose bodies in the knee are associated with OCD.
    2. **Natural history.** Most juvenile lesions (presenting before closure of growth plates) heal spontaneously. In the skeletally mature, higher incidence of cartilage trauma is evident. This cartilage damage exists in the area adjacent to the avascular bone and is thought to be altered because of reduced force transmission of bone below this cartilage. In its extreme form, the osteocartilaginous lesion can break away from the healthy bone, forming a loose body. Once the articular cartilage over the

OCD area becomes soft, symptoms increase and the involved fragment may become disengaged. The larger the defect, the more symptomatic the patient is and the more readily arthritic changes can occur locally.

   3. Treatment
   a. **Juvenile osteochondral** lesions can typically be treated nonsurgically with rest from high impact activities and observation. These patients should be followed up at regular intervals (3–6 months) until resolution of the lesion on roentgenogram is seen.
   b. Typically, surgical treatment for **adult OCD** (OCD after growth plate closure) is recommended. The type of surgical treatment depends on the degree of cartilage involvement and can include drilling, debridement, fixation, replacement, or excision (19).

V. Overuse syndromes
   A. **Definition.** Repetitive submaximal or subclinical trauma that results in macroscopic or microscopic damage to a structural unit that can result in pain or dysfunction. Although clinicians refer to it as an "itis," an inflammatory response is not always seen histologically. It is thought that damage to the structural unit or blood supply is a frequent cause of overuse injuries. The most common form of overuse injury is from an endogenous source, that is, mechanical circumstances in which the musculoskeletal tissue is subjected to greater tensile force or stress than it can effectively absorb.
   B. **History.** Overuse injuries are characterized by the absence of an acute injury, or at least no injury significant enough to explain the current clinical situation. The most important feature to look for in the patient's history is a "change" in functional demand. The patient is typically an athlete or worker who is undergoing change and who is considered a transitional person; these patients are at high risk for development of overuse injuries. A transitional athlete or worker is defined as a person with a change in his or her internal or external environment, such as the following:
      1. Change in intensity of repetitive activity (distance/time)
      2. Change in frequency or duration of repetitive activity
      3. Changes in equipment (footwear/surface changes including material composition or slope)
      4. Changes in competitive climate/work climate/activity level
      5. Changes in weather
      6. Changes in lifestyle (puberty, aging, significant weight gain, and, for women, pregnancy and menopause)
   C. **Physical examination**
      1. Inspection
         a. **Alignment** of the limb is necessary in evaluating any overuse injury of the lower extremity. This includes rotation of the pelvis, varus or valgus alignment of the knee, and pronation or supination at the foot. Any change in "normal alignment" can cause tissue overload anywhere along the kinetic chain. Some limb alignment features are constitutional and cannot be changed except by surgery; others can be modified. The two most common forms of modification include the following:
            (1) An **orthotic** can change the position of a flexible foot and thus can affect the entire kinematic chain. Particularly, a flexible pronated foot can be restored to normal alignment with the use of an orthotic.
            (2) An anteriorly tilted pelvis is associated with **increased internal femoral rotation** and **knee valgus.** This can frequently be altered by appropriate hip abductor and extensor strengthening exercises (28).
         b. **Redness or warmth** is not common in overuse injuries, but may indicate the presence of an acutely inflamed bursa or tendon.
         c. **Joint effusion** is not common in overuse injuries. It indicates an intraarticular source of pathology.

D. Investigational tests
1. **Strength tests.** These can include the following:
   a. **Weakness** compared with the contralateral limb
   b. **Concentric** (muscle shortens while contracting) muscle strength versus eccentric (muscle lengthens while contracting) muscle strength in the same muscle group (see **H.1.b.**)
   c. **Agonist** (joint motion in one plane resulting from muscle contraction) versus antagonist (the muscle group opposing or resisting joint motion caused by agonist muscle) strength in same limb (i.e., quadriceps to hamstring strength)
   d. **Absolute strength** and **peak torque** to body weight ratio compared with population norms
   e. **Endurance strength** with a measure of fatigability
2. Evaluation of **flexibility,** especially in key muscle groups, include quadriceps, hamstring, hip flexors, Achilles tendon.
E. Radiographs
1. **Plain radiographs** are infrequently necessary for evaluation of overuse injuries. Radiographic views of the patellofemoral joint, in particular axial views, may be helpful to assess patella position. Standing knee views show arthritic changes, including bone spurs and joint space narrowing.
2. **MRI.** The main advantage of an MRI scan is its ability to view intraarticular versus extraarticular pathology. Routine use of MRI to diagnose overuse injuries is not advantageous, although significant tendinitis and bursitis can be visualized by MRI.
F. Blood work. Evaluate for **systemic disease,** including collagen vascular disease and Lyme's disease.
G. Treatment
1. **Reduce inflammation with**
   a. **Nonsteroidal antiinflammatory medications**
   b. **Physical therapy** modalities
   c. **Rest or relative rest** of the injured part (reduce activities, substitute activities, and protect the injured part)
   d. **Ice**
   e. **Elevation** and **compression** if swelling is present
2. **Correct anatomic problems** when possible (patella sleeves, orthotics, braces, rarely surgery).
3. **Correct biomechanical errors** when possible (training sequence, sport style and form, strengthening and stretching of musculoskeletal units, evaluation of work station).
4. **Correct environmental concerns** when possible (new shoes, change to a more absorbent surface, adequate clothing).
H. Sports-specific rehabilitation
1. **Recovery** of strength
   a. **Closed chain exercises** of the lower extremity are those exercises in which the foot is supported or planted during the exercise, thus "closing the loop." Leg press or stand-up exercises such as partial squats are examples of closed chain lower leg exercises. For **lower extremity activities,** closed chained techniques are more functional and can obtain comparable gains in quadriceps strength with less overuse of the patellofemoral joint (28).
   b. **Concentric/eccentric** muscle strength
      (1) **Concentric** muscle contractions occur when a muscle shortens as it contracts. In an **eccentric** contraction, the muscle lengthens as contraction occurs.
      (2) **Eccentric** strengthening has long been favored for recovery of strength in the treatment of tendinitis. However, no studies have confirmed this scientifically. For the patellofemoral joint, eccentric muscle activity is an important part of functional use of the joint. Eccentric strength is the main decelerator of the body, an important function of the quadriceps complex.

I. **The physician's** role in diagnosing overuse injuries is to render an injury with its appropriate treatment as well as educating the patient. Patient education is the best treatment for the prevention of overuse injuries in the future.

J. The **patient's** role is to understand the causative factors in the injury and to understand the progression from injury to wellness. This includes activity modifications and their role in modifying their activities. The patient needs to implement a paced return to full activities.

VI. **Overuse injuries about the knee**

A. **Patella tendinitis**

1. Patella tendinitis is a common overuse injury that more typically affects the proximal attachment of the patella ligament to the inferior pole of the patella. It is also called a jumper's knee because it occurs most frequently in athletes who require repetitive eccentric quadriceps contractions, as is common in jumping athletes, and in athletes who frequently do heavy weight training.

2. The case of **patella tendinitis** is generally considered to be chronic stress overload resulting in microscopic tears of the tendon with incomplete healing.

3. **Treatment** is conservative for the main stage of early tendinitis. In addition to the general scheme of treatment of overuse syndromes outlined previously, the primary treatment emphasizes maximizing quadriceps strength and hamstring flexibility, reducing repetitive eccentric quadriceps contraction exercises, and adding them again in a paced fashion. Infrequently, surgery is necessary for the patient with recalcitrant disease. An MRI scan or ultrasound study can be used to define the area of the tendon affected by chronic tearing and subsequent degeneration. Excising this area of the tendon can be useful (27). Alternative schools of thought believe that the distal pole of the patella impinges on the patella tendon and that excision of the distal pole can be useful in treating this form of tendinitis (13).

B. **Iliotibial band syndrome**

1. **ITB syndrome (also known as ITB tendinitis)** is caused by excessive friction between the ITB and the distal lateral femoral condyle. The ITB functions as a weak extender of the knee in near full extension, and a more powerful knee flexor after 30 degrees of motion. The ITB is most stretched over the lateral femoral condyle at 30 degrees of knee flexion. This condition is common in runners and cyclists.

2. **Anatomic factors** have been implicated in ITB syndrome and include excessive foot pronation, genu varum at the knee, tight lateral patella retinacular structures, and an anterior tipped pelvis. Treatment is directed at modification of the initiating causative factors and reducing the inflammatory process. Stretching of the ITB, treating foot pronation with an orthotic, treating a tight lateral patella retinaculum with manual therapy, repositioning an anterior tilted pelvis, all can be useful interventions when the patient has these physical examination features.

C. **Tibial tubercle apophysis (Osgood-Schlatter's disease)**

1. **Clinical diagnosis.** This syndrome is usually seen in the rapidly growing athletic adolescent. It is characterized by point tenderness and enlargement of the tibial tubercle at the site of the patella tendon insertion. A constant traction to this location produces overgrowth of the tibial tubercle apophysis. Roentgenographic evaluation can be negative, or at times a prominent or irregular apophysis is seen. Once the apophyses have closed, there frequently can be a free bony particle anterior and superior to the tibial tubercle.

2. **Treatment.** The symptoms usually abate when the tibial tubercle fuses to the diaphysis, and, therefore, every effort should be made to quiet this injury down until full maturation is present in the developing adolescent. Treatment depends on the severity of the disease. Nearly all

cases are managed by the proper balancing of activities against the patient's symptoms. This can follow the general treatment pattern of overuse injuries as previously outlined. Surgical treatment is not indicated. Aggressive treatment might occasionally involve limited use of a knee immobilizer in recalcitrant cases in which the patient is dysfunctional in day-to-day activities.

D. **Patellofemoral pain syndrome**
   1. **Definition.** Patellofemoral pain syndrome is used to describe a constellation of symptoms that are related to the patellofemoral joint. Typically, this type of pain is considered an overuse syndrome, although the exact etiology and nature of pain continues to be poorly understood. Patellofemoral pain syndrome is that pain which originates in the anterior knee structures, in the absence of an identifiable acute injury (blunt trauma, dislocating or subluxing patella).
   2. **Chondromalacia patella** (CMP) is a term often used to describe anterior knee pain, although use of this term to describe clinical symptoms is not appropriate. CMP should be used only to describe the pathological entity of cartilage softening on the underneath side of the kneecap. Typically, this could only be diagnosed by surgical observation or MRI. The presence of cartilage softening does not always result in the clinical symptom of pain.
   3. **Preexisting conditions.** Anatomic factors that can predispose a patient to patellofemoral pain can include flexibility deficits, malalignment of the lower limbs, including excessive femoral anteversion, high Q-angle, rotation variations of the tibia, genu valgum at the knee, hindfoot valgus, and pes planus. Malalignment abnormalities have been implicated in the etiology of patellofemoral pain. However, there are a few population-based studies to support this. Any one abnormality may be trivial as a single entity. However, in combination with other anatomic variables and associated with overtraining and overuse, they frequently can lead to overuse injury (31).
   4. The role of **malalignment** and the etiology of patellofemoral pain continues to be debated. Radiographic imaging studies can reveal a patella that is malaligned within the trochlear groove, as evidenced by a patella tilt or subluxation. Some malalignment syndromes of the patella are residual from a previous subluxing or dislocating event. However, other malalignment syndromes can be present in the absence of an acute event and frequently are similar in both knees of the same person. It is thought that patella malalignment, when constitutional in a person, can become an overuse syndrome more readily and become a painful problem.
   5. **Clinical presentation.** The most common clinical presentation of a patellofemoral pain syndrome is pain on the anterior aspect of the knee that is aggravated by prolonged sitting and stair climbing. Because the retinacular structures of the patella extend both medially and laterally off the patella, pain can also be associated with either medial or lateral pain; therefore, it can create a very confusing clinical presentation. It is infrequently associated with swelling. Giving way episodes can be reported. Typically, the giving way episode is with straight-ahead activities, when one tries to engage the quadriceps, which then "fatigues." This should not be confused with giving way episodes associated with ligamentous instability, which typically occurs with planting, pivoting, or jumping activities. The patient may also have a catching or clicking phenomenon. This can occur because of irritation of the kneecap as it tracks in the trochlear groove. Another common patient complaint is that the knee "locks." When the knee "locks" in full extension, this is a manifestation of patellofemoral pain. The patient does not want to engage the kneecap in the groove because of pain, and, therefore, keeps the leg straight. If the knee is locked secondary to a loose body or meniscus, it is always locked in some degree of flexion.

6. **Treatment.** Historically, nonsurgical treatment has been the cornerstone for most patellofemoral pain disorders. The primary goal of patellofemoral rehabilitation is to reduce the symptoms of pain. This is done by a combination of reducing inflammation (antiinflammatory medications, physical therapy modalities) and improving quadriceps strength and endurance (see **V.H**). Other tools, such as orthotics, knee sleeves, and McConnell taping, can be used (20). Pelvic muscle strength, especially hip abductor and hip extensor strength, is essential for rotational control of the limb (28).

E. **Pes anserinus bursitis**
   1. **Definition.** The "pes" tendons are terminal insertions of three long thigh muscles, one from each muscle group. These tendons come together to insert on the anteromedial aspect of the proximal tibia, between the tibial tubercle and the distal (tibial) attachment of the medial (tibial) collateral ligament. The three tendons are sartorius (femoral innervation), gracilius (obturator innervation), and semitendonosis (sciatic innervation). They are powerful internal rotators of the leg (tibia) and aid in knee flexion.
   2. **Clinical presentation.** The patient has soreness just below the medial knee, which can be reproduced by direct palpation or resisted internal rotation of the leg. In middle age, it can represent a referred pain pattern as a result of medial knee arthritis.
   3. **Treatment.** In addition to the "rest, ice, compression, and elevation" principle, a steroid injection at the bursa site can be helpful.

HCMC Treatment Recommendations
Knee dislocation
  Diagnosis: Anteroposterior and lateral knee radiographs when the patient comes in with the knee dislocated; physical examination when this is not the case and after reduction of dislocated knees.
  Treatment: Closed reduction and careful assessment of the arterial supply to the distal limb with physical examination, duplex scan, and/or arteriogram. If the knee does not remain reduced after closed reduction, a temporary external fixator across the knee joint may be required to hold the joint reduced. MRI is helpful for surgical planning.
  Indications for surgery: Unstable knee (nearly all patients) in a patient with moderate functional demands
  Recommended technique: Open reduction and internal fixation of all associated fractures; ligament reconstruction with allograft or autograft tissues

---

References
   1. American Medical Association. *Standard nomenclature of athletic injuries.* Chicago: American Medical Assocation, 1966.
   2. Arendt EA. Assessment of the athlete with a painful knee. In: Griffin LU, ed. *Rehabiliation of the injured knee.* St. Louis: Mosby, 1990.
   3. Canale ST. Physeal injuries. In: Green NE, Swiontkowski MF, eds. *Skeletal trauma in children.* Philadelphia: WB Saunders, 1998:17–58.
   4. Cannon WDJ, Vittori JM. The incidence of healing in arthroscopic meniscal repairs in anterior cruciate ligament-reconstructed knees versus stable knees. *Am J Sports Med* 1992;20:176–181.
   5. Carson WG, James SL, Larson RL, et al. Patellofemoral disorders—physical and radiographic examination. Part II, radiographic examination. *Clin Orthop* 1984; 185:178–186.
   6. Cheung LP, Li KC, Hollett MD, et al. Meniscal tears of the knee: accuracy of detection with fast spin-echo MR imaging and arthroscopic correlation in 293 patients. *Radiology* 1997;203:508–512.
   7. DeHaven K. Diagnosis of acute knee injuries with hemarthrosis. *Am J Sport Med* 1980;8:9.

8. Fithian DC, Meier SW. The case for advancement and repair of the medial patellofemoral ligament in patients with recurrent patellar instability. *Operative techniques in sports medicine* 1999;7:81–89.
9. Friedman MJ. Tibial tubercle transfer technique. In: Fox JM, Del Pizzo W, eds. *The patellofemoral joint*. New York: McGraw-Hill, 1993:325–332.
10. Green NE, Allen BL. Vascular injuries associated with dislocation of the knee. *J Bone Joint Surg (Am)* 1977;59:236.
11. Hughston JC, Deese M. Medial subluxation of the patella as a complication of lateral retinacular release. *Am J Sports Med* 1988;16:383–388.
12. Indelicato PA. Non-operative treatment of complete tears of the medial collateral ligament of the knee. *J Bone Joint Surg (Am)* 1983;65:323–329.
13. Johnson DP, Wakele CJ, Watt I. Magnetic resonance imaging of patellar tendonitis. *J Bone Joint Surg (Br)* 1996;78:452–457.
14. LaPrade RF. The medial collateral ligament complex and the posterolateral aspect of the knee. In: Arendt EA, ed. *Orthopaedic knowledge update*. Rosemont, IL: American Academy of Orthopaedic Surgeons, 1999:327–340.
15. LaPrade RF, Terry GC. Injuries to the posterolateral aspect of the knee: association of anatomic injury patterns with clinical instability. *Am J Sports Med* 1997; 25:433–437.
16. Laurin CA, et al. The abnormal lateral patellofemoral angle. *J Bone Joint Surg (Am)* 1978;60:55.
17. Laurin CA, Dussault R, Levesque HP. The tangential x-ray investigation of the patellofemoral joint: x-ray technique, diagnostic criteria and their interpretation. *Clin Orthop* 1979;144:16.
18. Losee RR, Johnson TR, Southwick WO. Anterior subluxation of the lateral tibial plateau. *J Bone Joint Surg (Am)* 1978;60:1015.
19. Mandelbaum BR, Seipel PR, Teurlings L. Articular cartilage lesions: current concepts and results. In: Arendt E, ed. *Orthopaedic knowledge update*. Rosemont, IL: American Academy of Orthopaedic Surgeons, 1999:19–28.
20. McConnell J. The management of chondromalacia patellae: a long-term solution. *Aust J Physiother* 1986;32:215–223.
21. Merchant AC, Mercer RL, Jacobsen RH, et al. Roentgenographic analysis of patellofemoral congruence. *J Bone Joint Surg (Am)* 1974;56:1391–1396.
22. Miller MD, Harner CD, Koshiwaguchi S. Acute posterior cruciate ligament injuries. In: Fu FH, Harner CD, Vince KG, eds. *Knee surgery*. Philadelphia: Williams & Wilkins, 1994:749–767.
23. Minas T, Nehrer S. Current concepts in the treatment of articular cartilage defects. *Orthopaedics* 1997;20:525–538.
24. Moore TM. Fracture-dislocaton of the knee. *Clin Orthop* 1981;156:128.
25. Mueller ME, et al. *Manual of internal fixation,* 2nd ed. Berlin: Springer-Verlag, 1979.
26. Polly OW, et al. The accuracy of selective magnetic resonance imaging compared with the findings of arthroscopy of the knee. *J Bone Joint Surg (Am)* 1988;70:192.
27. Popp JE, Yu JS, Kaeding CC. Recalcitrant patellar tendinitis: magnetic resonance imaging, histologic evaluation, and surgical treatment. *Am J Sports Med* 1997; 25:218–222.
28. Powers C. Rehabilitation of patellofemoral joint disorders: a critical review. *Am J Sports Med* 1998;28:345–354.
29. Rappeport ED, Wieslander SB, Stephensen S, et al. MRI preferable to diagnostic arthroscopy in knee joint injuries. A double-blind comparison of 47 patients. *Acta Orthop Scand* 1997;68:277–281.
30. Sisto JD, Warren RF. Complex knee dislocations. A follow-up study of operative treatment. *Clin Orthop* 1985;198:94.
31. Timm K. Randomized controlled trial of protonics on patellar pain, position, and function. *Med Sci Sports Exerc* 1998;30:665–670.
32. Torg JS, Conrad W, Kalen V. Clinical diagnosis of anterior cruciate ligament instability in the athlete. *Am J Sports Med* 1976;4:84.
33. Wilkinson J. Fracture of the patella treated by total excision. *J Bone Joint Surg (Br)* 1977;59:352–354.

25. FRACTURES OF THE TIBIA

I. **Fractures of the tibial plateau (6,12,13,18)**
   A. For practical purposes, fractures of the tibial plateau are classified as follows:
      1. **Undisplaced** (a vertical fracture of the plateau)
      2. **Split** (a split fracture with displacement, with or without slight comminution)
      3. **Depressed** (centrally depressed fracture)
      4. **Split and depressed** with an intact tibial rim
      5. **Any of 1–4 with metaphyseal or even diaphyseal extension.** The elements of these descriptions are contained within **Schatzker's system** (Fig. 25-1).
   B. **Examination** is different from that for other knee injuries. It is wise to carry out a definitive examination only after roentgenographs have been obtained. Differential diagnosis includes a major ligamentous injury or knee dislocation (9,26,27). The examination should include inspection for wounds, evaluation of the distal circulation (pulses and capillary refill), and neurologic (motor or sensory) function. Motion and stability should not routinely be assessed in these injuries; however, this type of injury can be associated with ligamentous or meniscal damage (6).
   C. **Roentgenograms.** Oblique films in addition to the routine anteroposterior and lateral roentgenograms are often helpful in identifying fracture lines and articular displacement. Computed tomography demonstrates minor fractures and accurately depicts the degree of depression of the tibial plateau; axial cuts with sagittal reconstruction are the routine.
   D. Magnetic resonance imaging (MRI) can be helpful when there is clinical concern for associated ligamentous injury. The functional results of **treatment** are often better than the routine roentgenograms seem to predict. Early motion of the knee joint and delayed full weight bearing are the keys to maximum restoration of joint function (12,13,18).
      1. **Undisplaced fractures.** In some settings, especially when multiple injuries are involved, fixation with two percutaneous cannulated cancellous lag screws is advisable to ensure maintenance of reduction. Generally, nonoperative management is selected. A splint is applied, and the leg is elevated for the first 24–48 hours. Knee aspiration is carried out if a significant hemarthrosis is present, and knee motion is started with continuos passive motion (CPM) if available. As soon as the patient is comfortable and the range of motion is increasing, he or she can be followed up as an outpatient. Follow-up radiographs should be obtained shortly after motion is instituted to ensure that the fracture remains nondisplaced. Touch-down weight bearing should be maintained for 8 weeks to prevent displacement from shear forces.
      2. **Displaced fractures**
         a. **Split fracture.** Open reduction and fixation, if technically possible, is done if there is a significant widening (lateral or medial displacement of more than 3–5 mm) of the plateau (34,35). The internal fixation must be rigid enough to allow movement of the joint as soon as there is soft-tissue healing. In this situation, the authors prefer to use the Association of the Study of Internal Fixation (ASIF) buttress plate (Fig. 25-2) or dynamic compression plate when the patient is osteoporotic (18). Recently, there has been a move toward use of smaller implants for all tibial plateau fixation. Specialized 3.5-mm T- and L-buttress plates allow the placement of more screws under the articular surface. If the patient is young and has dense bone, then multiple percutaneous cannulated lag screws can be inserted under fluoroscopic control. Percutaneous placement of a large reduction clamp is often successful in providing

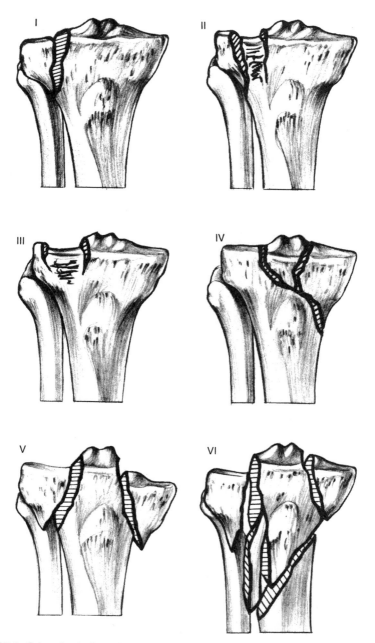

FIG. 25-1. Schatzker's classification system. I, split; II, split with depression; III, depression; IV, medial condyle; V, bicondylar; VI, bicondylar with shaft extension. (From Hansen ST, Swiontkowski MF. *Orthopaedic trauma protocols.* New York: Raven, 1993:315.)

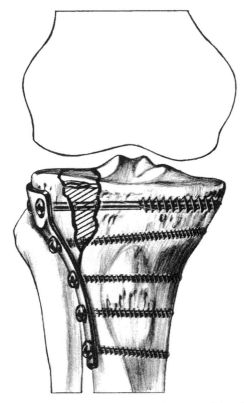

FIG. 25-2. Internal fixation of a split depression fracture of the tibial plateau using L-buttress plate fixation with bone grafting of the elevated segment. (From Hansen ST, Swiontkowski MF. *Orthopaedic trauma protocols.* New York: Raven, 1993:318.)

reduction of the fracture. If open reduction and internal fixation are not feasible, then treatment should be as for comminuted fractures.

b. **Central depression of the plateau.** If depression is greater than 3–5 mm, especially with valgus stress instability of the knee greater than 10 degrees in full extension, then most authors currently recommend elevation with bone grafting and fixation (12,13,16,25). More recently, articular reductions have been done with arthroscopic visualization with percutaneous technique for elevation of the segment. Autogenous bone graft remains the treatment of choice, but allograft and cancellous substitutes such as corallin hydroxyapatite have been successfully used (35). Generally, percutaneous lag screws are adequate for support of the elevated joint surface pieces and bone graft.

c. **Split-depressed fractures** with a displacement/depression of more than 3–4 mm are treated with reduction, fixation, and early motion in most young patients. Generally, this reduction is done with an open technique with an anterior or anterolateral approach, elevation, and bone grafting using buttress plates for older patients (Fig. 25-2) and lag screws or 3.5-mm small fragment T- or L-plates or one-third tubular plates (as washers) in younger patients. These fractures may be managed with arthroscopic reduction in skilled hands. Secure fixation is critical so that early motion with CPM can be initiated. Patients are generally limited to touch-down weight bearing for 12 weeks to prevent late fracture settling. If the patient's limb is stable to varus and valgus stress in an examination under anesthesia shortly after injury, then traction treatment with a tibial pin and early motion is an option (16,25). The patient is placed in a cast-brace (as described in Chap. 7, **III.H**) for 4 weeks (6). This treatment is not currently recommended on a routine basis. If the instability exceeds 10 degrees, then reduction and fixation as described earlier is indicated (25).

- d. **Fractures with metaphyseal/diaphyseal extension** are treated similarly to split-depressed fractures if the joint extension is significant. Generally, buttress plate fixation and bone grafting are required. When the injury is bicondylar, stripping the soft tissues off both condyles from an anterior approach should be avoided; this results in a high incidence of non-union and deep infection. Instead, the most unstable condyle (usually lateral) is selected for the buttress fixation via an anterolateral approach and the other condyle is stabilized by percutaneous screw fixation, fixation with a posterior medial incision and small buttress plate, or neutralization with an external fixator for 4–6 weeks while motion is limited. With all tibial plateau fractures treated with operative stabilization, it is important to examine the knee for ligamentous stability after completing the fixation in the operating room to rule out ligamentous injury (see **II**) (6).
  - (1) Apply a **cast-brace** as described in Chap. 7, **III.H,** off the self-hinged knee braces, which are lightweight and limit varus and valgus stress are more widely used. The same ambulation protocol, touch-down weight bearing is followed.
  - (2) In special situations, the patient is placed in a **long-leg cast** until the fracture is healed. Then the patient is placed in a rehabilitation program to regain full extension and flexion of the knee to beyond 90 degrees. The patient is kept on protected weight bearing for at least 6 months. This treatment is generally limited to patients with a severe neurologic condition or massive osteopenia.

E. **Complications**
  1. Significant **loss of range of motion** may occur, particularly if early movement is not instituted.
  2. **Early degenerative joint changes** with pain can occur regardless of the degree of joint reconstruction. In some instances, the pain may be severe enough to require arthroplasty or arthrodesis (34).
  3. The **infection rate** following operative treatment is reduced in experienced hands. Most infections occur because of excessive soft-tissue stripping.
  4. **Nerve and vascular injuries** that occur at the time of injury or subsequent to treatment are not uncommon (7). Nerve injuries are usually traction injuries, and recovery is unpredictable. Compartmental syndrome may be present and should be treated as described in Chap. 2, **III.**

II. **Fracture-dislocations of the knee**
  A. **Definition.** Injuries that appear to be plateau fractures can also involve significant ligament disruption. In the past, there has been no specific classification for these injuries, not only with significant ligament disruption but also with **arterial injury** (9,17,19).
  B. **Classification** is based on the experience of Moore (see Selected Historical Readings).

1. A **large-fragment, medial plateau fracture** may have the medial capsule completely avulsed from the posterior portion of the fragment, leading to rotatory instability after fracture fragment reduction and healing.
2. A **fracture involving either the medial or lateral plateau** may be associated with rupture of the collateral ligament and one or both of the cruciate ligaments (6).
3. A **lateral fracture** may be an avulsion injury with or without an associated anterior or posterior cruciate ligament tear.
4. A **rim compression fracture** may be associated with ligament disruption on the opposite side of the knee.
5. A **four-part fracture** of both condyles with separation of the medial eminence may signify a knee dislocation that has been reduced.

C. When evaluating plateau fractures that are known to be associated with ligament injury, it is important to obtain an MRI scan or careful stress **roentgenograms** to determine the full extent of the ligamentous damage. Concern about making the fracture worse is not justified in light of the potential gain from accurate diagnosis and appropriate treatment.

D. **Treatment** is based on accurate diagnosis, with internal fixation of the fracture fragments to reconstruct the joint surface and primary repair or reconstruction of the torn ligaments. A high index of suspicion for popliteal artery injuries must be maintained with diagnostic studies (arteriogram or duplex studies) when indicated (7).

E. **Postoperative care** is the same as for collateral or cruciate ligament repairs. Weight bearing is limited until the fractures are healed, generally at 12 weeks.

III. Diaphyseal fractures

A. **Examination.** Document soft-tissue injuries, including the neurologic and vascular status distal to the site of the injury. The examination must be repeated frequently. If the patient has significant or increasing pain after fracture reduction, then the possibility of compartmental syndrome must be ruled out. Ischemia can occur while the patient maintains excellent peripheral pules. Persistent complaints of pain with exacerbation by passive flexion and extension of the toes when there is not pressure from the cast supports the diagnosis. Decompression must be done early to prevent tissue loss (see Chap. 2).

B. **Treatment.** The selection of nonoperative or operative management must involve the consideration of many factors, including associated skeletal and ligamentous injuries, the degree of soft-tissue injury, injuries to other organs systems, the general condition of the patient, the skill and experience of the treating physician, and the resources of the facility. For the isolated closed tibial fracture with minimal shortening, most physicians recommend closed treatment with casting or fracture bracing (29,30). When compartmental syndrome, open fracture, or multiple injuries (other fractures or organ system damage) are also present, or when the displacement and initial shortening are excessive, the majority of experienced fracture surgeons recommend internal fixation. When the fracture is closed and shortening is 1–1.5 cm, the patient should be allowed to make an informed choice. Operative management involves a small increase in the risk of an infection versus early motion of the knee and ankle with a more accurate anatomic result. Over the past 15 years, the trend has been in favor of operative stabilization, generally with interlocking nails (1,4,11,21,29). A recent meta-analysis of the literature suggests overall higher rates of non-union, but there are no single randomized trials of significant statistical power (14,21). Interlocking nails are usually placed after reaming in closed fractures and in all but higher grade open fractures.

1. **Closed fractures/closed treatment.** Dehne advocated using a long-leg cast with the knee at 0 degrees. Sarmiento (29,30) developed a below-the-knee cast and prefabricated functional brace that allowed

knee motion while maintaining stability and length in the affected leg. This cast is generally applied after 2–3 weeks in the long-leg bent knee cast applied following a closed reduction. Prefabricated braces are the most widely used. One of these two treatment methods should be chosen, and the particular technique should be strictly adhered to if the same excellent results reported in the literature are to be expected. These cast techniques are described in detail in Chap. 4. It must be reemphasized that a below-the-knee total contact cast may not be applied immediately after the fracture; one must wait until the swelling has diminished. The authors suggest using a modified Robert Jones compression long-leg splint during the period of acute swelling. When the patient is ready for casting and following an appropriate spinal or general anesthetic, nearly all tibial fractures can be reduced by placing the leg over the end of the table. Adequate reduction and alignment are maintained in this position while the cast is applied. If shortening is minimal, then analgesia may suffice. The average healing time with closed treatment is approximately 18 weeks (range 14.5–21 weeks). One of Sarmiento's principles is that, in general, the amount of shortening is demonstrated on the initial radiograph, and the patient should be so informed. Good functional outcomes can be expected in 90% of cases (8,10,23). Closed treatment is recommended for children's fractures except when the physis or joint is involved (5,32).

2. **Closed fractures/open treatment.** After comparison of the results of treatment of intramedullary (IM) nailing versus plating, an IM nail is usually the internal fixation device of choice; flexible reamers and prebent nails are used for fractures of the middle and third tibia. For example, some authorities using Kuntscher blind IM technique report no nonunions, a 0%–1.5% infection rate, and a healing time of 17–18 weeks (4). The results using plate fixation are in the range of a non-union rate of 4%–6%, an infection rate of 6%–8%, but an excellent healing time of 14 weeks. If a midshaft tibial fracture is to be internally fixed, the authors suggest using an interlocking IM nail (Fig. 25-3). If the fracture is comminuted or in the metaphyseal/diaphyseal transition region, then an interlocking nail is mandatory. If it is anticipated that a patient will not ambulate on the affected leg within the first 2 months after injury, then the dynamic compression plate is indicated, not only to achieve rigid stabilization but also to compress the fragments and to maximize the chances for bony union in this particular situation. Plates are routinely used for metaphyseal fractures and in closed fractures associated with compartmental syndrome (1,21). Without weight bearing, the many advantages of closed IM nailing (e.g., improved blood supply, compression at the fracture site) with early ambulation are not obtained. Tourniquets should not be used in general for operative management of tibia fractures (28).

3. **Open fractures.** Stability of fracture fragments is required to enhance revascularization and minimize infection. Therefore, cast treatment is not recommended for the vast majority of open fractures. The exception may be a grade I–II injury in a child with a stable fracture pattern in whom closed reduction is successful. External fixation techniques have been vastly improved in the past 10 years. Development of half-pin fixators has allowed excellent wound access without limiting adjacent joint motion. External fixation remains a reliable treatment for open fractures; excellent results have been reported (2,11,33). When compared with interlocking nails, there is a higher rate of malunion and non-union, and pin tract infection is common. Where bone loss is present, posterolateral bone grafting at 4–6 weeks is recommended, and repeated grafting may be needed to achieve union (2). Plate fixation results in a higher rate of deep infection (1). Unreamed, flexible nails (Enders) and solid nails (Lottes) have equal rates of associated deep infection in similarly designed trials (11,33). Because unreamed nails minimize the endosteal damage to the remaining diaphysis, their use

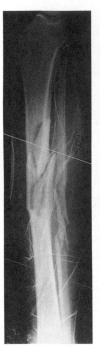
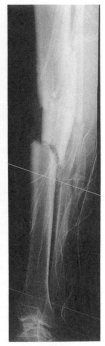

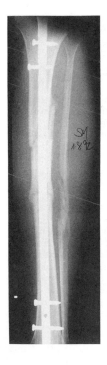
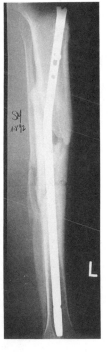

FIG. 25-3. Displaced closed fractures of the tibia shaft, when shortened more than 1 cm or considered to be unstable, are best treated with interlocking nails. **A and B:** Preoperative radiographs of a shortened, unstable segmental fracture of the tibia shaft. **C and D:** The interlocking nail in place. The screws placed through the holes in the nail proximal and distal to the fracture provide length and rotational stability for the fracture. Nearly all fractures of the femoral shaft in skeletally mature individuals are treated with similar interlocking nails, allowing mobilization of the patient and early range of motion of adjacent joints.

was previously preferred over reamed nails. Reamed nails, because of their larger diameter, result in lower rates of implant failure without a concomitant increase in deep infection (33). Interlocking nails, because of their ability to control fracture length and rotation, are currently favored for the management of most grade I, II, and IIIa open tibial shaft fractures. Because debridement must be aggressive and may possibly result in bone loss, posterolateral bone grafting is often required (2). These devices have been proven to be efficacious in randomized trials. For grade IIIb open fractures of the tibial shaft, external fixation remains an option to consider. In severe grade IIIc open fractures, amputation should be considered because of the consequences of prolonged surgical procedures and residual disability (3). Factors such as transection of the tibial nerve, degree of muscle damage, hypotension from associated injury, and age should be considered first.

C. **Complications.** Most patients experience some residual disability after a tibial fracture (15,23,24).

1. **Compartmental syndrome** has been discussed previously (see Chap. 2, III).

2. **Joint stiffness** can be largely prevented by aggressive treatment to achieve early union. Flexion and extension exercises to the toes must not be neglected because these joints frequently stiffen and produce considerable postcasting dysfunction.

3. **Delayed union and non-union** (2,31)
    a. These complications can be minimized by adequate immobilization, early weight bearing (which is often delayed for 2 months if a dynamic compression plate is used), and early bone grafting where delayed union appears certain. The **following factors are related to delayed union or non-union:**
        (1) **Severe initial displacement** of the fracture fragments (probably indicating significant soft-tissue injury)
        (2) **Significant comminution**
        (3) **Associated soft-tissue injuries or open fractures**
        (4) **Infection**
        (5) **Open management with inadequate stability**
    b. **There is fair documentation that pulsed, electromagnetic field stimulation** can heal delayed unions and non-unions, thus avoiding open grafting in many patients (2,31).

4. **Infection** is a complication of open fractures or the opening of a closed fracture. The risk of infection is minimized by efficient surgical technique, by the proper use of antibiotics, and by a delayed primary closure for open fractures. For the most severe soft-tissue injuries, aggressive debridement and coverage with free or rotational muscle flaps minimizes this complication. Pin tract infection is common with the use of external fixators.

5. **Angulation** can be prevented by proper casting followed by wedging as necessary or by surgical stabilization. Some degree of anterior angulation, usually no more than 5–7 degrees, is acceptable. Medial and lateral angulation should be within 5 degrees of neutral because of the risk of ankle arthritis (20,22–24). Patients tolerate a few degrees of external rotational malalignment but no abnormal internal rotation. These recommendations are widely accepted, but it seems that greater degrees of deformity are tolerated with little functional loss (23).

6. With use of a cast treatment regimen (even with early weight bearing of comminuted fractures), significant further shortening after proper cast application usually is not a problem. **Shortening** of up to 1 cm is common with closed management and of little consequence (29). Shortening beyond 1 cm is considered significant and should be avoided if possible (8,10).

HCMC Treatment Recommendations

Tibial Plateau Fractures

Diagnosis: Anteroposterior and lateral radiographs and physical examination. Computed tomography scans are helpful for assessment of displacement and for surgical planning.

Treatment: Open reduction and internal fixation or percutaneous reduction with lag screw fixation aided by arthroscopy for fractures displaced more than 2 mm (depression or gapping). Knees that remain stable to varus/valgus stress in full extension may be treated nonoperatively.

Indications for surgery: Knees with more than 10 degrees of instability in extension and/or joint displacement of greater than 2 mm

Recommended technique: Joint visualization via open reduction or arthroscopy, reduction and fixation with lag screws and/or low profile plates and bone graft or bone graft substitute, early range-of-motion therapy and limited weight bearing for 8–12 weeks

---

HCMC Treatment Recommendations

Tib-Fib Fractures

Diagnosis: Anteroposterior and lateral radiographs of the leg and clinical examination. In 10%–20% cases there is an open wound communicating with the fracture.

Treatment: Nonoperative care for fractures that are isolated and not shortened more than 1 cm on initial radiographs, long leg splint for 2–3 weeks followed by fracture brace until fracture is united, operative stabilization for length unstable and/or open fractures. Interlocking nail, inserted with reaming is the procedure of choice.

Indications for surgery: Fractures close to the joint or shortened on initial radiographs greater than 1 cm or failure to control angulation with nonoperative technique or open fracture

Recommended technique: Interlocking nailing, statically locked. Insert with reaming: more reaming for larger diameter nails with closed fractures, less reaming for open fractures

---

References

1. Bach AW, Hansen ST Jr. Plate versus external fixation in severe open tibial shaft fractures. A randomized trial. *Clin Orthop* 1989;241:89.
2. Blick SS, et al. Early prophylactic bone grafting of high-energy tibial fractures. *Clin Orthop* 1989;240:21.
3. Bondurant FJ, et al. The medical and economic impact of severely injured extremities. *J Trauma* 1988;28:1270.
4. Bone LB, Johnson KD. Treatment of tibial fractures by reaming and intramedullary nailing. *J Bone Joint Surg (Am)* 1986;68:877.
5. Cooperman DR, Spiegel PG, Laros GS. Tibial fractures involving the ankle in children. *J Bone Joint Sug (Am)* 1978;60:1040.
6. Delamarter RB, Hohl M, Hopp E. Ligament injuries associated with tibial plateau fractures. *Clin Orthop* 1990;250:226–233.
7. Dennis JN, Jagger C, Butcher JL, et al. Reassessing the role of arteriograms in the management of posterior knee dislocations. *J Trauma* 1993;35:692–697.
8. Faergemann C, Frandsen PA, Rock ND. Expected long-term outcome after a tibial shaft fracture. *J Trauma* 1999;46:683–686.
9. Frassica FJ, Sim FH, Staehl JW, et al. Dislocation of the knee. *Clin Orthop* 1991;263:200–205.

10. Gaston P, Will E, Elton RA, et al. Fractures of the tibia; can their outcome be predicted? *J Bone Joint Surg (Br)* 1999;81:71–76.
11. Holbrook JL, Swiontkowski MF, Sanders R. Treatment of open fractures of the tibial shaft: ender nailing versus external fixation. A randomized prospective comparison. *J Bone Joint Surg (Am)* 1989;71:1231.
12. Honkonen SE. Degenerative arthritis after tibial plateau fractures. *J Orthop Trauma* 1995;9:273–277.
13. Honkonen SE. Indicators for surgical treatment of tibial condyle fractures. *Clin Orthop* 1994;302:199–205.
14. Hooper GJ, Keddel RG, Penny ID. Conservative management or closed nailing for tibial shaft fractures: a randomized prospective trial. *J Bone Joint Surg (Br)* 1991;73;83–85.
15. Horne G, et al. Disability following fractures of the tibial shaft. *Orthopedics* 1990;13:423.
16. Jensen DB, Rude C, Duus B, et al. Tibial plateau fractures: a comparison of conservative and surgical treatment. *J Bone Joint Surg (Br)* 1990;72:49–52.
17. Johansen K, Lynch K, Paun M, et al. Non-invasive vascular tests reliably exclude occult arterial trauma in injured extremities. *J Trauma* 1991;31:515–522.
18. Keating JF. Tibial plateau fractures in the older patient. *Bull Hosp Joint Dis* 1999;58:19–23.
19. Kendall RW, Taylor DC, Salvian AI, et al. The role of arteriography in assessing vascular injuries associated with dislocations of the knee. *J Trauma* 1993;35: 875–878.
20. Kettelkamp DB, Hillberry BM, Murrish DE, et al. Degenerative arthritis of the knee secondary to fracture malunion. *Clin Orthop* 1988;234:159–169.
21. Littenberg B, Weinstein LP, McCarren M, et al. Closed fractures of the tibial shaft. A meta-analysis of three methods of treatment. *J Bone Joint Surg (Am)* 1998;80:174–183.
22. McKellop HA, Sigholm G, Redfern FC, et al.. The effect of simulated fracture-angulation of the tibia on cartilage. Pressures in the knee joint. *J Bone Joint Surg (Am)* 1991;73:1382–1391.
23. Merchant TC, Dietz FR. Long-term follow-up after fractures of the tibial and fibular shafts. *J Bone Joint Surg (Am)* 1989;71A:599.
24. Puno RM, Vanghan JJ, Stetten ML, et al. Long-term effects of tibial angular motion on the knee and ankle joints. *J Orthop Trauma* 1991;5:247–251.
25. Rasmussen PS. Tibial condyle fractures: impairment of knee joint stability as an indication for surgical treatment. *J Bone Joint Surg (Am)* 1973;55:1331.
26. Rasul AT, Fischer DA. Primary repair of quadriceps tendon rupture; results of treatment. *Clin Orthop* 1993;289:205–207.
27. Rougraff BT, Reeck CC, Essenmacher J. Complete quadriceps tendon ruptures. *Orthopedics* 1996;19:509–514.
28. Salam AA, Fenres KS, Cleary J, et al. The use of a tourniquet when placing tibial fractures. *J Bone Joint Surg (Br)* 1991;73:86–87.
29. Sarmiento A, Gersten LM, Sobol PA, et al. Tibial shaft fractures treated with functional braces. Experience with 780 fractures. *J Bone Joint Surg (Br)* 1989;71:602.
30. Sarmiento A, McKellop HA, Liinas A, Parck SH, et al. Effect of loading and fracture motion in diaphyseal tibial fractures. *J Orthop Res* 1996;14:80–84.
31. Sharrard WJW. A double blind trial at pulsed electromagnetic fields for delayed union of tibial fractures. *J Bone Joint Surg (Br)* 1990;72B:347.
32. Spiegel PG, Cooperman DR, Laros GS. Epiphyseal fractures of the distal ends of the tibia and fibula. *J Bone Joint Surg (Am)* 1978:60:1046.
33. Tornetta P, Beroman M, Watnik N, et al. Treatment of grade IIIb open tibial fractures—a prospective randomized comparison of external fixation and non-reamed locked nailing. *J Bone Joint Surg (Br)* 1992;76:13–19.
34. Volpin G, Dowd GSE, Stein H, et al. Degenerative arthritis after intra-articular fractures of the knee; long-term results. *J Bone Joint Surg (Br)* 1990;72:634–638.
35. Weale AE, Bannister GC. The management of depressed tibial plateau fractures. A comparison of non-operative with operative treatment using allograft and autograft. *J Orthop Trauma* 1994;4:61–64.

Selected Historical Readings

Bassett CAL, Mitchell SN, Gaston SR. Treatment of ununited tibial diaphyseal fractures with pulsing electromagnetic fields. *J Bone Joint Surg (Am)* 1981;63:511.

Burwell HN. Plate fixation of tibial shaft fractures. *J Bone Joint Surg (Br)* 1971;53:258.

Clancey GJ, Hansen ST Jr. Open fractures of the tibia. *J Bone Joint Surg (Am)* 1978;60:118.

Dehne E. Treatment of fractures of the tibial shaft fractures. *Clin Orthop* 1969;66:159.

Fernandez-Pallazzi F. Fibular resection in delayed union of tibial fractures. *Acta Orthop Scand* 1969;40:105.

Hohl M. Tibial condylar fractures. *J Bone Joint Surg (Am)* 1967;49:1455.

Karlstrom G, Olerud S. External fixation of severe open tibial fractures with the Hoffmann frame. *Clin Orthop* 1983;180:68.

Lottes JO: Medullary nailing of the tibial with the triflange nail. *Clin Orthop* 1974;105:253.

Moore TM. Fracture dislocation of the knee. *Clin Orthop* 1981;156:128.

Nicoll EA: Fractures of the tibial shaft. *J Bone Joint Surg (Br)* 1964;46:373.

Olerud S, Karlstrom G. Secondary intramedullary nailing of tibial fractures. *J Bone Joint Surg (Am)* 1972;54:1419.

Pare A. Compound fracture of leg. Pare's personal care (MII, 328). In: Hamby WB, ed. *The case reports and autopsy records of Ambrose Pare.* Springfield, IL: Charles C. Thomas, 1960;82–87.

Parkhill C. A new apparatus for the fixation of bones after resection and in fractures with a tendency to displacement. *Trans Am Surg Assoc* 1897;15:251.

Sarmiento A. Functional bracing of tibial fractures. *Clin Orthop* 1974;105:202.

Schatzker J, McBroom R, Bruce D. The tibial plateau fractures. The Toronto experience. *Clin Orthop* 1979;138:94.

Sorensen KH. Treatment of delayed union and nonunion of the tibia by fibular resection. *Acta Orthop Scand* 1969;40:92.

26. ANKLE INJURIES

I. **Fracture and fracture-dislocations**
   A. **Classification.** Ankle fractures are intraarticular injuries, and accurate reduction as well as maintenance of the reduction is required for a satisfactory long-term result. To achieve reduction by closed manipulation, it is necessary to know the direction of the forces producing the fractures. It must be emphasized that fractures about the ankle usually are not isolated injuries but have significant associated ligamentous ruptures. Ankle fractures may be classified by the Lauge-Hansen scheme as follows (Fig. 26-1):
   1. **Supination, lateral rotation.** The term **supination** defines the position of the foot at the time the lateral rotation force is applied. The sequence of events is as follows:
      a. **Rupture of the anterior tibiofibular ligament** with foot in inversion
      b. **Spiral fracture of the lateral malleolus** about the level of the ankle joint
      c. **Rupture of the posterior tibiofibular ligament or, occasionally, fracture of the posterior malleolus of the tibia**
      d. **Rupture of the deltoid ligament or avulsion of the medial malleolus**
   2. **Pronation, lateral rotation.** In this injury, the foot is pronated while the lateral force is applied. Consequently, the medial ligament is tight at the beginning of the injury and the sequence then is as follows:
      a. **Rupture of the deltoid ligament or avulsion fracture of the medial malleolus**
      b. **Rupture of the anterior tibiofibular ligament plus the tibiofibular interosseous ligament**
      c. **A short spiral fracture of the fibula** (several inches above the ankle joint)
      d. **Rupture of the posterior tibiofibular ligament and fracture of the posterior malleolus of the tibia**
   3. **Supination, adduction.** The foot is inverted on the leg. The talus moves and tilts medially. The series of events is as follows:
      a. **An avulsion fracture of the lateral malleolus** at or below the level of the ankle joint **or rupture of the talofibular ligament**
      b. **A near-vertical fracture of the medial malleolus,** which can be associated with an osteochondral fracture of the talus
   4. **Impaction or posterior dislocation.** This injury is associated either with a fall from a height or with a sudden deceleration injury in a vehicle. It may take several forms based on the direction of the force applied and the position of the talus in flexion and extension. The common injuries seen are as follows:
      a. **An impaction fracture (usually comminuted) of the tibial plafond (roof of the mortise) with or without an oblique fracture of the medial malleolus.** This is termed the pilon fracture.
      b. **A classic trimalleolar fracture** (fracture-dislocation), with fracture of the posterior malleolus of the tibia, fracture of the medial and lateral malleoli, and disruption of the anterior capsule of the ankle joint
   5. **The Danis-Weber or AO classification** system concentrates on the pattern of the fibular fracture (Fig. 26-2). The type A fracture is below the level of the joint and frequently transverse, the type B fracture is a spiral oblique fracture at the level of the joint, and the type C fracture is high above the mortise.
   6. **Fibular fracture.** In general, the criteria for open reduction includes any lateral shifting of the talus on the mortise roentgenogram.

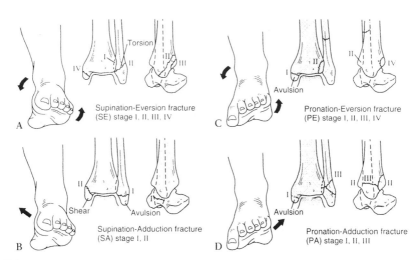

FIG. 26-1. The Lauge-Hansen classification of ankle fractures. **A:** The supination-eversion fracture. Stage I: The avulsion of the anterior talofibular ligament from the tibia or simple rupture of the ligament. Stage II: The classic oblique fracture of the distal fibula, beginning anteriorly at the joint line and extending obliquely and posteriorly toward the shaft of the bone. Stage III: Avulsion or rupture of the posterior tibiofibular ligament. Stage IV: Avulsion fracture of the medial malleolus. **B:** The supination-adduction fracture. Stage I: Avulsion of the tip of the lateral malleolus or rupture of the associated ligaments. Stage II: Vertical fracture of the medial malleolus, usually beginning at the plafond. **C:** The pronation-eversion fracture. Stage I: Avulsion of the medial malleolus or ruptured deltoid ligament. Stage II: Rupture or avulsion of the anterior tibiofibular ligament. Stage III: A high short oblique fracture of the fibula. Stage IV: A posterior lip fracture of the tibia. **D:** The pronation-abduction fracture. Stage I: Avulsion of the medial malleolus or ruptured deltoid ligament. Stage II: Rupture or avulsion of the syndesmotic ligaments. Stage III: A short, oblique fracture of the distal fibula at about the level of the ankle joint. (From Weber MJ. Ankle fractures and dislocations. In: Chapman MW, Madison M, eds. *Operative orthopaedics,* 2nd ed. Philadelphia: JB Lippincott, 1993:731–745.)

B. Examination. Inspection of the entire surface of the ankle to check for abrasions or lacerations that may communicate with the fracture surfaces is critical. Carefully identify points of tenderness. If there is tenderness over the ligament, a ligamentous or capsular injury is probably present.

C. Roentgenograms. Anteroposterior, lateral, and oblique films (the mortise view), the last obtained with the malleoli equidistant from the roentgenographic film, are essential for evaluating any ankle injury. Occasionally, axial tomography or computed tomography (CT) scanning is useful to assess the degree of injury of the tibial plafond, particularly with medial malleolus impaction fractures. A clearer delineation of the medial malleolar fractures may be achieved by an additional view obtained with the foot in 45 degrees of internal rotation.

D. Treatment. The success of treatment is dependent on accurate and stable reduction of the ankle mortise. If only one side of the ankle joint is disrupted, then treatment may be carried out by a closed reduction and cast immobilization (e.g., an intact deltoid ligament should not allow the talus to shift laterally in the mortise) (6). If both sides of the ankle are injured, then the joint is unstable; although closed reduction may be achieved, it is difficult to maintain. For this reason, the treatment of choice for such an injury is open reduction and internal fixation (ORIF). Always obtain postreduction roent-

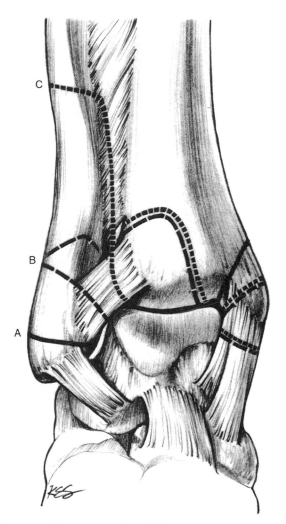

FIG. 26-2. Diagrammatic representation of the Danis-Weber classification system. **A:** Transverse fracture of the distal malleolus. **B:** Spiral fracture at the level of the mortise. **C:** Fractures above the mortise with disruption of the syndesmosis. (From Hansen ST, Swiontkowski MF. *Orthopaedic trauma protocols.* New York: Raven, 1993:340.)

genograms in three planes to verify an anatomic reduction. Analysis of functional outcome of patients with operative management reveals continued improvement throughout the first 6 months after fracture with mild residual disability (2,18).

1. A **stable injury.** Elevate, reduce, and immobilize as soon as possible to reduce swelling. The reduction maneuver for most oblique fractures of the fibula is plantar flexion and internal rotation. This can often be achieved by lifting the patient's limb (in the supine position) by the great toe. Immobilize the patient's leg in a short leg cast in this position. The patient should be advised in non-touch or toe-touch weight bearing until there are roentgenographic signs of callus and lack of tenderness to pressure

(3–4 weeks). Further protect the injury in a short leg cast with the foot in neutral position for another 3–4 weeks. Stable ankle fractures have equivalent results when treated nonoperatively (1).

2. **Unstable fractures**

   a. These fractures should be reduced and internally fixed as an urgent procedure if the patient is seen **before significant swelling is apparent** (7,17). Preoperative planning is essential to minimize soft-tissue stripping and maximize fixation. Patients with open fractures should be managed with wound debridement and internal fixation; the results are generally equivalent to those for closed fractures (11).

   (1) Medial malleolar fragments should be reattached with screws for larger fragments and with Kirschner wires with supplemental tension band wires for smaller fragments. With screw fixation, a length of 35–40 mm is appropriate so that the metaphyseal bone is engaged and the medullary canal is avoided with loss of screw purchase.

   (2) Posterior malleolar fragments are stabilized with screw fixation if they involve more than one fourth of the articular surface. Generally these fragments are inadvertently reduced by reduction of the distal fibula. The lag screw placement can be from the anterior to posterior direction (frequently percutaneously). Formal open reduction, if required, must be done before definitive fixation of the lateral malleolus, which may limit the surgical exposure; the incision must be well posterior to the fibula.

   (3) Lateral malleolar fractures of the avulsion type may be reduced as medial malleolar fractures. If possible, an attempt should first be made to reduce and fix the fracture with a lag screw. Fractures with disruption of both anterior and posterior tibiofibular ligaments can be held with a "position" (or syndesmosis) screw inserted parallel to the plafond into the tibia. This screw is generally placed after anatomic reduction of a type B or C fibula fracture, with the foot maximally dorsiflexed (to prevent narrowing of the ankle mortise), through the plate, and after gaining purchase on one or both of the tibial cortices. See **(4).** Spiral or oblique fractures with the tibiofibular ligament intact may be reapproximated by oblique lag screws with a small, one-third tubular plate. Prophylactic antibiotics should be utilized (16). These plates could be placed on the posterior aspect of the fibula to prevent skin irritation from the plate when in the lateral, more subcutaneous position (22). More recently, success has been achieved with bioabsorbable implants (4,8). Repair to the deltoid ligament avulsion is not necessary (21). Postoperatively, the leg may be treated in a short-leg compression dressing with a plaster or fiberglass splint to control the position of the foot. As soon as the swelling is controlled, at 5–7 days, a removable splint can be used and early active motion started. The patient should remain partial weight bearing for 4–6 weeks. If the patient is unable to cooperate with the early, active range-of-motion protocol, then a short-leg cast is applied for 4–6 weeks (12,20). Weight bearing and strengthening exercises are initiated following this period.

   (4) If the tibiofibular syndesmosis is widened, associated with a very high fibula fracture (the Maisonneuve fracture), then the lower interosseous membrane is torn. Authorities who report the best results treat this injury with a suture repair of a ligamentous rupture when feasible and with one or two position (or syndesmosis) screws placed parallel to the plafond. Some authors record the use of 4.5-mm cortical screws; we favor the use of one or two 3.5-mm screws put in as four cortex screws (exit the tibia slightly to allow removal if they break. Care must be taken to maintain the normal fibular length and, by keeping the foot in neutral, the proper mortise width. Some authorities recommend delaying full weight bearing until the position screws are removed. However, the authors have seen many more problems following removal of the syndesmosis screws and recorded leaving them in as weight bearing is progressed. The patient should be advised that the screws may break.

   b. **When swelling is already significant,** any gross malalignment should be corrected. Then the leg should be placed in a compression dressing with splints and elevated until the swelling has receded sufficiently for a safe open reduction. In order to avoid wound healing complications, patients should be seen and surgically treated as soon after the injury as possible (7). The complication rate is very high for diabetic and obese patients managed operatively (3,14).

E. **Complications**

   1. **Incomplete reduction** is associated with a higher incidence of ankle joint symptoms than are seen when anatomic restitution is achieved. This situation can be improved by osteotomy and internal fixation even years after the fracture occurs (13).

   2. **Non-union,** although rare, can occur and is usually symptomatic. On the medial side, it may be associated with interposition of the posterior tibial tendon. Non-union of either malleolus should be managed with internal fixation and bone grafting.

II. **Pilon fractures.** Fractures of the articular surface of the tibia are generally high-energy injuries from axial loads. They occur from high-speed vehicular trauma and falls from heights (15).

A. **Diagnosis** is confirmed by roentgenograms—as for ankle fractures. The history of high-energy trauma or fall from a significant height should prompt a thorough examination of the heel, foot, and ankle, observing for swelling and tenderness. If the plain roentgenograms do not sufficiently document the intraarticular fracture pattern, then CT or plain tomography may be indicated.

B. **Treatment.** Fractures of the joint surface with more than 2–3 mm of gap or depression are generally managed with reduction, fixation, and bone grafting. Significant swelling occurs rapidly with these injuries, so operative management must be emergent or, otherwise, it is frequently delayed for 7–10 days until the swelling subsides. Plating of an associated fibular fracture, application of external fixation across the ankle joint, or calcaneal pin traction on a Böhler frame is indicated in the interim to achieve indirect reduction of the joint fragment; this limits the amount of subsequent stripping of the fragments required at surgery. Compartmental syndrome is not uncommon with these fractures, and if fasciotomy is performed, then fibular plating is indicated. Because of a high incidence of wound complication and deep infection, there is a trend toward limited fracture exposure, reduction and fixation of the joint surface with lag screws, and definitive treatment with external fixation. Bone grafting may not be required if the fracture is not exposed but should be carried out if there is any doubt.

C. **Complications.** Deep infection can require debridement, hardware removal, and muscle flap (often free) coverage (15). If the problem is identified early, then hardware can be generally left in place. Pilon fractures are associated with chronic swelling, loss of motion, and degenerative arthritis; ankle arthrodesis is frequently required.

III. **Sprains**

A. **Diagnosis.** The grading or severity of sprains is described in Chap. 1, **V.D.1.** A third-degree sprain is a complete rupture of a ligament and is often only one stage short of a dislocation. A complete ligamentous rupture allows roentgenographic evidence of talar instability with stressing of the ankle joint after pain is relieved by local, spinal, or general anesthesia. Rupture of the lateral ligaments is diagnosed when the amount of talar inversion on the affected side is at least 6 degrees. Third-degree ankle sprains are associated with high morbidity. For example, the average duration of disability has been reported to be from 4.5 to 26 weeks, and only 25%–60% of patients are symptom-free 1–4 years after injury. Therefore, these so-called minor injuries deserve careful treatment.

B. **Examination.** All of the ankle ligaments should be palpated for point tenderness, including the distal tibia-fibular ligaments, the deltoid and talonavicular ligaments, as well as the anterior capsule. One should look for a positive anterior drawer sign of the talus within the mortise. This test is accomplished by holding the leg in one hand and grasping the heel in the other hand. By pulling anteriorly on the heel, the examiner attempts to subluxate the talus from within the mortise. A positive anterior drawer sign of the ankle indicates a third-degree sprain of the anterior talofibular ligament. If this sign is present, then an anteroposterior roentgenogram of the ankle should be obtained using anesthesia—a local intravenous anesthetic is expedient—while an inversion stress is applied to the ankle. This instability cannot occur, however, if the drawer test is negative, because the anterior talofibular ligament is always the first of the lateral collateral ligaments injured. The course of the peroneal tendons as they curve behind the lateral malleolus should also be carefully palpated to rule out subluxating peroneal tendons. If this subluxation is present, then usually a small flake of bone from an avulsion of the superior peroneal retinaculum is seen roentgenographically behind the lateral malleolus. Suture repair of the retinaculum is then indicated (9). The importance of a proper examination is explained in the following paragraphs, and it is also critical for prognosis. For example, an isolated talonavicular ligament sprain can have marked swelling initially, but this injury heals very quickly.

C. **Treatment.** Surgical repair of ruptured ankle ligaments does not appear warranted (except in grossly unstable ankles), both in terms of the reported results and in terms of the security achieved by the repair (10,19). There are physicians, however, who do advocate surgical repair of certain ankle sprains. We usually use the following approach for treatment of ankle sprains:

1. **If the anterior talofibular ligament is intact** as demonstrated by a negative anterior drawer test of the ankle, then protective strapping (see Chap. 7) is often used; this is followed by early mobilization and range-of-motion exercises. Initially, a cane or crutches are often needed for ambulation assistance.

2. Frequently, the physician does not wish to subject the patient to an anesthetic and stress roentgenograms to rule out ankle joint instability. **If there is significant tenderness of the deltoid ligament or anterior capsule,** then assume that a severe sprain has occurred and lateral joint instability is likely. In our experience, immobilization in a commercial fracture boot or short-leg walking cast until there is no pain or tenderness has produced good clinical results. **If stress roentgenograms do confirm lateral instability,** then anticipate that a fracture boot or short-leg walking cast is required for 6–8 weeks before there is no pain or tenderness about the ankle. We have found this treatment program to be successful. Studies of different approaches to this common problem show that there is no advantage to operative treatment over cast immobilization. Furthermore, a recent study evaluating cost-effectiveness of the various diagnostic approaches—(1) wrapping without stress roentgenograms, (2) casting, (3) stress roentgenograms followed by appropriate treatment (wrapping, casting or surgery), (4) arthrography and appropriate treatment, and (5) stress films and arthrography with appropriate treatment—indicated the high probability (79%) of eventual ankle stability regardless of the treatment protocol. Therefore, the wrapping strategies were clearly more cost-effective. Use of an air-filled stirrup aids patients who have high functional demands to return to activity earlier.

D. Complication. The most common long-term complication of an ankle sprain is lateral talar instability within the mortise. Isometric peroneal muscle exercises often are recommended to help improve dynamic stability for the lateral side of the ankle joint. A ¼-inch laterally based heel and sole wedge is also helpful for mild chronic instability. If nonoperative measures do not improve the lateral instability or if stress mortise films demonstrate more than 6 degrees of talon tilting, then do not hesitate to perform a surgical reconstruction.

IV. Achilles tendon (tendo calcaneus) rupture

A. The **history** associated with an Achilles tendon rupture is often diagnostic. Usually the patient was running or jumping when a sudden severe pain was felt behind the ankle, almost as if it had been struck by something. The patient can then walk but usually with a limp.

B. Examination is most easily accomplished with the patient prone. By inspection and palpation, the defect in the Achilles tendon can be documented. Squeezing the calf in this position with an intact Achilles tendon causes passive plantar flexion to occur; this response is absent with tendon rupture (Thompson's test). Do not be misled by the patient's ability to plantar flex the ankle actively, because this can be done with the toe flexors.

C. Treatment

1. Patients with low functional demands may undergo **nonoperative** treatment. The foot is held in equinus for 8 weeks in a short-leg cast. Ambulation with crutches using an elevated heel on the shoe for 8–12 weeks then follows. Finally, rehabilitation exercises are begun to increase strength and range of motion.

2. **Operative treatment** may be recommended, especially for the young, competitive athlete. The advantages of open treatment are that the proper strength-length relationship of the musculotendinous unit is reestablished, the internal repair probably adds extra strength to the ruptured tendon, and immobilization can be limited. The risk of re-rupture of the tendon is lower with operative management (5). The incision should be made to one side of the tendon (not directly posteriorly) and should not extend distally into the flexor creases posterior to the ankle; this helps minimize adhesions of the tendon to the skin. A careful repair of the tendon sheath also limits these adhesions. The actual type of tendon repair is left to the discretion of the surgeon; numerous materials and patterns of suture repair have been discussed. The plantaris tendon may be used to augment the repair. Postoperatively, the ankle is kept in an equinus position with a short-leg cast for 8 weeks. Ambulation and physical therapy are then allowed as tolerated to increase strength and range of motion.

D. The **late complication** of a second or repeat rupture has been reported to be a significant problem with both methods of treatment but it is possibly more common with the nonoperative method. A large randomized study demonstrated little difference in outcome or complication rate, however.

HCMC Treatment Recommendations

Ankle Fractures

Diagnosis: Lateral and mortise radiographs of the ankle, clinical examination

Treatment: Splint application, acutely followed by walking orthoses or cast at 1–2 weeks; progressive weight bearing as tolerated for stable fractures

Indications for surgery: Trimalleolar or bimalleolar fractures, Weber B fractures with widening of the medial mortise and medial tenderness, high fibular fractures with widening of the syndesmosis

Recommended technique: Small fragment lag screws for medial malleolus; one-third tubular fixation for Weber B fractures, placed posteriorly in the "antiglide" position where possible; fixation of posterior fragments greater than 25% of the transverse diameter of the tibia with lag screws; fixation of syndesmosis with four cortex non-lag screws for syndesmosis disruption; limited weight bearing for 4–6 weeks for operatively treated fractures and early AROM

HCMC Treatment Recommendations

Pilon Fractures

Diagnosis: Lateral and mortise radiographs of the ankle, clinical examination. CT scan can be helpful for preoperative planning.

Treatment: Irrigation and debridement for open wounds followed by stabilization of the fibula to establish length and indirect reduction of the articular surface and external fixation for the tibia. Select fractures can be treated with ORIF/plate fixation in experienced hands.

Indications for surgery: Open fractures, fractures with >2 cm of joint gap or impaction

Recommended technique: ORIF of fibula followed by definitive or temporary external fixation of the tibia, eventual ORIF of articular surface and stabilization with plate or thin-wire external fixator (generally with half pins for the tibial shaft)

HCMC Treatment Recommendations

Ankle Sprains

Diagnosis: Tenderness over lateral ligament complex and/or deltoid with negative ankle radiographs

Treatment: Ice acutely followed by AROM and progressive weight bearing as tolerated

Indications for surgery: Unstable ankle with recurrent sprains

Recommended technique: Reconstruction with a portion of the peroneus brevis tendon

---

References

1. Bauer M, Bergstrom B, Hemborg A, et al. Malleolar fractures: nonoperative versus operative treatment: a controlled study. *Ankle Fractures* 1985;199:17–27.
2. Belcher GL, Radomisli TE, Abate JA, et al. Functional outcome analysis of operatively treated malleolar fractures. *J Orthop Trauma* 1997;11:106–109.
3. Bostman OM. Body-weight related to loss of reduction of fractures of the distal tibia and ankle. *J Bone Joint Surg (Br)* 1995;77:101–103.
4. Bostman OM. Osteoarthritis of the ankle after foreign-body reaction to absorbable pins and screws: a three to nine year follow-up study. *J Bone Joint Surg (Br)* 1998; 80:333–338.
5. Bowler J, Sturup J. Achilles tendon rupture. An 8-year follow-up. *Acta Orthop Belg* 1989;55:307.
6. Brink O, Staunstrup H, Sommer J. Stable lateral malleolar fractures treated with aircast ankle brace and DonJoy ROM–walker brace: a prospective randomized study. *Foot Ankle Int* 1996;17:679–684.
7. Carragee EJ, Csongradi TZ, Bleck EE. Early complications in the operative treatment of ankle fractures; influence of delay before operation. *J Bone Joint Surg (Br)* 1991;73:79–82.
8. Dijkema ARA, van der Elst M, Breederveld RS, et al. Surgical treatment of fracture-dislocations of the ankle joint with biodegradable implants: a prospective randomized study. *J Trauma* 1993;34:82–84.
9. Escalas F, Figueras JM, Merino JA. Dislocation of the peroneal tendons. *J Bone Joint Surg (Am)* 1980;62:451.
10. Evans GA, Hardcastle P, Frenyo AD. Acute rupture of the lateral ligament of the ankle: to suture or not to suture? *J Bone Joint Surg (Br)* 1984;66:209.
11. Franklin JL, Johnson KD, Hansen ST. Immediate internal fixation of open ankle fractures. *J Bone Joint Surg (Am)* 1984;66:1349.
12. Hedstrom M, Ahl T, Dalen N. Early postoperative ankle exercise. *Clin Orthop Rel Res* 1994;300:193–196.

13. Marti RK, et al. Malunited ankle fractures. The late results of reconstruction. *J Bone Joint Surg (Br)* 1990:72:709.
14. McCormack RG, Leith JM. Ankle fractures in diabetics: complications of surgical management. *J Bone Joint Surg (Br)* 1998;80:689–692.
15. Ovadia DN, Beals RK. Fractures of the tibial plafond. *J Bone Joint Surg (Am)* 1986; 68:543.
16. Paiement GD, Renaud E, Dagenais G, et al. Double-blind randomized prospective study of efficacy of antibiotic prophylaxis for open reduction and internal fixation of closed ankle fractures. *J Orthop Trauma* 1994;8:64–66.
17. Phillips WA, et al. A prospective, randomized study of the management of severe ankle fractures. *J Bone Joint Surg (Am)* 1985;67:67.
18. Ponzer S, Nasell H, Bergman B, et al. Functional outcome and quality of life in patients with type B ankle fractures: a two year follow-up study. *J Orthop Trauma* 1999;13:363–368.
19. Povacz P, Salzburg FU, Wels KM, et al. A randomized, prospective study of operative and non-operative treatment of injuries of the fibular collateral ligaments of the ankle. *J Bone Joint Surg (Am)* 1998;80:345–351.
20. Sondenaa K, Hoigaard U, Smith D, et al. Immobilization of operated ankle fractures. *Acta Orthop Scand* 1986;57:59–61.
21. Stromsoe K, Hoqevold HE, Skjeldal S, et al. The repair of a ruptured deltoid ligament is not necessary in ankle fractures. *J Bone Joint Surg (Br)* 1995;77:920–921.
22. Winkler B, Weber BG, Simpson LA. The dorsal antiglide plate in the treatment of Danis-Weber type-B fractures of the distal fibula. *Clin Orthop Rel Res* 1990;259: 204–209.

Selected Historical Readings

Block HM, Brand RL, Eichelberger MR. An improved technique for the evaluation of ligamentous injury in severe ankle sprains. *Am J Sports Med* 1978;6:276.
Brantigan JW, Pedegana LR, Lippert FG. Instability of the subtalar joints. *J Bone Joint Surg (Am)* 1977;59:321.
Goergen TG, et al. Roentgenographic evaluation of the tibiotalar joint. *J Bone Joint Surg (Am)* 1977;59:874.
Martens DJM, et al. Comparison of conservative and operative treatment of Achilles tendon rupture. *Am J Sports Med* 1978;6:107.
Mast JW, Spiegel PG, Pappas JN. Fractures of the tibial pilon. *Clin Orthop* 1988;230:68.
Nistor L. Surgical and nonsurgical repair of Achilles tendon rupture. *J Bone Joint Surg (Am)* 1981;63:394.
Ramsey P, Hamilton W. Changes in tibiotalar area of contact caused by lateral talar shift. *J Bone Joint Surg (Am)* 1976;58:356.
Yablon IG, Keller FG, Shouse L. The key role of the lateral malleolus in displaced fractures of the ankle. *J Bone Joint Surg (Am)* 1977;59:169.

27. FRACTURES AND DISLOCATIONS OF THE FOOT

I. **Fractures of the calcaneus**
   A. **Mechanism of injury.** Calcaneal fractures are more frequent than any other fracture of the tarsal bones and comprise 1%–2% of all fractures. These fractures, which are often bilateral, are likely to occur when a person falls from a height and lands on the heels. Associated injuries include compression fractures of the lumbar spine and, occasionally, fractures about the knee or pelvis.
   B. **Classification.** Although there are many classification systems, a description of the fracture location provides the most information.
      1. **Avulsion fractures** occur in the posterior process of the tubercle as a result of increased tension in the Achilles tendon. This tension causes a fracture of the calcaneus rather than a ruptured tendon. If the avulsion fracture is large and runs into the body of the calcaneus (into or beyond the posterior facet), it is termed a *tongue-type fracture* (Fig. 27-1).
      2. **Fractures into the body of the calcaneus**
         a. **Fractures not involving the subtalar joint,** with or without disruption of the plantar surface of the calcaneus, can result in heel shortening and varus.
         b. **Fractures involving the subtalar joint** typically involve a triangular-shaped subarticular fragment that remains in place medially, the fractured and impacted posterior facet (generally the anterior portion is driven down into the body of the calcaneus to a greater degree than the posterior portion), and displacement of the lateral wall under the fibula. This is termed a *joint depression fracture* (Fig. 27-1).
   C. **Examination.** Pain and tenderness in the heel are present, with associated broadening of the heel and ecchymosis. Ecchymosis on the posterior sole of the foot with calcaneal tenderness is nearly diagnostic of a calcaneal fracture. When open fractures are occurring, the wound is most often medial near the sustentaculum talus. A foot compartmental syndrome can occur in 2%–5% of patients and must be treated with urgent decompression (see Chap. 2). Because of the risk of associated injuries, the spine and pelvis must be thoroughly evaluated.
   D. **Roentgenograms.** Fractures are identified on roentgenograms by a fracture line of increased (impaction) or decreased bone density. Consideration must be given to any distortion of the normal shape of the calcaneus. In addition to the lateral roentgenograms, calcaneal (axial) views and computed tomography (CT) are valuable to clarify the fracture pattern and to assess any increased width of the calcaneus. As with any severe fracture, analgesics often are required for the patient's comfort during the roentgenographic examination.
   E. **Treatment.** All fractures should initially be treated in a well-padded splint for the first 7–10 days until the swelling begins to resolve.
      1. **Isolated avulsion fractures** do not usually involve the subtalar joint.
         a. Those with **minimal displacement** may be treated by a short-leg, non–weight-bearing cast with the ankle in a neutral position for 4–6 weeks (12). The lack of displacement should be confirmed by a roentgenogram after the cast is applied.
         b. Avulsion fractures (tongue type) with **major displacement** require reduction and internal fixation of the displaced bone to reattach the Achilles tendon. This procedure, generally accomplished with two lag screws, is followed by non–weight-bearing immobilization in a short-leg cast. The foot is held in slight equinus for the first 3–4 weeks and then in a neutral position for an additional 3–4 weeks. Alternatively, a percutaneous reduction maneuver as described by Essex-Lopresti provides excellent reduction (18).

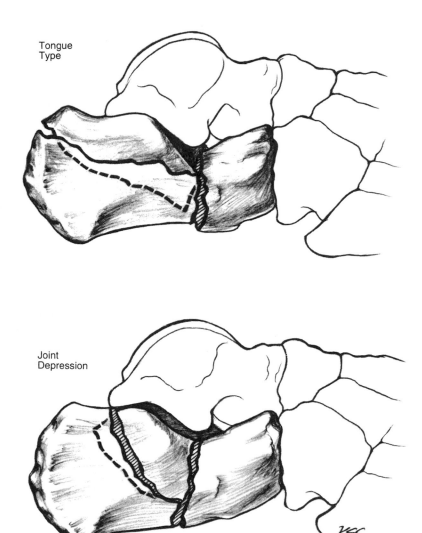

FIG. 27-1. Diagrammatic representation of tongue-type and joint depression-type calcaneal fractures. (From Hansen ST, Swiontkowski MF. *Orthopaedic trauma protocols.* New York: Raven, 1993:355.)

2. **Fractures into the body of the calcaneus**
   a. **Treatment**
      (1) The **tuber (Böhler) angle should be restored** with treatment whenever possible. The tuber angle, which is established by the lateral roentgenogram, is formed by the intersection of one line along the superior aspect of the tuber of the calcaneus with a second line along the superior aspect of the middle and anterior portions of the calcaneus. The angle is normally 30 degrees.
      (2) **With conservative treatment, restoration** of this angle is thought to be **unnecessary,** and **treatment consists of**

compression to prevent edema and decrease hemorrhage, **followed by early subtalar motion** and 6–12 weeks of no weight bearing.

(3) **Open reduction** for anatomic restoration is desirable to re-align articular fragments and prevent peroneal impingement while allowing for normal shoe wear (Fig. 27-2). There is no solid evidence to suggest that patients who have open reduction and internal fixation (ORIF) have better functional results (2,9,16). Most experienced surgeons believe that the risk of infection that accompanies ORIF is outweighed by better foot shape and heel position.

(4) **Early subtalar arthrodesis** may be appropriate; such treatment is rarely advocated.

b. The **authors advocate** a surgical reduction for intraarticular fractures only when the fracture can be anatomically reduced and held in that reduced position (9). The calcaneus is cancellous bone, and fractures of the calcaneus usually are comminuted. Attempts at reconstruction require a great deal of operative skill and knowledge of internal fixation with specialized implants. Referral to an experienced surgeon is recommended. When the surgeon is inexperienced and referral is not possible, these fractures should be treated by compression and early motion under proper supervision (2,12,16). Early motion should be started within the first 72 hours. Short-term hospital treatment appears to be worth the cost in improving the end result and shortening the period of disability following this serious and frequently disabling injury (11). The **authors recommend the following treatment program:**

(1) The **patient is admitted to the hospital** when necessary for adequate pain medication, elevation of the foot, and a proper compression dressing.

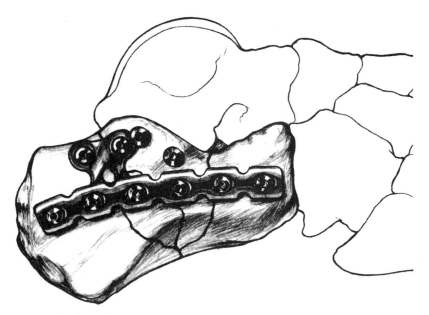

FIG. 27-2. Postoperative view of standard internal fixation for a joint depression fracture. (From Hansen ST, Swiontkowski MF. *Orthopaedic trauma protocols.* New York: Raven, 1993:359.)

(2) After control of pain and **within 2–3 days, motion** is begun, with emphasis on inversion and eversion. Once the patient is comfortable with the therapy and after outside follow-up therapy is arranged, the patient is discharged.

(3) **Weight bearing** may be started as soon as the fracture is consolidated (usually 8–10 weeks). When partial weight bearing is begun, a sponge placed in the heel is helpful. A wheelchair is generally required for 8–12 weeks for patients with bilateral fractures.

F. **Complications**

1. **Fracture blisters** and skin loss can occur.
2. Persistent pain can arise from swelling (the **sequela of a compartmental syndrome**), deformity, and stiffness.
3. **Problems with shoe fitting** occur because of heel widening and varus. A pedorthotist should be consulted for specialized shoes and inserts.
4. **Persistent pain,** usually associated with loss of subtalar motion, can be severe enough to require a triple arthrodesis. This procedure does not always produce a pain-free foot and should be undertaken with caution (13). Pain frequently occurs beneath the lateral malleolus because of widening of the calcaneus with impingement of the peroneal tendons and loss of heel height. Surgical relief involving the decompression of the peroneal tendons can improve symptoms and should be considered.

G. **Calcaneal fractures in children** (19)

1. Calcaneal fractures in children follow the same pattern and are caused by the **same mechanisms as in adults.**
2. The **treatment** program follows the same general plan as for the adult.
3. Unreduced intraarticular fractures persist in limiting subtalar joint motion but have **minimal symptoms** in short-term follow-up.

II. **Subtalar and talar dislocations**

A. **Definition**

1. A **subtalar dislocation** occurs through the subtalar joint with the ankle and foot displaced medially or laterally. The talus can snap back by itself inside the mortise, leaving the foot displaced medially or laterally relative to the toes (4,8).
2. In a **talar dislocation,** the talus is completely dislocated from its position within the mortise and tarsus. This is a rare injury.

B. **Mechanism of injury.** Progressive degrees of inversion forces applied to the foot cause rupture of progressively more ligaments around the talus, resulting in a subtalar-talonavicular or a complete talar dislocation. Inversion, internal rotation, and equinus forces cause rupture of the talonavicular ligament. More displacement ruptures the medial, interosseous, and lateral talocalcaneal ligaments; finally, the lateral ligaments (anterior talofibular, calcaneal-fibular, and posterior talofibular ligaments) can rupture. The talus can ultimately be forced from its major attachments and dislocate. The skin often breaks; in this event, the talus may extrude from the foot. This injury can also be associated with a fracture of the neck of the talus, which is also commonly an open injury (3,13).

C. **Examination**

1. A **subtalar dislocation** shows a classic positioning of the foot medially or laterally on the ankle. There is always marked tenting of the skin on the side opposite the foot.
2. With a closed **talar dislocation,** the talus comes to rest under the skin on the dorsolateral aspect of the ankle.
3. With both injuries, swelling is always severe. These are **true emergencies.**

D. **Roentgenograms.** The diagnosis may be made on physical examination, but the extent of injury and the exact position of the involved bones should be confirmed by multiple roentgenographic views. Do not delay. Arrange for anesthesia even before obtaining roentgenograms.

E. **Treatment**
  1. It may be advisable to carry out a **manual reduction** by slow but firm traction in the line of the deformity with analgesia, but only if there are delays with gaining access to the operating room for anesthesia services. Reduction is easy unless there is trapping of the posterior tibial tendon around the neck of the talus in a lateral subtalar dislocation where open reduction is necessary.
  2. **After reduction,** a short-leg Jones compression splint is applied until swelling is controlled. Then active range-of-motion exercises are begun.
  3. An **associated fracture must be reduced anatomically** and the reduction rigidly maintained, preferably with small fragment lag screws. Where fixation is stable, early active motion may be started using a removable posterior splint.
F. **Complications**
  1. **Ischemic skin loss** can be seen.
  2. **Avascular necrosis of the body of the talus** can occur with a talar dislocation (3,5).
  3. **Pain and stiffness** can ensue.
III. **Fracture of the talus**
  A. **Neck of the talus** (3). Talus neck fractures are generally classified by the Hawkins' system (Fig. 27-3). Type I is nondisplaced and type II is displaced with associated subtalar joint subluxation. In type III, the talar body is dislocated from the ankle mortise, and in type IV the talonavicular joint is also subluxated.
    1. **Mechanism of injury.** This injury is most commonly the result of forceful ankle dorsiflexion. Historically, it occurred with biplanes impacting the ground (the "aviator's astralagus"). The talus impinges on the anterior portion of the tibia, causing a fracture through the talar neck. The fracture, which may not be displaced, is easily overlooked without adequate roentgenograms.
    2. **Treatment.** Accurate reduction and rigid immobilization are important. To preserve the function of the hind foot joints, open anatomic reduction and internal fixation are recommended. Placement of small fragment lag screws across the fracture site is advisable. Because posttraumatic avascular necrosis of the body of the talus occurs commonly, most surgeons recommend waiting for subchondral resorption of the body of the talus to be apparent in the mortise roentgenogram before allowing full weight bearing (Hawkins' sign). This complication is less frequent with emergent reduction and fixation of widely displaced fractures.
    3. **Complications**
      a. **Dislocation of the peroneal tendons** occurs as an associated injury that should be ruled out and treated if present (see Chap. 26, **III.B**).
      b. **Avascular necrosis** is the most serious complication. Ankle arthrodesis can be difficult in this setting and specialized techniques must be used (18).
  B. **Other talar fractures.** Fractures may involve the body of the talus as well as the neck. Anatomic reduction is necessary for fractures involving the articular surfaces (10). Whenever the fragments are large enough and it is technically possible, ORIF usually is required. See the foregoing discussion of Hawkins' sign.
IV. **Fractures of the navicular, cuneiform, and cuboid bones** occur rarely as isolated injuries; the navicular is the most common. Whenever there is displacement of greater than 2 mm, the authors recommend open anatomic reduction and screw fixation (14). When associated with midfoot fractures or subluxations, reduction and fixation can be difficult. Referral to a surgeon experienced in the management of the fractures should be considered. Swelling can be severe, as with calcaneus fractures, so the procedure may be delayed 7–10 days while swelling subsides. Postoperative treatment involves 6 weeks in a non–weight-bearing cast or brace followed by 6 weeks in a short-leg weight-bearing boot or cast.

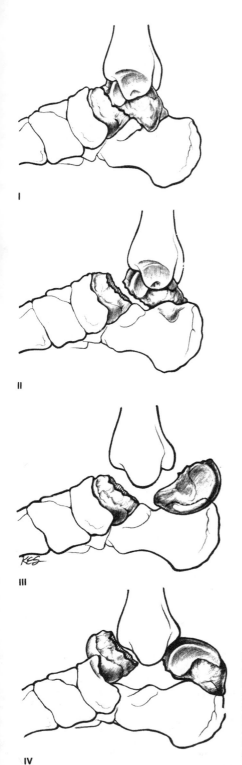

I

II

III

IV

FIG. 27-3. Diagrammatic representation of Hawkins' classification of talar neck fractures. I, nondisplaced; II, displaced with associated subtalar joint subluxation; III, talar body dislocated from the ankle mortise; IV, talonavicular joint subluxated also. (From Hansen ST, Swiontkowski MF. *Orthopaedic trauma protocols.* New York: Raven, 1993:340.)

V. **Subluxation, dislocation, and fracture-dislocation of the midtarsal, tarsal-metatarsal, or phalangeal joints** (1,6)
   A. **Roentgenograms.** The usual deformities can be masked in massive swelling. Anteroposterior, lateral, and oblique roentgenograms of the foot are essential. It is frequently helpful to compare these with films of the normal foot. Midfoot subluxations can be subtle, and a high index of suspicion is necessary when there is a history of axial loading of the foot and midfoot tenderness. Stress roentgenographs of the midfoot are indicated when the diagnosis is not clear.
   B. **Treatment.** Manipulative reduction is done; **anesthesia** is usually used for **forefoot** dislocations. If reduction is possible and if stability is sufficient, plaster immobilization for 4 weeks is adequate. If reduction is incomplete or if there is instability, then displacement may occur, leading to malunion, persistent subluxation, and a painful planovalgus forefoot. If the reduction is unstable, then open reduction may be required and internal fixation is generally necessary.
      1. For **midtarsal dislocations and subluxations (Lisfranc's joint injury),** accurate anatomic reduction is required to prevent the sequelae of forefoot abduction and collapse of the medial arch. Open reduction and fixation with screws is recommended (1). This allows arthrofibrosis of the injured joints, which preserves the normal slope of the foot. Although screw breakage can occur, it is generally advisable to leave the screws in place because removal can lead to planovalgus deformity. Although nearly all patients experience long-term discomfort and swelling, the normal shape of the foot makes the management of these complaints easier.
      2. **Phalangeal dislocations** require only reduction and symptomatic treatment. Stiff-soled shoes are often helpful for 4–6 weeks postinjury. Taping of injured toes to the adjacent uninjured toe can be helpful.
VI. **Fractures of the forefoot**
   A. The **diagnosis** of a forefoot fracture is usually suspected when localized bony tenderness or deformity is found.
   B. Anteroposterior, oblique, and lateral **roentgenograms** of the foot generally confirm the diagnosis.
   C. **Treatment**
      1. **Metatarsals**
         a. **Avulsion fractures of the base of the fifth metatarsal** (the insertion of the peroneus brevis) should be treated symptomatically unless there is gross displacement, in which case the treatment of choice is ORIF. Symptomatic treatment usually consists of a compression dressing and elevation until the swelling is controlled, followed by a short-leg weight-bearing cast with a well-molded arch. This fifth metatarsal proximal neck shaft *junction* fracture (Jones fracture) is prone to delayed union and non-union (7,17). Therefore, no weight bearing for 10–12 weeks is indicated. Open reduction and bone grafting is required for non-union (7); intramedullary screw fixation is preferred.
         b. **Fractures of the metatarsal shaft** are caused by a crushing injury. As a rule, the soft-tissue injury is more severe than the fracture. Initial treatment should include a compression dressing and elevation to control swelling, which is followed by reduction if the fracture is displaced. If the great toe remains cocked up or the first web space remains widened with **fractures to the first metatarsal,** then the reduction is incomplete or unstable. Open reduction with small fragment plates for this type of unstable first metatarsal fracture is recommended. If the second through fifth metatarsal fractures are seen to have the metatarsal heads at the same level without excessive (more than 5 mm) shortening, then the reduction is satisfactory. If displacement is more severe, then closed reduction with axial Kirschner wire fixation may be necessary to prevent long-term

transfer metatarsalgia. After proper reduction, the foot is placed in a short-leg plaster cast with well-contoured longitudinal and metatarsal arches. No weight bearing is allowed on the affected foot for 4–6 weeks. An additional 6 weeks is spent in a walking cast or fracture boot. Open reduction rarely is indicated for lesser metatarsal fractures unless there is marked shortening or plantar angulation.

c. **Fractures of the metatarsal necks** can be associated with displacement of the metatarsal head toward the weight-bearing surface of the foot, which disrupts the normal mechanics of proper weight bearing.

   (1) **Fractures of the first metatarsal neck or of multiple metatarsal necks** must be reduced and are usually held with some type of percutaneous wire fixation, because they are often unstable. Pins can be placed through the plantar surface of the foot, through the metatarsal heads, and into the shaft of the metatarsals. Roentgenographic image intensification aids in the placement of these pins, but with proper palpation and anesthesia, it can ordinarily be accomplished percutaneously.

   (2) **An isolated metatarsal neck fracture** should be grossly aligned to avoid abnormal pressure of the metatarsal head on the sole of the foot (transfer metatarsalgia) and to avoid forcing the toe against the top of the shoe. Immobilize in a short-leg walking cast for 6–10 weeks.

2. **Toes**

   a. **Fractures of the toes** are treated by taping them to the adjacent toe, which acts as an adequate splint. Avoid maceration by using dry cotton or Webril between the toes.

   b. A **fracture of the great toe** often requires a short-leg cast with a platform under the toes for comfort as well as immobilization.

   c. **Fractures of the sesamoids of the great toe**

   (1) **Mechanism of injury.** These fractures are usually the result of a direct force applied to this area of the foot either from a fall with landing on the metatarsal heads or from a weight being dropped on the foot. Occasionally, these injuries occur as avulsion fractures from forceful hyperextension of the great toe or from traction injuries to the flexor hallucis brevis. The fractures are usually transverse.

   (2) **Examination.** The patient experiences localized pain over the area. Differential diagnosis takes into account a congenital bipartite sesamoid. Local pain and irregular surfaces on the roentgenogram are the distinguishing features for a fracture.

   (3) **Treatment.** No weight bearing is allowed as long as the area is painful. After initial treatment, a metatarsal pad can help relieve pressure. Occasionally, pain persists; sesamoid resection and reconstitution of the tendon are then indicated.

HCMC Treatment Recommendations

Calcaneus Fractures

   Diagnosis: Lateral and axial views of the heel, CT scan, clinical examination

   Treatment: Non–weight bearing for 12 weeks with early subtalar motion where nonoperative treatment is selected, ORIF with non–weight bearing and passive subtler motion for 12 weeks where ORIF indicated

   Indications for surgery: Significant widening of the heel with lateral wall "blow out," depression or gapping of the subtalar joint more than 2–3 mm

   Recommended technique: ORIF via lateral incision

HCMC Treatment Recommendations

Talus Fractures

   Diagnosis: Lateral and mortise radiographs, clinical examination

   Treatment: ORIF for any displaced fracture

   Indications for surgery: Fractures with >2-mm gapping, loose osteochondral fragment

   Recommended technique: ORIF with small fragment lag screws via medial and lateral approaches; subtalar joint must be debrided of bone/cartilage fragments; non–weight bearing for 8–12 weeks

---

HCMC Treatment Recommendations

Subtalar Dislocations

   Diagnosis: Lateral and axial views of the hindfoot, clinical examination

   Treatment: Closed reduction with follow-up radiographs with or without CT scan

   Indications for surgery: Irreducible dislocation, significant debris in subtalar joint

   Recommended technique: Incision on the side of the deformity, exploration of the subtalar joint after removing tissue blocking reduction—ORIF with small or minifragment screws of larger fragments

---

HCMC Treatment Recommendations

Tarsometatarsal (Lisfranc's) Fracture / Dislocations

   Diagnosis: Lateral, oblique anteroposterior radiographs of the foot; clinical examination

   Treatment: ORIF of displaced fractures

   Indications for surgery: Displacement of first, second, third metatarsal bases with ligament disruption or major displacement of base of the first, second, third, metatarsals

   Recommended technique: ORIF with small fragment screws, K-wire fixation for displaced base of fifth metatarsal ligament disruptions

---

HCMC Treatment Recommendations

Metatarsal Fractures

   Diagnosis: Anteroposterior, lateral, oblique foot radiographs; clinical examination

   Treatment: 4–6 weeks of limited weight bearing

   Indications for surgery: Open fractures, shortening/comminution of first metatarsal or fifth metatarsal, multiple metatarsal fractures

   Recommended technique: ORIF with small or minifragment plates, K-wires for metatarsal neck fractures

HCMC Treatment Recommendations
Toe Fractures
  Diagnosis: Anteroposterior, lateral, oblique foot radiographs; clinical examination
  Treatment: Protective orthosis or shoe wear for 6–8 weeks, progressive weight bearing as tolerated, buddy taping of lesser toe fractures
  Indications for surgery: Open fractures, displaced intraarticular fracture of the great toe
  Recommended technique: ORIF with K-wires or minifragment screws

References
 1. Arntz LT, Veith RG, Hansen S T. Fractures and fracture-dislocations of the tarsometatarsal joint. *J Bone Joint Surg (Am)* 1988;70:173.
 2. Buckley RE, Meek RN. Comparison of open versus closed reduction of intraarticular calcaneal fractures: a matched cohort in workmen. *J Orthop Trauma* 1992;6:216–222.
 3. Canale ST, Kelly FB. Fractures of the neck of the talus: long-term evaluation of seventy-one cases. *J Bone Joint Surg (Am)* 1978;60:143.
 4. DeLee JC, Curtis R. Subtalar dislocation of the foot. *J Bone Joint Surg (Am)* 1982; 64:433–437.
 5. Goldner JL, Polett SC, Gates HS III, et al. Severe open subtalar dislocations–long-term results. *J Bone Joint Surg (Am)* 1995;77:1075–1079.
 6. Hardcastle PH, et al. Injuries to the tarsometatarsal joint. *J Bone Joint Surg* 1982;64B:439.
 7. Kavanaugh JH, Brower TD, Mann RV. The Jones fracture revisited. *J Bone Joint Surg (Am)* 1978;60:776.
 8. Monson ST, Ryan JR. Subtalar dislocations. *J Bone Joint Surg (Am)* 1981;63: 1156–1158.
 9. Parmar HV, Triffitt PD, Gregg PJ. Intra-articular fractures of the calcaneum treated operatively or conservatively—a prospective study. *J Bone Joint Surg (Br)* 1993;75:932–937.
10. Pettine KA, Morrey BF. Osteochondral fractures of the talus. *J Bone Joint Surg (Br)* 1987;69:89–92.
11. Pozo JL, Kirwan EOG, Jackson AM. The long-term results of conservative management of severely displaced fractures of the calcaneus. *J Bone Joint Surg (Br)* 1984;66:386.
12. Sanders R. Current concepts review—displaced intra-articular fractures of the calcaneus. *J Bone Joint Surg (Am)* 2000;82:225–249.
13. Sanders R, Pappas J, Mast J, et al. The salvage of open grade IIIB ankle and talus fractures. *J Orthop Trauma* 1992;6:201–208.
14. Sangeorzan BJ, et al. Displaced intraarticular fractures of the tarsal navicular. *J Bone Joint Surg (Am)* 1989;71:1504.
15. Stephenson JR. Treatment of displaced intraarticular fractures of the calcaneus using medial and lateral approaches, internal fixation and early motion. *J Bone Joint Surg (Am)* 1987;69:115.
16. Thordarson DB, Krieger LE. Operative vs. non-operative treatment of intraarticular fractures of the calcaneus: a prospective randomized trial. *Foot Ankle Int* 1996;17:2–9.
17. Torg JS, et al. Fractures of the base of the fifth metatarsal distal to the tuberosity. *J Bone Joint Surg (Am)* 1984;66:209.
18. Tornetta P. The Essex-Lopresti reduction for calcaneal fractures revisited. *J Orthop Trauma* 1998;12:469–473.
19. Wiley JJ, Profitt A. Fractures of the os calcis in children. *Clin Orthop* 1984; 188:131.

Selected Historical Readings

Barnard L, Odegard JK. Conservative approach in the treatment of fractures of the calcaneus. *J Bone Joint Surg (Am)* 1970;52:1689.

Canale T, Belding RH. Osteochondral lesions of the talus. *J Bone Joint Surg (Am)* 1980;62:97.

Essex-Lopresti P. The mechanism, reduction technique and results in fractures of the os calcis. *Br J Surg* 1952;39:395.

Hawkins LG. Fractures of the talus. *J Bone Joint Surg (Am)* 1970;52:991.

Mindell ER, et al. Late results of injuries to the talus. *J Bone Joint Surg (Am)* 1963;45:221.

Noble J, McQuillan WM. Early posterior subtalar fusion in the treatment of fractures of the os calcis. *J Bone Joint Surg (Br)* 1979;61:90.

28. OVERUSE AND MISCELLANEOUS CONDITIONS OF THE FOOT AND ANKLE

I. **Achilles tendinitis**
  A. **Insertional** type may be associated with a Haglund's deformity or retrocalcaneal bursitis. This is a typical overuse injury caused by accumulated impact load (2), which occurs most often in runners and repetitive jumpers. Insertional type occurs more in the older age group than does noninsertional tendinitis.
    1. **Treatment** should be **conservative** in 95% of cases. Rest, nonsteroidal antiinflammatory drugs (NSAIDs), cross training, physiotherapy orthotics, and occasionally casting should be used. No steroid treatment is necessary (12,19).
    2. **Surgery** is indicated after 6–12 months of failed conservative treatment. Surgery consists of the following: excise retrocalcaneal bursa, resect superior prominence, and debride diseased or calcified portion of tendon. Reattach if necessary. The patient should be non–weight bearing for 6–8 weeks. Rehabilitation is resumed but recovery might take up to 1 year. Success rate is 70%–86%.
  B. **Noninsertional** type is associated with typical hypovascular zone 2–6 cm proximal to insertion. The etiologic profile includes repetitive micro trauma, more common in males, older athletes, tight gastrosoleus and hamstrings, functional over pronation. Extrinsic factors include improper training, improper shoe wear, systemic or injected steroids, and fluoroquinolone antibiotics (10). There are various classification systems that could be simplified into peritendinitis (sheath only), tendinosis (tendon only), or pantendinitis (sheath and tendon) (3). Diagnosis is primarily by history and clinical evaluation and is confirmed with ultrasound (operator dependent) or magnetic resonance imaging (MRI). Typical signs and symptoms are morning stiffness or pain, start-up pain, postexercise pain, and tendon fullness or nodule.
    1. **Treatment** in **acute** situations includes pain relief, reduction of inflammation (NSAIDs, ice), and restriction of activities. A heel lift or boot brace can be used until symptoms subside (12), followed by a rehabilitation program (6). Other measures include stretching and strengthening of the Achilles and gastrosoleus, review and modification of training regimens (frequency, duration, intensity), correction of structural abnormalities (overpronation), and modifications in foot wear. Treatment is 90%–95% successful.
    2. **Treatment** of **chronic** cases (>3 months) depends on severity. Peritendinitis is treated with mechanical "brisement" or surgical debridement followed by an early rehabilitation program (6). Chronic pantendinitis is treated with debridement, longitudinal tenotomy (8), or tendon transfer depending on clinical situation. It appears from the literature that surgical treatment of chronic tendinitis might do better than nonoperative treatment.
II. **Plantar heel pain** is a common foot problem in the athlete. Running and jumping place repetitive stress on the heel and create an overuse syndrome with chronic inflammation.
  A. **Differential diagnosis.** To differentiate, a thorough history and examination is required. This should include exact location and duration of pain and the relationship to athletic activity. Chronic pain at rest is unusual and might be due to a tumor. The differential diagnosis includes the following:
    1. Plantar fasciitis
    2. Nerve entrapment
    3. Fat pad atrophy
    4. Heel bruise
    5. Tendinitis of flexor hallucis longus or flexor digitorum brevis

6. Stress fracture
7. Tumor

B. Plantar fasciitis could be at insertion into medial calcaneal tuberosity or midfoot and may be due to repetitive traction and microtears. Usually, plantar fasciitis has an insidious onset as an overuse condition in long distance runners. Midfoot plantar fasciitis is more common in sprinters who run on their toes.

1. **Symptoms and signs** include pain during the first minutes of walking, especially when first getting out of bed. Athletic activities intensify pain.
2. Always evaluate for **leg length discrepancy**. Heel pain is more common in the shorter leg and may be treated with an appropriate lift. Also inquire about a functional short leg syndrome from running on the same tilt of the road. Plantar fasciitis is frequently caused by a tight Achilles tendon, because limited ankle dorsiflexion increases the stress on the plantar fascia. Fasciitis at the insertion has localized deep tenderness. It is usually not associated with increased pain or with passive dorsiflexion of the toes (windlass mechanism). Midfoot fasciitis has tenderness in midfoot and increased pain with passive dorsiflexion of the toes. Passive dorsiflexion of the big toe aggravates both plantar fasciitis and flexor hallucis longus tendinitis. Resisted flexion of the big toe is painful only with involvement of the tendon.

C. Treatment

1. **Conservative.** The cornerstone of treatment is modification in training, for example, reducing mileage, shortening workouts, and alternating activities such as low resistance cycling and swimming pool running (14). There is not a single entity that works for everyone, but conservative measures usually include the following:
   a. A shock-absorboing heel cup for heel pain, or a full length orthotic or UCBL (University of California Berkley laboratory) orthotic for mid-sunstance pain.
   b. Oral non-steroid anti-infammatory agents.
   c. Physical therapy to unclude Achilles and plantar fascia stretching, hindfoot taping, contrast baths and ultrasound treatment.
   d. A night splint might help to keep the fascia under tension to reduce early morning weight bearing pain.
   e. Steroid injection may be used in refractory cases and should be injected deep to the plantar fascia to avoid fat pad necrosis.
   f. shockwave therapy might proof to be helpful in future.
   The heel spur seen on roentgenograms is seldom, if ever, the cause of heel pain.
2. **Surgical.** Plantar fascia release should be avoided in competitive athletes because it may increase the compressive forces to the dorsal aspect of the midfoot and decrease flexion forces on the metatarsophalangeal joint complex (4). When indicated, the plantar fascia is released from the calcaneus through a medial incision. The patient is allowed to bear weight as tolerated with crutches and rehabilitation is started after 2 weeks.

D. Calcaneal fat pad trauma. The patient complains of diffuse plantar heel pain that is exacerbated with weight bearing and with activities on hard surfaces.

1. **Examination** reveals diffuse tenderness localized to the fat pad. There is no radiation of the pain. The heel pad feels soft and thin, and the underlying calcaneus is palpable.
2. **Treatment** is nonsurgical. A cushioned heel cup and shock-absorbing shoes might help. The patient should reduce activities and avoid hard running surfaces.

E. Nerve entrapment syndromes

1. Entrapment of the **first branch of the lateral plantar nerve** is a common cause of chronic heel pain in athletes (1). The site of compres-

sion is between the deep fascia of the abductor hallucis muscle and the medial margin of the quadratus plantae muscle. This injury is more common in athletes who spend a significant amount of time on their toes such as ballet dancers, figure skaters, and sprinters.

a. **Diagnosis** is made on clinical grounds. Exclude the more common reasons for heel pain. Early morning pain is less problematic; the pain increases as the day goes on. Tenderness is specific over the area of compression.

b. **Treatment** is similar to that for other causes of heel pain. If conservative treatment fails, a release of the nerve may be done through a medial incision.

2. **Tarsal tunnel syndrome** could also be a source of heel pain. Compression of the posterior tibial nerve within the tarsal tunnel results in tenderness over the area. Excessive pronation in long-distance runners may place repeated stress on the medial structures of the heel.

a. On **examination,** there might be burning, pain, or tingling on the plantar aspect of the foot. Pain is more diffuse than with the other causes of heel pain. Electromyography and nerve conduction studies can be helpful but are not always sensitive enough.

b. **Treatment.** A medial heel wedge decreases the tension on the medial side of the ankle and therefore the nerve. Steroid injection into the tarsal tunnel might give short-term pain relief. Tarsal tunnel release is helpful in recalcitrant cases.

3. **Metatarsalgia**

a. Metatarsalgia is the most common forefoot problem and can have numerous etiologies.

(1) A **tight Achilles tendon** limits ankle dorsiflexion, which, in turn, increases the forces on the forefoot. A person compensates by using the long toe extensors to augment dorsiflexion power, but this pulls the plantar fat pad away from the weight bearing surface under the metatarsal heads, further aggravating forefoot pain.

(2) Similarly, **idiopathic claw toe deformities** could displace the fat pad and cause metatarsalgia.

(3) **Metatarsophalangeal joint capsulitis** might cause pain over the plantar aspect of the joint. This is more common at the second metatarsophalangeal joint and is associated with a long second metatarsal or instability of the first ray.

(4) A **Morton's (or common digital nerve) neuroma** causes pain in the web space and is most common in the third web space. Stress fractures of the metatarsals could also cause forefoot pain.

b. **Treatment.** The goal is to unload the metatarsal area. Orthotics, metatarsal bars, cushioned shoes, NSAIDs, and Achilles stretching are the cornerstones of initial management. If conservative management does not help, surgical correction of claw toes or excision of neuroma might be indicated.

III. **Tibialis posterior dysfunction syndrome.** Rupture of the tibialis posterior (TP) tendon is a cause of a painful, acquired flatfoot deformity in adults. It is more common in women 40 years of age and older (7,16,20). Numerous reports describing the condition have been published over the past 20 years, but it still remains a condition that is not commonly recognized. This could be due to the insidious nature of the condition, usually without a history of acute trauma (7).

A. **Anatomy.** By virtue of its lever arm length and muscle strength, the TP tendon is the main dynamic stabilizer of the hind foot against valgus deformity. It also plays a major role in maintaining the medial longitudinal arch. Insufficiency of the TP results in excessive strain on the static ligament-bone hind and midfoot constrains. The soft tissue gradually elongates, the arch flattens, and the pers longus and brevis have an unopposed abduction force on the forefoot.

B. Etiology of TP tendon rupture. To understand the etiology of TP tendon tears, it is important to remember its function. It resists considerable forces in maintaining the medial longitudinal arch. It also helps lock the mid and hind foot to allow a solid lever arm during the push-off part of the gait cycle. Approximately 20% of TP ruptures are associated with rheumatic conditions (7). An estimated 80% of TP tendon ruptures develop spontaneously. There are several theories to explain this phenomenon.

   1. **Mechanical.** The acute angle around the medial malleolus could lead to excessive friction that leads to slow deterioration over many years. This also explains the age predilection of this condition.
   2. **Vascular.** Laboratory studies have identified an area of poor blood supply to the tendon behind the medial malleolus. This could lead to a decrease in healing potential after minor trauma.
   3. **Achilles tendon contracture.** Either due to gastrocnemius alone or in combination with soleus, a longstanding (hereditary) tightness increases the workload and force on the TP during the gait cycle.

C. Clinical presentation. Contrary to popular belief, TP tendon rupture or insufficiency is common in American society. A proper history and thorough physical examination is usually all that is needed to make this a straightforward diagnosis.

   1. **History.** Onset is insidious, with discomfort reported on the medial side of the foot without any preceding acute trauma. Women are affected more often then men, and persons in their 40s are most often affected. There is not necessarily a relation to activity level.
   2. **Symptoms.** Initially, patients complain of only mild to moderate pain and of swelling and discomfort on the medial side of the foot and ankle. It is usually not incapacitating; rather, there is a chronic medial weight-bearing ache that limits physical activities. Without treatment, the symptoms might increase over a variable length of time. In a late stage, the patient might complain of additional weight-bearing pain on the lateral aspect of the ankle, a progressive deformity, and an abnormal gait.
   3. **Signs**
      a. In an early stage, one can see and palpate the swelling behind the medial malleolus and over the course of the TP tendon to its insertion in the navicular. The tenderness is usually over the same area.
      b. In a more advanced stage, the hallmark deformity becomes apparent. This is a combination of hind foot valgus, forefoot abduction, and flattening of the medial longitudinal arch.
      c. Much information can be gathered by observing the patient. When viewed from posterior, the amount of heel valgus above the normal neutral to 5 degrees in the weight-bearing position can be noted. The "too many toes" sign is indicative of forefoot abduction. The patient is also asked to raise on the toes. A normal TP locks the hind foot in varus to give a solid lever for push-off. With an insufficient TP, the heel does not move into varus, and it is impossible to raise oneself on the toes.
      d. Frontal and side views confirm the forefoot abduction and loss of medial arch. An apropulsive, antalgic gait is usually noticed if the patient is asked to walk at a rapid pace.
      e. Physical examination further confirms the clinical suspicion. Tendon and muscle power around the ankle is tested. The TP is evaluated with the foot in plantar flexion, and the patient is asked to invert the foot against resistance. Look for recruitment of the tibialis anterior to augment this action.
      f. The excursion of the ankle is tested with the knee first extended to determine the role of the gastrocnemius in possible tightness, and then with the knee flexed to isolate the soleus by eliminating the influence of the gastrocs.
      g. Range of movement of the ankle, especially the subtalar joint, is evaluated, and any pain is noted. In advanced cases, there might be ten-

derness on the lateral aspect of the ankle as a result of impingement
of the fibula on the calcaneus.
4. **Diagnostic workup.** Thorough history and clinical examination is
usually all that is needed to make the diagnosis.
   a. **Plain roentgenographs.** In most cases beyond stage 1, weight-
   bearing radiographs show specific changes. The most obvious is the
   change in the talo–first metatarsal alignment on the anteroposterior
   and lateral views. In a normal foot, the talo–first metatarsal alignment is in a straight line. In TP tendon ruptures, the alignment is
   altered to varying degrees because of the peritalar subluxation.
   b. **MRI** confirms a tear or degeneration in the TP tendon and shows the
   abnormal alignment of the bony elements, but it is costly and usually
   unnecessary. It is helpful in early, subtle injuries of the tendon.
   c. **Computed tomography** (CT) also is not necessary as a primary
   diagnostic tool, but it can be helpful to determine the integrity of the
   peritalar joints and, therefore, in **planning** the surgical procedure.
   It is of great value in the continuing study of the changes in the foot
   secondary to TP tendon ruptures.
5. **Classification**
   a. **Stage 1a: mild, occult (13%).** Symptoms last less than 1 year, there
   is mild swelling and tenderness over the TP tendon and slight weakness in inversion power, and there is minimal hind foot valgus on
   weight bearing.
   b. **1b: moderate (44%).** Symptoms last up to 18 months, and there is
   definite tenderness, swelling, and weakness of the TP tendon. Moderate pes planus and heel valgus occur as a result of dorsolateral
   peritalar subluxation.
   c. **Stage 2: advanced (17%).** Symptoms last for 1.5–2.5 years. There
   is more pronounced flatfoot deformity caused by peritalar subluxation, and there is considerable heel valgus and moderate prominence
   of the talar head medially. The subtalar joint is usually still mobile
   and the deformities passively correctable.
   d. **Stage 3a: complete (15%)**
   e. **3b: Peritalar dislocation (11%).** Progressive dorsolateral peritalar subluxation reaches the point of dislocation in the neglected
   case. Symptoms last between 4 and 20 years. Pain occurs also on the
   lateral side as a result of impingement of the calcaneus on the distal fibula. The fibula takes an increasing amount of load on weight
   bearing. It becomes hypertrophic, and stress fractures are not uncommon. The talocalcaneal relation is completely distorted, with
   minimal actual articular contact. The majority of these deformities
   are fixed and not passively correctable.
6. **Treatment**
   a. Nonsurgical. Other than certain grade 1a tears, nonsurgical management of TP tendon tears is essentially palliative. In most cases,
   it will neither result in healing of the tendon nor correction of the deformity. Noninvasive means are therefore only useful if there are factors present that contraindicate surgical intervention. This includes
   advanced age, significant medical problems, low activity level, and
   minimal discomfort. It is still advisable to start most patients on conservative treatment before electing to do surgery. Treatment should
   be directed to control pain, inflammation, and development of deformity. Options include the use of crutches, minimal weight bearing,
   or casting in a recent onset case. NSAIDs might help relieve pain and
   swelling. In more advanced cases, orthotics come into play. These include heel or sole lifts, inserts, UCBL type heel cups, and modified,
   accommodative shoes. In severe deformities, shoe modifications that
   incorporate calipers could be used.
   b. **Surgical.** Surgical treatment options include tendon repair, tendon
   augmentation, and bony stabilization of both nonessential and essential joints.

    (1) Stage 1. A tendon repair is still feasible. The TP tendon is usually augmented with a second tendon. A multitude of augmenting techniques have been described (7,20). This includes the use of the flexor digitorum longus, flexor hallucis longus, or peroneus longus that serve as dynamic stabilizers. Free tendon grafts are also used to repair the TP tendon, although the results are variable. It is of utmost importance to evaluate for tightness of the Achilles tendon and to lengthen it if necessary.

    (2) Stage 2. In more advanced cases, tendon repair and augmentation is usually not sufficient to relieve pain and prevent deformity. The surgical option is dependent upon the degree and mobility of the deformity. If the peritalar subluxation is still correctable, the bony stabilization is done in nonessential joints. This includes the lateral column distraction fusion that reduces the peritalar subluxation and heel valgus without compromising the important subtalar and talonavicular movement. Other options include a medial column or a subtalar fusion, with or without an Achilles lengthening.

    (3) Stage 3. The surgical treatment of subtotal peritalar dislocation with a fixed hind foot deformity (grade 3b) usually requires a triple arthrodesis.

IV. Stress fractures

A. Description. The foot and ankle are the most common areas for stress fractures. A stress fracture is defined as a partial or complete fracture resulting from its inability to withstand repetitive stress applied in a repeated, subthreshold manner. It is, therefore, a series of events causing stress fractures. Ninety-five percent of stress fractures are in the lower extremities, +/− 50% are of the foot and ankle. All the bones of the foot and ankle can sustain stress fractures. The metatarsals, though, are involved in 55% of cases, whereas the sesamoids and talus are involved in less than 1%. Stress fractures occur in all sports but especially in running and running-based sports. Sedentary people starting a fitness program are more prone to stress fractures. This is a well-demonstrated phenomenon in new military recruits. Stress fractures are more likely to develop in women. Leg length discrepancy, malalignment, prior injury as well as poor physical condition predispose to stress fracture.

B. Diagnosis

    1. The history is fairly typical, with pain being intensified by ongoing training. There might be an association with a recent increase in duration and intensity of training. It is usually insidious with an increase of pain over a period of time.

    2. There should always be a high index of suspicion for stress fractures with insidious onset of pain. This is especially true of the history correlated with the possibility of a stress fracture. Physical examination should localize the involved area.

    3. The gold standard for recognizing a stress reaction in bone used to be a Technisium bone scan. The bone scan becomes positive after a week of ongoing stress reaction in the bone. A negative bone scan effectively rules out a stress fracture (17).

    4. MRI can be extremely helpful in the diagnosis and grading of stress fractures. It is the most sensitive and specific method of diagnosing and grading stress fractures (22).

    5. Standard radiographs are still the most reliable and convenient tool for differential diagnosis, diagnosis, and follow-up (17).

    6. The combination of a negative roentgenogram and positive bone scan represents an early fracture, and treatment at this stage may prevent longstanding problems. CT scan has a place in diagnosing talus and midfoot fractures because these bones are cancellous in structure and stress fractures are difficult to identify on plain radiographs.

7. The most critical or at-risk stress fractures of the foot are of the navicular, proximal second metatarsal (11) and intraarticular fractures, and the great toe sesamoids. The navicular is particularly difficult to diagnose (18). Workup should include plain films, MRI bone scan, and CT scan. Significant disability can result from delayed diagnosis.

C. Treatment
1. Treatment should include 6 weeks of casting followed by verification of union by CT. Resumption of leg-based athletics is at 12–18 weeks after initiation of treatment. Custom orthotics should be used when the patient returns to athletics (17).
2. Noncritical fractures include distal metatarsals 2, 3, 4, and 5, the lateral malleolus, and the calcaneus (5). Treatment should be aimed at keeping the level of activity below that which causes pain. This implies decreasing the level of activity or substituting swimming, biking, circuit training, or other low impact activities. Orthotics within shoes can limit stress in the involved area (18).

V. First tarsometatarsal joint problems
A. Turf toe is a general term used for injuries around the first metatarsophalangeal joint. Differential diagnosis includes injury to the medial or lateral ligamentous structures, the phalangeal sesamoid ligament, a fractured sesamoid, osteochondral or chondral injury, chondral contusion caused by direct linear impact, and dislocations and injury to the interphalangeal joint (15). This injury is common in football players but is also seen in basketball and track athletes. Careful history and clinical evaluation is necessary to localize injury. Anteroposterior, lateral, oblique, and sesamoid views should be obtained.
1. Initial **conservative treatment** consists of the general approach: rest, ice, compression, and elevation. A postoperative shoe with firm sole to limit movement helps in ligamentous injuries. The patient's foot is immobilized for 3 weeks and rehabilitation is started as tolerated. Sesamoid fractures are treated with a cast shoe with the great toe in 10 degrees of flexion for 8–10 weeks.
2. **Surgical treatment** consists of debridement and drilling of articular surface if pain persists in a case of chondral fracture. Partial excision or internal fixation of sesamoid fracture is undertaken when the fracture does not heal.

B. Hallux rigidus. Degenerative arthritis of the first metatarsophalangeal joint. In most cases, there is no specific predisposing factor.
1. Possible etiologies include congenital flattening of the metatarsal head, metatarsus primus elevatus, osteochondritis of the head, a long hallux, pes planus, and osteochondral injuries (turf toe).
2. Hallux rigidus presents a significant problem for an athlete. Dorsiflexion of the big toe plays an important role in activities such as accelerating and jumping. Compensation by rolling onto the lateral aspect of the foot might cause stress and strain on the ankle, knee, and hip.
3. **Diagnosis.** Enlargement around the metatarsophalangeal joint is usually obvious. This is due to a combination of bony prominences and synovitis. Dorsiflexion is limited and reproduces the patient's pain. Radiographic findings might be minimal in early stages. With time, obvious degenerative changes and osteophytes within the joint become apparent. Sesamoids are generally not involved.
4. Differential diagnosis includes gout, or other inflammatory arthritis.
5. **Treatment**
   a. **Conservative.** Pressure against the toe is alleviated by modifying foot wear, incorporating a higher and wider toe box, a stiffer shoe, a rigid insert, or a rocker bottom sole. NSAIDs or injected steroids might give symptomatic relief.
   b. **Surgical.** Fusion is a good option in older people but would significantly impair athletic performance. In athletes, a cheilectomy with or

without a dorsiflexion osteotomy of the proximal phalanges (Moberg procedure) is preferred (9,13). The patient is permitted to ambulate weight bearing as tolerated in a postoperative shoe. Rehabilitation starts 7–10 days after surgery with active and passive range-of-motion exercises. The patient should wear a soft shoe to allow motion at the metatarsophalangeal joint with walking. Athletes could resume cycling, swimming, and any activity that avoids significant impact against the metatarsophalangeal joint but should avoid running, jumping, and similar activities for 10–12 weeks. Metatarsophalangeal joint arthroplasties (excision or prosthetic replacement) has very limited application in the young, active population.

References

1. Baxter DE, Pfeffer GB. Treatment of chronic heel pain by surgical release of the first branch of the lateral plantar nerve. *Clin Orthop* 1992;279:229.
2. Clain MR. Baxter DE. Achilles tendinitis. *Foot Ankle Int* 1992;13:482–487.
3. Clement DB, Taunton JE, Smart GW. Achilles tendinitis and peritendinitis: etiology and treatment. *Am J Sports Med* 1984;12:179–184.
4. Daly PJ, Kitaoka HB, Chao EYS. Plantar fasciotomy for intractable plantar fasciitis: clinical results and biomechanical evaluation. *Foot Ankle* 1992;13:188.
5. DeLee JC, Evans JP, Julian J. Stress fracture of the fifth metatarsal. *Am J Sports Med* 1992;35:697.
6. Johnston E, Scranton P, Pfeffer GB. Chronic disorders of the Achilles tendon: results of conservative and surgical treatments. *Foot Ankle Int* 1997;18:570–574.
7. Johnson KA. Tibialis posterior tendon rupture. *Clin Orthop* 1983;177;140–147.
8. Maffulli N, Testa V, Capasso G, et al. Results of percutaneous longitudinal tenotomy for Achilles tendinopathy in middle-and long-distance runners. *Am J Sports Med* 1997;25:835–840.
9. Mann RA, Clanton TO. Hallux rigidus: treatment by cheilectomy. *J Bone Joint Surg (Am)* 1988;70:400.
10. McCarvey WC, Singh D, Trevino SG. Partial Achilles tendon rupture associated with fluoroquinolone antibiotics: a case report and literature review. *Foot Ankle Int* 1996;17:496–498.
11. Micheli LJ, Sohn RS, Solomon R. Stress fractures of the second metatarsal involving Lisfranc's joint in ballet dancers. *J Bone Joint Surg (Am)* 1985;67:1372.
12. Mohr RN. Achilles tendonitis—rationale for use and application or orthotics. *Foot Ankle Clin* 1997;2:439–456.
13. Mulier T, Steenwerckx A, Thienpont E, et al. Result after chcilectomy in athletes with hallux rigidus. *Foot Ankle Int* 1999;20(4):232–237.
14. Pfeffer G, Bacchetti P, Deland J, et al. Comparison of custom and prefabricated orthotics in the initial treatment of proximal plantar fasciitis. *Foot Ankle Int* 1999; 20(4):214–221.
15. Rodeo SA, et al. Turf-toe: an analysis of metatarsophalangeal joint sprains in professional football players. *Am J Sports Med* 1990;18:280.
16. Sangeorzan BJ, Smith D, Veith R, et al. Triple arthrodesis using internal fixation in treatment of adult foot disorders. *Clin Orthop* 1993;294;299–307.
17. Santi M, Sartoris DJ. Diagnostic imaging approach to stress fractures of the foot. *J Foot Surg* 1991;30:85.
18. Schwellnus MP, Jordaan G, Noakes TD. Prevention of common overuse injuries by the use of shock absorbing insoles. *Am J Sports Med* 1990;18:636.
19. Shrier I, Matheson GO, Kohl HW 3rd. Achilles tendonitis: are corticosteroid injections useful or harmful? *Clin J Sports Med* 1996;6:245–250.
20. Thordarson DB, Schmotzer H, Chon J. Reconstruction with tenodesis in an adult flatfoot model. A biomechanical evaluation of four methods. *J Bone Joint Surg (Am)* 1995;77: 1557–1567.
21. Ting A, et al. Stress fractures of the tarsal navicular in long-distance runners. *Clin Sports Med* 1988;7:89.
22. Arendt EA, Griffiths HJ. Use of MR imaging in the assessment and clinical management of stress reactions of bone in high-performance athletes. *Clin Sports Med* 1997;16:291–306.

Selected Historical Readings

Anzel SH, Covey KW, Weiner AD, et al. Disruption of muscle and tendons. An analysis of 1,014 cases. *Surgery* 1959;45:406–414.

Astrom M, Gentz CF, Nilsson P. Imaging in chronic Achilles tendinopathy: a comparison of ultrasonograpy, magnetic resonance imaging and surgical findings in 27 histologically verified cases. *Skeletal Radiol* 1996;25:615–620.

Bennett GL, Graham CE, Mauldin DM. Triple arthrodesis in adults. *Foot Ankle* 1991;12(3):138–143.

Bonney G, McNag I. Hallux valgus and hallux rigidus. *J Bone Joint Surg (Br)* 1952; 34:366.

Dameron TB Jr. Fractures and anatomical variations of the proximal portion of the fifth metatarsal. *J Bone Joint Surg (Am)* 1975;57:788.

Key JA. Partial rupture of the tendon of the posterior tibial muscle. *J Bone Joint Surg (Am)* 1953;35:1006–1008.

Leach RE, Seavey NS, Salter DK. Results of surgery in athletes with plantar fasciitis. *Foot Ankle* 1986;7:155.

Lehman RC, et al. Fractures of the base of the fifth metatarsal distal to the tuberosity: a review. *Foot Ankle* 1987;7:245.

Lutter LD. Surgical decisions in athletes' subcalcaneal pain. *Am J Sports Med* 1986; 14:481.

Puddu G, Ippolito E, Postacchini F. A classification of Achilles tendon disease. *Am J Sports Med* 1976;4:145–150.

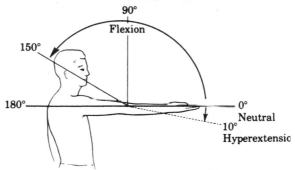

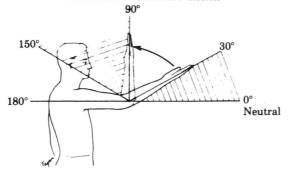

FIG. A-1. Elbow.

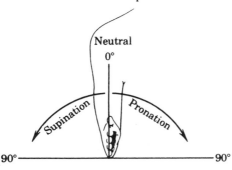

FIG. A-2. Forearm.

Flexion and extension

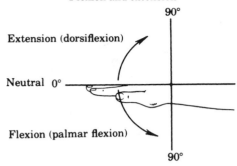

Radial and ulnar deviation

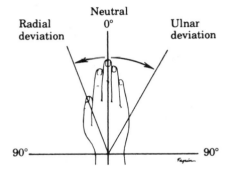

FIG. A-3. Wrist.

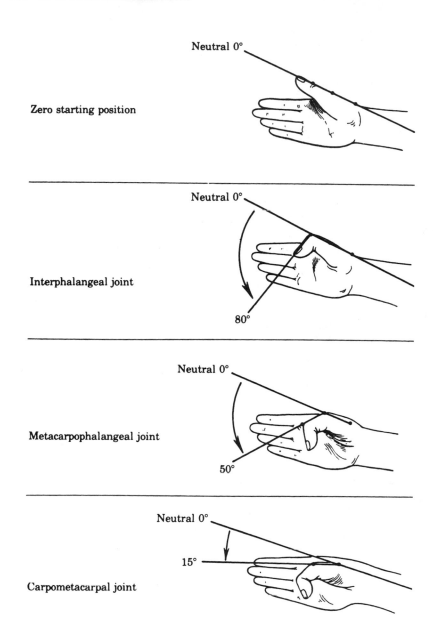

Neutral 0°

Zero starting position

Neutral 0°

Interphalangeal joint

80°

Neutral 0°

Metacarpophalangeal joint

50°

Neutral 0°

15°

Carpometacarpal joint

FIG. A-4. Thumb (flexion).

Measurement of limitation of opposition

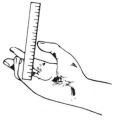

By distance between thumbnail and top of little finger

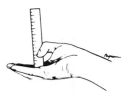

By distance between thumb and base of little finger

(Advice: Use fifth finger when present.)

FIG. A-5. Thumb (opposition).

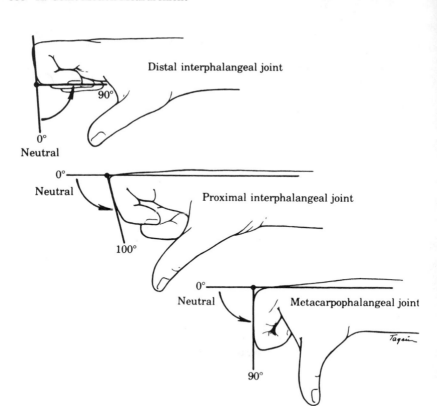

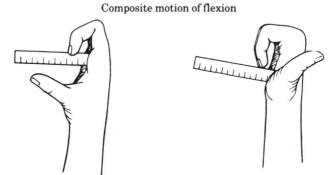

Fingertip to distal palmar crease   Fingertip to proximal palmar crease

FIG. A-6. Fingers (flexion).

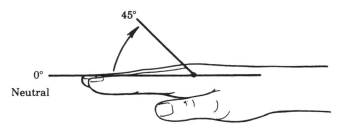

Extension—metacarpophalangeal joint

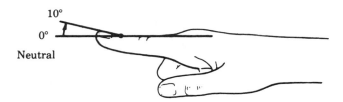

Hyperextension—distal interphalangeal joint

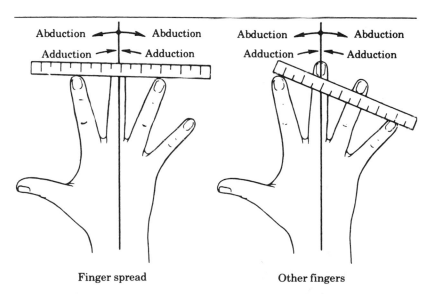

FIG. A-7. Fingers (extension, abduction, and adduction).

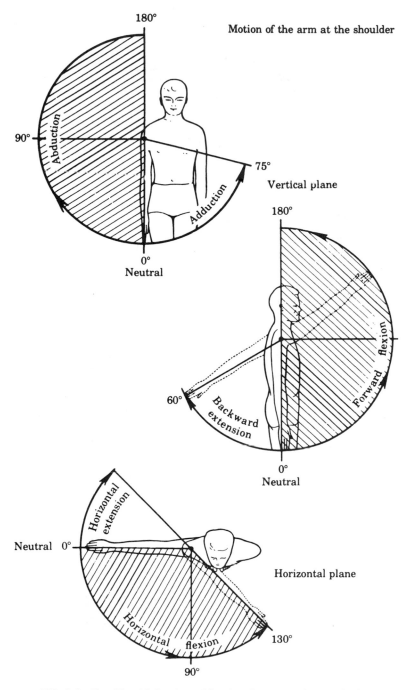

FIG. A-8. Shoulder (abduction, adduction, flexion, and extension).

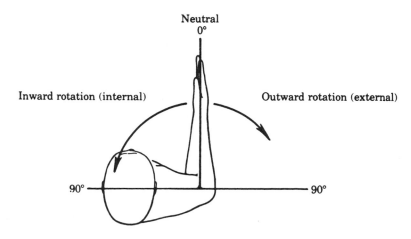

Rotation with arm at side

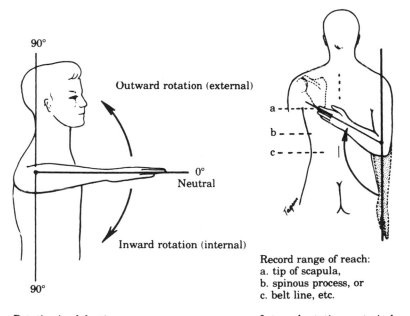

Rotation in abduction

Record range of reach:
a. tip of scapula,
b. spinous process, or
c. belt line, etc.

Internal rotation posteriorly

FIG. A-9. Shoulder (rotation).

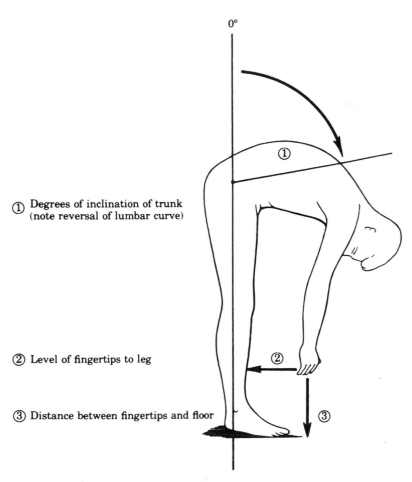

0°

① Degrees of inclination of trunk
(note reversal of lumbar curve)

② Level of fingertips to leg

③ Distance between fingertips and floor

FIG. A-10. Methods of measuring spinal flexion.

④ The steel tape measuring method

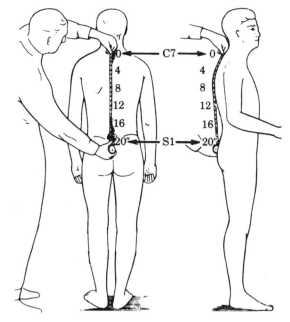

The patient standing erect

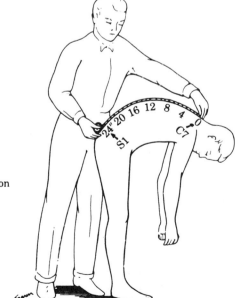

Note the 4″ in motion
(20″ to 24″)

The patient bending forward

FIG. A-10. *Continued*

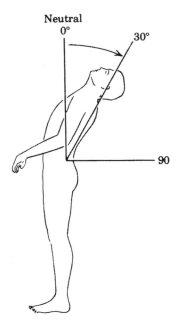

FIG. A-11. Thoracic and lumbar spine (extension).

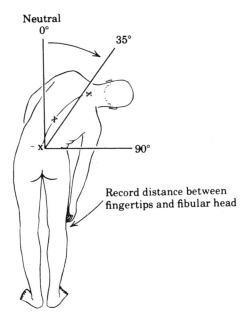

FIG. A-12. Thoracic and lumbar spine (lateral bending).

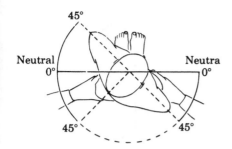

FIG. A-13. Spine (rotation).

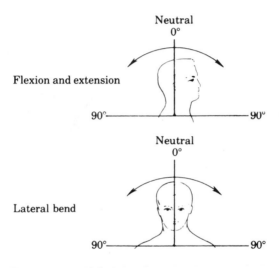

Flexion and extension

Lateral bend

Rotation

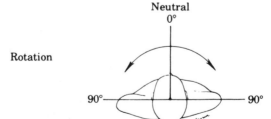

FIG. A-14. Cervical spine.

Zero starting position

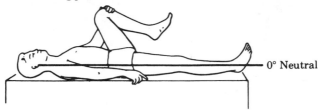

Flexion

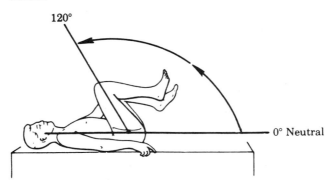

Limited motion in flexion

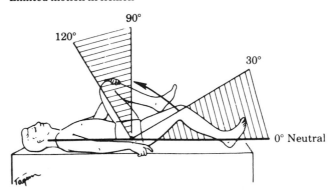

FIG. A-15. Hip (flexion). Always keep opposite hip flexed to flatten lumbar spine.

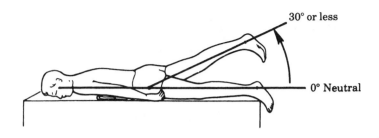

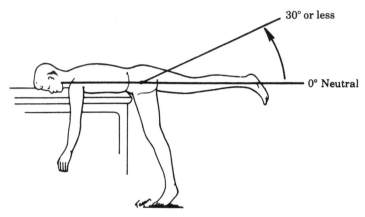

FIG. A-16. Hip (extension).

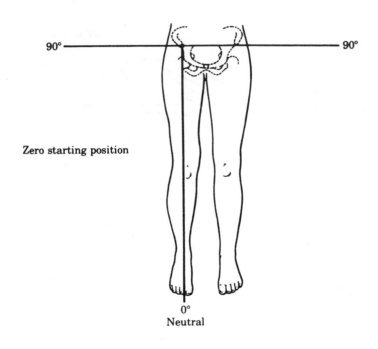

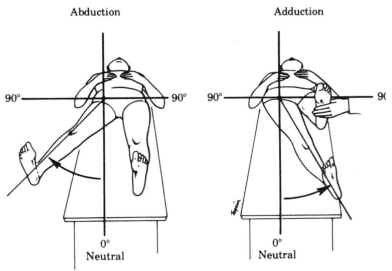

FIG. A-17. Hip (abduction and adduction).

Rotation in flexion

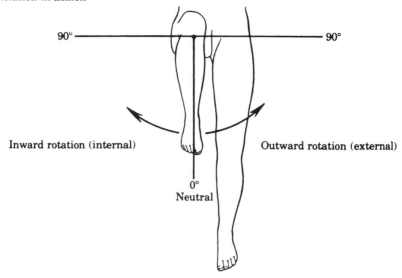

Rotation in extension

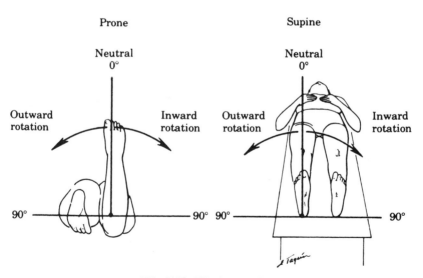

FIG. A-18. Hip (rotation).

Flexion and hyperextension

Hyperextension

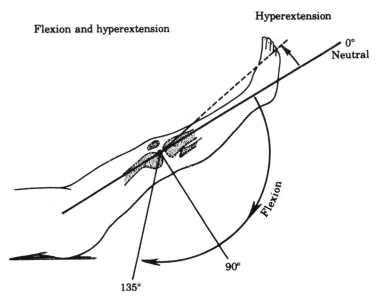

FIG. A-19. Knee.

Flexion and extension

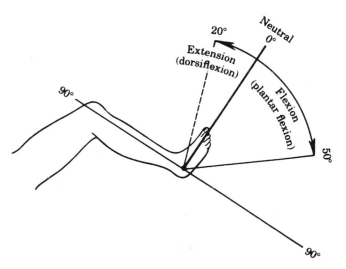

FIG. A-20. Ankle. Always note position of knee when recording ankle extension and flexion.

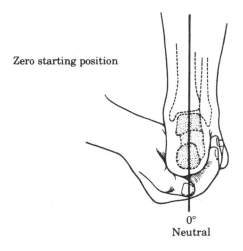

Zero starting position

0°
Neutral

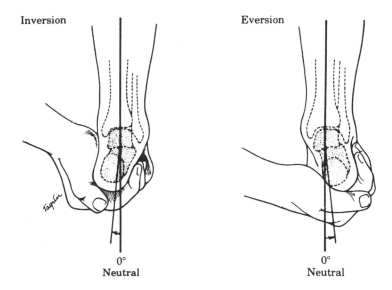

Inversion

0°
Neutral

Eversion

0°
Neutral

FIG. A-21. Hind part of the foot (passive motion).

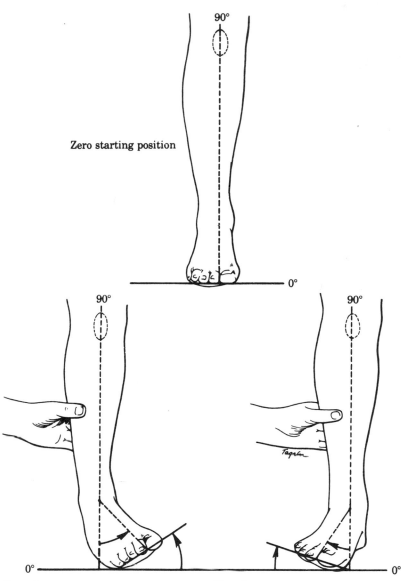

FIG. A-22. Forepart of the foot.

Table A-1. Normal range of joint motion in male subjects: Comparison of estimated ranges of motion (degrees)

Joint	Average ranges of joint motion[a]	This study[b,c] (N = 109)	This study < 19 years[b,c] (N = 53)	This study > 19 years[b,c] (N = 56)
SHOULDER				
Horizontal flexion	135	140.7 ± 5.9	140.8 ± 6.8	140.7 ± 4.9
Horizontal extension		45.4 ± 6.2	47.3 ± 6.1[d]	43.7 ± 5.8[d]
Neutral abduction	170	184.0 ± 7.0	185.4 ± 3.6	182.7 ± 9.0
Forward flexion	158	166.7 ± 4.7	168.4 ± 3.7[d]	165.0 ± 5.0[d]
Backward extension	53	62.3 ± 9.5	67.5 ± 8.0[d]	57.3 ± 8.1[d]
Inward rotation	70	68.8 ± 4.6	70.5 ± 4.5[d]	67.1 ± 4.1[d]
Outward rotation	90	103.7 ± 8.5	108.0 ± 7.2[d]	99.6 ± 7.6[d]
ELBOW				
Flexion	146	142.9 ± 5.6	145.4 ± 5.3[d]	140.5 ± 4.9[d]
Extension	0	0.6 ± 3.1	0.8 ± 3.5	0.3 ± 2.7
FOREARM				
Pronation	71	75.8 ± 5.1	76.7 ± 4.8	75.0 ± 5.3
Supination	84	82.1 ± 3.8	83.1 ± 3.4[d]	81.1 ± 4.0[d]
WRIST				
Flexion	73	76.4 ± 6.3	78.2 ± 5.5[d]	74.8 ± 6.6[d]
Extension	71	74.9 ± 6.4	75.8 ± 6.1[d]	74.0 ± 6.6[d]
Radial deviation	19	21.5 ± 4.0	21.8 ± 4.0	21.1 ± 4.0
Ulnar deviation	33	36.0 ± 3.8	36.7 ± 3.7	35.3 ± 3.8
HIP				
Beginning position flexion	113	2.1 ± 3.6	3.5 ± 4.3[d]	0.7 ± 2.1[d]
Flexion		122.3 ± 6.1	123.4 ± 5.6	121.3 ± 6.4
Extension	28	9.8 ± 6.8	7.4 ± 7.3[d]	12.1 ± 5.4[d]
Abduction	48	45.9 ± 9.3	51.7 ± 8.8[d]	40.5 ± 6.0[d]
Adduction	31	26.9 ± 4.1	28.3 ± 4.1[d]	25.6 ± 3.6[d]

(continued)

Table A-1. (*Continued*)

Joint	Average ranges of joint motion[a]	This study[b,c] (N = 109)	This study < 19 years[b,c] (N = 53)	This study > 19 years[b,c] (N = 56)
Inward rotation	45	47.3 ± 6.0	50.3 ± 6.1[d]	44.4 ± 4.3[d]
Outward rotation	45	47.2 ± 6.3	50.5 ± 6.1[d]	44.2 ± 4.8[d]
KNEE				
Beginning position flexion		1.6 ± 2.7	2.1 ± 3.2[d]	1.1 ± 2.0[d]
Flexion	134	142.5 ± 5.4	143.8 ± 5.1[d]	141.2 ± 5.3[d]
ANKLE				
Flexion (plantar)	48	56.2 ± 6.1	58.2 ± 6.1[d]	54.3 ± 5.9[d]
Extension (dorsiflexion)	18	12.6 ± 4.4	13.0 ± 4.7	12.2 ± 4.1
FOREPART OF THE FOOT				
Inversion	33	36.8 ± 4.5	37.5 ± 4.7[d]	36.2 ± 4.2[d]
Eversion	18	20.7 ± 5.0	22.3 ± 4.6[d]	19.2 ± 4.9[d]

[a] Averages of estimates from four sources used by The American Academy of Orthopaedic Surgeons.
[b] Mean ± one standard deviation (S.D.).
[c] Average age (± S.D.) = 22.4 ± 2.7, 9.2 ± 1.7, and 34.9 ± 3.4 years, respectively; average leg length (± S.D.) = 81.2 ± 5.6, 68.7 ± 7.1, and 93.1 ± 3.6 cm, respectively.
[d] Significant differences, $p < 0.01$.
From Boone DC, Azen SP. Normal range of motion of joints in male subjects. *J Bone Joint Surg* 1979;61A:756.

Appendix B. MUSCLE STRENGTH GRADING

Grade 5. Normal Normal power is present. The muscle can move the joint through a full range of motion against full resistance applied by the examiner or by any other test methods.

Grade 4. Good The muscle can move the joint through a full range of motion against gravity and against some resistance but cannot overcome normal resistance.

Grade 3. Fair The muscle can move the joint through a full range of motion only against gravity.

Grade 2. Poor The muscle can move the joint through a complete range only when gravity is eliminated.

Grade 1. Trace Contraction of the muscle is felt but no motion of the joint is produced.

Grade 0. Zero Complete paralysis is present with no visible or palpable contractions.

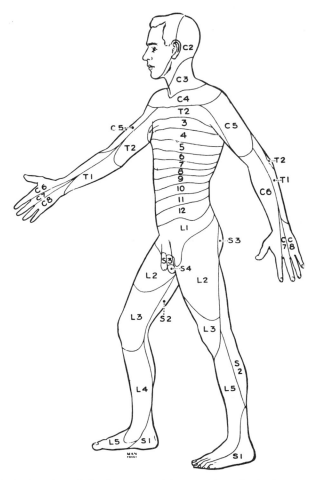

FIG. C-1. Anterior view of the dermatomal innervation of spinal segments. (From Haymaker W, Woodhall B. *Peripheral nerve injuries,* 2nd ed. Philadelphia: WB Saunders, 1953:26.)

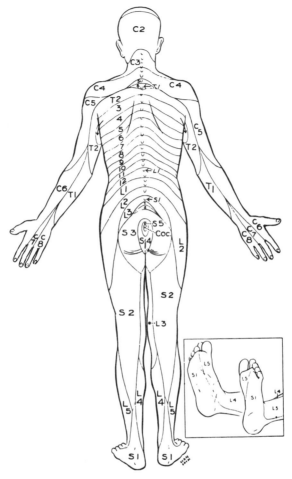

FIG. C-2. Posterior view of the dermatomal innervation of spinal segments. (From Haymaker W, Woodhall B. *Peripheral nerve injuries,* 2nd ed. Philadelphia: WB Saunders, 1953:27.)

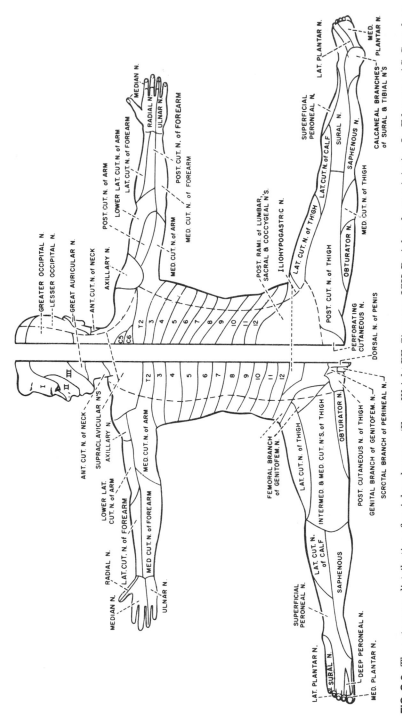

FIG. C-3. The cutaneous distribution of peripheral nerves. (From Wright PE, Simmons JCH. Peripheral nerve injuries. In: Edmonson AS, Crenshaw AH, eds. *Campbell's operative orthopaedics*, 6th ed. St. Louis: Mosby, 1980:1644.)

Appendix D. DESIRABLE WEIGHTS OF ADULTS

Table D-1. Height (ft) and weight (lb) tables[a]

Men					Women				
Height		Small frame[b]	Medium frame	Large Frame	Height		Small Frame	Medium frame	Large frame
Feet	Inches				Feet	Inches			
5	2	128–134	131–141	138–150	4	10	102–111	109–121	118–131
5	3	130–136	133–143	140–153	4	11	103–113	111–123	120–134
5	4	132–138	135–145	142–156	5	0	104–115	113–126	122–137
5	5	134–140	137–148	144–160	5	1	106–118	115–129	125–140
5	6	136–142	139–151	146–164	5	2	108–121	118–132	128–143
5	7	138–145	142–154	149–168	5	3	111–124	121–135	131–147
5	8	140–148	145–157	152–172	5	4	114–127	124–138	134–151
5	9	142–151	148–160	155–176	5	5	117–130	127–141	137–155
5	10	144–154	151–163	158–180	5	6	120–133	130–144	140–159
5	11	146–157	154–166	161–184	5	7	123–136	133–147	143–163
6	0	149–160	157–170	164–188	5	8	126–139	136–150	146–167
6	1	152–164	160–174	168–192	5	9	129–142	139–153	149–170
6	2	155–168	164–178	172–197	5	10	132–145	142–156	152–173
6	3	158–172	167–182	176–202	5	11	135–148	145–159	155–176
6	4	162–176	171–187	181–207	6	0	138–151	148–162	158–179

Table D-1. (*Continued*) Elbow measurements for medium frame

Men		Women	
Height in 1" heels	Elbow breadth	Height in 1" heels	Elbow breadth
5'2" – 5'3"	2 1/2" – 2 7/8"	4'10" – 4'11"	2 1/4" – 2 1/2"
5'4" – 5'7"	2 5/8" – 2 7/8"	5'0" – 5'3"	2 1/4" – 2 1/2"
5'8" – 5'11"	2 3/4" – 3"	5'4" – 5'7"	2 3/8" – 2 5/8"
6'0" – 6'3"	2 3/4" – 3 1/8"	5'8" – 5'11"	2 3/8" – 2 5/8"
6'4"	2 7/8" – 3 1/4"	6'0"	2 1/2" – 2 3/4"

[a] Weights at ages 25–29 years based on lowest mortality rate. Weight in lb according to frame (in indoor clothing weighing 5 lb for men and 3 lb for women; shoes with 1 inch heels).

[b] To approximate frame size: Bend forearm upward at a 90-degree angle. Keep fingers straight and turn the inside of the wrist toward body. Place thumb and index finger of other hand on the two prominent bones on either side of the elbow. Measure space between fingers on a ruler. (A physician uses a caliper.) Compare with elbow measurements for *medium-framed* men and women. Measurements lower than those listed indicate small frame. Higher measurements indicate large frame. From Metlife Height and Weight Tables. Reprinted courtesy of Metropolitan Life Insurance.

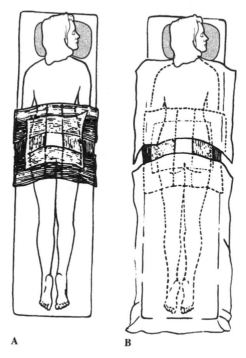

A   B

FIG. E-1. A back drape. **A:** Four towels are used to square off the operative site. A plastic adherent sheet is then applied to the skin and towels. **B:** One sheet is placed over the superior portion of the body. A lap or split sheet is used last. An easier alternative is to use a commercially available impervious sheet after toweling off the operative area.

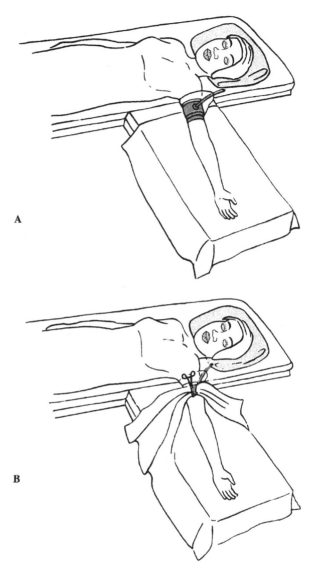

A

B

FIG. E-2. An extremity drape. **A:** Place a small waterproof sheet under the extremity. If a cloth or nonwaterproof sheet is used, place a plastic or waterproof sheet over the first sheet. **B:** A second small sheet is placed under the extremity with the proximal edge brought around the extremity and clipped just distal to the tourniquet. **C:** If the skin has been prepared with a germicidal antiseptic, two layers of tubular stockinet are rolled over the extremity up to the tourniquet, but any unprepared skin must also be wrapped with sterile bias-cut stockinet. The third small sheet is placed proximal to the extremity and is clipped beneath the extremity just distal to the tourniquet. **D:** A lap or split sheet is applied last. Commercial extremity sheets with a tight waterproof rubberized cuff to seal off the extremity are now available.

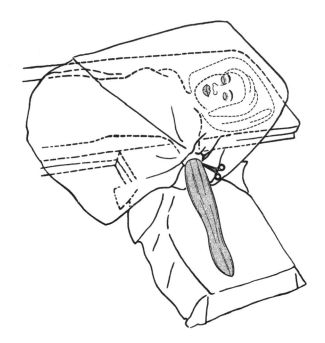

C

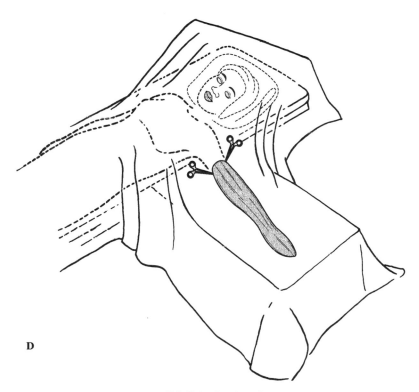

D

FIG. E-2. *Continued*

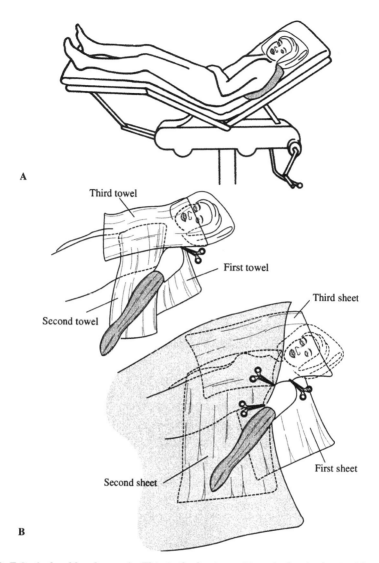

FIG. E-3. A shoulder drape. **A:** This is the basic position. A plastic sheet with an adherent edge may be placed just inferior to the hairline. A sandbag is placed under the appropriate shoulder. A neurologic headrest may be used. If necessary, the surgical table can be adjusted to make the upper body more upright. **B:** The arm is squared off with towels that are clipped to each other. A plastic split sheet with an adherent edge may be placed over the towels. Two layers of tubular stockinet are rolled up the arm. Three or four small sheets are placed over the towel edges and are clipped, or a split sheet may be used. The head and neck need to be properly sealed off. One large sheet is placed over the inferior portion of the body. The stockinet can be kept secure by overwrapping with a sterile 4-inch elastic compression (Ace) wrap.

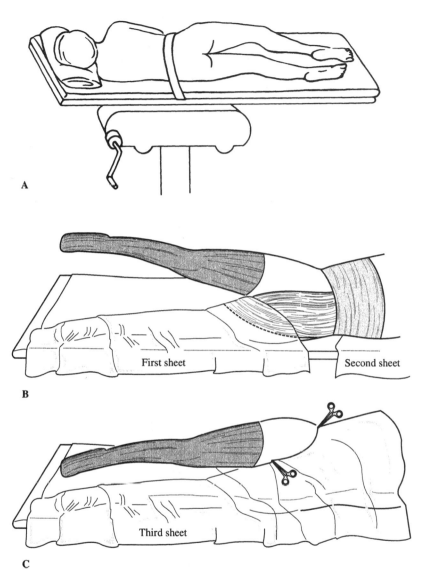

FIG. E-4. A lateral hip drape. **A:** The patient is carefully positioned lateral on the table (perpendicular to the table). **B:** Three towels are used to drape the hip and are clipped together. The anterior and posterior towels must cover the pubic area. The first sheet is placed between the legs, and two layers of stockinet are rolled up the leg, which has been prepared first with a germicidal antiseptic, and overwrapped with a 6-inch elastic compression (Ace) wrap. A split sheet with an adhesive edge is applied next, sealing off the perineum snugly, but allowing for proper posterior exposure. **C:** An adhesive plastic sheet is placed over the exposed skin. The completed draping system must have two layers of sterile sheets superior, inferior, and around the hip.

I. Electromyography

A. Usage. An electromyelogram (EMG) assists in the differential diagnosis of diseases affecting the lower motor neuron and its motor unit. The muscle action potentials are picked up by three electrodes—a recording or positive electrode, an indifferent electrode, which subtracts out extraneous electrical disturbances, and a ground. The electrical activity is displayed on an oscilloscope, as shown in Fig. F-1, and is played through a loudspeaker. It takes 7–21 days for denervation to occur, and studies performed during the first week following injury or onset of symptoms are usually unrevealing.

B. Findings

1. **When denervated, a muscle at rest has fibrillation potentials and positive "sharp waves."** Both potentials are shown in Fig. F-2. The fibrillation potentials have a voltage of 10–300 μV, a duration of 1–5 msec, and a frequency of 1–30/second. They sound like raindrops falling on a tin roof. The positive sharp waves have a great variability of voltage, a duration exceeding 10 msec, and a frequency of 2–100/second. The sound is that of a dull, loud thumping.

2. **In partially denervated muscles under voluntary contraction, a polyphasic unit** (highly complex motor unit voltages) often develops. It has a voltage of 50–500 μV, a duration of 5–25 msec, and usually six or more spikes (Fig. F-3).

3. The **nascent** (just born) **motor unit activity** (Fig. F-4) **is the early evidence of nerve regeneration.**

4. **Myotonia dystrophica and myotonia congenita produce high-frequency discharges** that sound like a dive bomber in the loudspeaker. They are precipitated by needle insertion, percussion, or voluntary contraction (Fig. F-5). **Pseudomyotonic potentials** have no waxing or waning of the sound and are found in **polymyositis, alcoholic neuropathy,** and so on.

5. **In primary muscle disease,** voluntary contraction produces small polyphasic units of short duration (Fig. F-6).

6. A **complete nerve lesion** has **no action potentials;** a **partial lesion** has at least **a few action potentials with voluntary contraction.**

7. The localization of a nerve lesion is made by the application of a thorough knowledge of neuromuscular anatomy. A **summary of EMG findings and their interpretation is found in Table F-1.**

II. Nerve conduction studies

are done by stimulating a nerve trunk at two points with an electrical pulse strong enough to activate all of the motor axons. The pulse required is 0.1–0.5 msec in duration with 60–300 V. The sweep of the oscilloscope is calibrated so the time between each shock and the beginning of each evoked muscle action potential (picked up by another set of electrodes) can be measured. By dividing the distance between the two stimulating points by the difference in time to activate the muscle, the motor conduction velocity is obtained:

$$\text{Conduction velocity} = \text{distance}/\text{latency}_2 - \text{latency}_1$$

A. Motor

1. In general, **motor conduction velocities in excess of 45 m/second in the arms and in excess of 40 m/second in the legs are considered normal.** Conduction velocity of a nerve increases 2.4 m/second/1°C elevation in temperature. This increase must be considered when studying a limb with impaired vascularity. Also, conduction velocities are faster in the proximal segments of a nerve than in the distal segments. This difference is a function of temperature and of the diameter of the

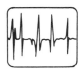

FIG. F-1. Normal innervated muscle contracted. Action potential 5–10 msec, 500–2000 µV.

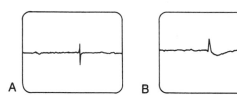

A   B

FIG. F-2. Denervation. **A:** Fibrillation potential. **B:** Positive sharp wave.

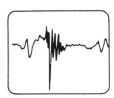

FIG. F-3. Complex polyphasic motor unit.

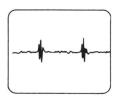

FIG. F-4. Nascent motor unit activity.

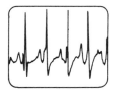

FIG. F-5. Myotonia.

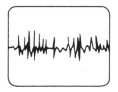

FIG. F-6. Myopathic activity.

Table F-1. Presumptive diagnoses from EMG findings

EMG Findings	Presumptive diagnoses
Fibrillation potentials with the muscle at rest	Muscle at least partially denervated
Positive sharp waves	Muscle at least partially denervated
Polyphasic motor unit voltages	Chronic denervation
Nascent motor units	Nerve regeneration
Myotonic voltage discharges	Myotonia dystrophica or myotonia congenita
Pseudomyotonic discharges	Polymyositis, alcoholic neuropathy, etc.
Small polyphasic units	Primary muscle disease
No action potential	A complete nerve lesion

nerve. The newborn has conduction velocities of one half the adult value, with the adult range reached by age 3 years. Conduction velocity gradually decreases with aging, slowing by 6% between the third and seventh decades.

    2. Distal motor latencies are normally lower than 5 msec except in the posterior tibial and peroneal nerves where latency should be less than 7 msec.

  B. Sensory nerve conduction studies are often the most sensitive to detect nerve abnormalities. They are done by stimulating the sensory fibers of a digit and recording the sensory nerve's electrical activity with electrodes placed more proximally on the extremity so as to measure both the conduction velocity and latency. An absent response is a positive finding and indicates significant abnormality. The sensory nerve conduction studies require more expertise by the examiner.

    1. Sensory nerve conduction velocities in the upper extremities are normally greater than 35 m/second in the wrist to elbow segment.

    2. The upper limit for normal distal sensory latencies is 4 msec.

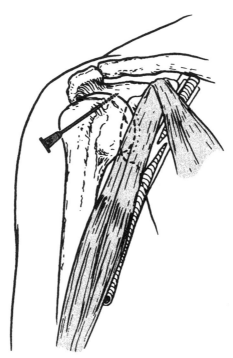

FIG. G-1. Aspiration of the shoulder. The shoulder may be aspirated anteriorly, posteriorly, or laterally. Because the fluctuant area is usually palpable anteriorly and the bony landmarks identified easily, the needle is inserted here most often. The aspiration site is located one half the distance between the coracoid process and the anterolateral edge of the acromion. The needle is directed posteriorly through the joint capsule, and the joint is aspirated. (After Warner WC Jr. Infectious arthritis. In: Crenshaw AH, ed. *Campbell's operative orthopaedics,* 8th ed, vol. 1. St. Louis: Mosby–Year Book, 1992.)

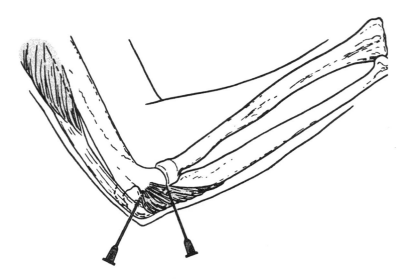

FIG. G-2. Aspiration of the elbow. The elbow is flexed and the needle is inserted on the posterior aspect just lateral to the olecranon. The needle is advanced through the skin and joint capsule and the joint is aspirated. (After Warner WC Jr. Infectious arthritis. In: Crenshaw AH, ed. *Campbell's operative orthopaedics,* 8th ed, vol. 1. St. Louis: Mosby–Year Book, 1992.)

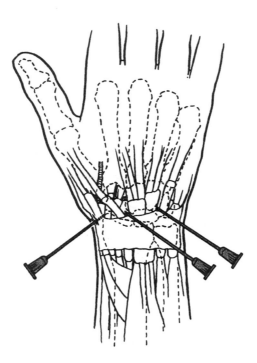

FIG. G-3. Aspiration of the wrist. Aspiration is performed on the dorsal side of the wrist. Several aspiration sites on the dorsum of the wrist may be used. The most common site of aspiration is between the first and second extensor compartments at the radiocarpal level, immediately adjacent to the point where the extensor pollicis longus crosses the extensor carpi radialis longus. Other aspiration sites are between the third and fourth or the fourth and fifth extensor compartments. (After Warner WC Jr. Infectious arthritis. In: Crenshaw AH, ed. *Campbell's operative orthopaedics,* 8th ed, vol. 1. St. Louis: Mosby–Year Book, 1992.)

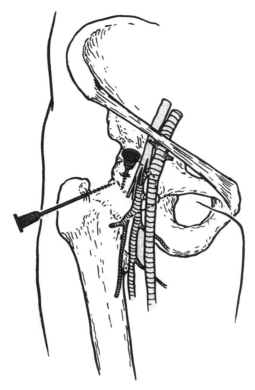

FIG. G-4. Aspiration of the hip, lateral and anterior approaches. A medial approach can also be used to aspirate the hip joint. The use of image intensification makes needle placement more certain. At times, pus cannot be aspirated, although later it is proved to be present by open drainage. In these circumstances, the hip should be explored if local and systemic symptoms cannot be otherwise controlled. (After Warner WC Jr. Infectious arthritis. In: Crenshaw AH, ed. *Campbell's operative orthopaedics,* 8th ed, vol. 1. St. Louis: Mosby–Year Book, 1992.)

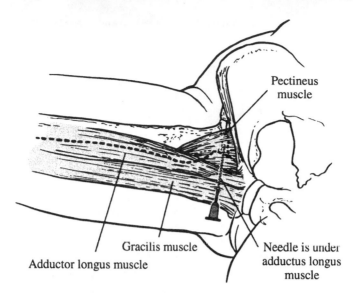

FIG. G-5. Aspiration of the hip, medial approach. (After Warner WC Jr. Infectious arthritis. In: Crenshaw AH, ed. *Campbell's operative orthopaedics,* 8th ed, vol. 1. St. Louis: Mosby–Year Book, 1992.)

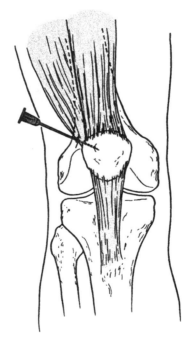

FIG. G-6. Aspiration of the knee, anteroposterior view. The knee is a superficial joint, and it may be easily aspirated. The needle is inserted on the lateral side at the level of the superior pole of the patella. It is then advanced through the lateral retinaculum and into the joint. (After Warner WC Jr. Infectious arthritis. In: Crenshaw AH, ed. *Campbell's operative orthopaedics,* 8th ed, vol. 1. St. Louis: Mosby–Year Book, 1992.)

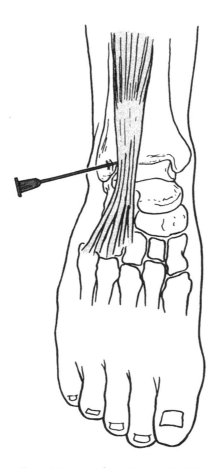

FIG. G-7. Aspiration of the ankle, anterolateral view. Swelling about the ankle often makes fluctuation difficult to locate. To avoid injuring important structures, the needle is inserted 2.5 cm proximal and 1.3 cm medial to the tip of the lateral malleolus. This is just lateral to the peroneus tertius tendon. (After Warner WC Jr. Infectious arthritis. In: Crenshaw AH, ed. *Campbell's operative orthopaedics,* 8th ed, vol. 1. St. Louis: Mosby–Year Book, 1992.)

Table G-1. Approaches for injection and aspiration

Joint	Common approach	Other approaches
Ankle	Anterolateral—1 inch proximal and ½ inch medial to tip of lateral malleolus	
Knee	Lateral—into the suprapatellar pouch at the level of the superior patellar pole	
Hip	Anterior—insert needle perpendicular to the skin at a point 1 inch inferior and 1 inch lateral from the center of a line drawn from the anterior superior iliac spine to the symphysis pubis	Lateral—insert needle just anterior and inferior to the greater trochanter; then, while angling the tip 45 degrees superiorly, walk the needle tip gently over the bone and into the joint
Shoulder	Anterior—insert needle ½ inch inferior and ½ inch lateral to the coracoid process	
Elbow	Lateral—hold the elbow in flexion and insert needle just proximal to the radial head; or, if an effusion is present, insert the needle just anterior to the olecranon where the effusion is usually most easily palpated	
Wrist	Dorsal—insert needle just medial to the anatomic snuffbox	
Fingers	Dorsolateral corner of joint	

From Anderson LD. Infections. In: Edmonson AC, Crenshaw AH, eds. *Campbell's operative orthopaedics*, 6th ed. St Louis; Mosby, 1980:1031–1099, with permission.

SUBJECT INDEX

Pages followed by *f* indicate figures; pages followed by *t* indicate tables.

A

Abdominal injuries, 5, 6*f*
Acetabulum
  dysplasia of, 65–67
  fractures of, 271–272, 273
    examination in, 267, 268*f*, 271
    heterotopic ossification in, 27, 272
    with posterior hip dislocation,
      269–270
    sciatic nerve injuries in, 20, 270
    without posterior hip dislocation,
      271–272
Acetaminophen, 108*t*
Achilles tendon
  in calcaneus fractures, 334
  in metatarsalgia, 347
  rupture of, 331
  tendinitis of, 345
  in tibialis posterior rupture, 348, 350
Acromioclavicular joint, 185, 187–191
  anatomy of, 187–188, 188*f*
  arthritis of, 200
  classification of injuries, 188, 189*f*
  in osteolysis of clavicle, 200
Acromion morphology, 197, 198*f*
Adam's forward bending test in
  scoliosis, 73
Adhesive capsulitis, 199–200
Adhesive strapping in athletic injuries,
  100–101
Adolescents. *See* Children
AIDS, 32, 47
Air splints, 81, 84
Airway management in initial resuscitation, 1
Allopurinol in gout, 53
Ampicillin, 34*t*
Amputation, traumatic, 14
  of hand, 14, 236, 237*f*, 238
Analgesics, 107, 108*t*, 109*t*
Anesthesia, 132
  malignant hyperthermia in, 137–139
  in shoulder dislocation, 193
  in skeletal traction, 116
Ankle, 325–332
  Achilles tendon injuries of, 331, 345
  aspiration and injection of, 395*f*,
    396*t*
  emergency splinting of, 81, 83*f*, 84
  fractures and fracture-dislocations
    of, 325–329, 331–332
    classification of, 325, 326*f*, 327*f*
    stress, 350

  range of motion measurements,
    370*f*, 374*t*
  sprains of, 329–331, 332
  in tibialis posterior rupture, 348
Ankylosing spondylitis, 40, 48, 48*t*, 54
Anterior cord syndrome, 168
Antibiotic therapy, 32–33, 34*t*–36*t*, 38
  in avascular necrosis, 30
  in femoral fractures, 283
  in gas gangrene, 37
  in open fracture and soft tissue
    wounds, 8–9
  in orthopaedic unit, 107
  in osteomyelitis, 30, 31, 32, 36*t*
    in children, 71
  preoperative, 131–132, 133*t*
  in puncture wounds of foot, 32, 36*t*
  selection of drugs in, 33, 36*t*
  in septic arthritis, 36*t*, 49*t*, 52
    in children, 72–73
Antiinflammatory drugs
  in knee injuries, 300
  in rheumatoid arthritis, 48–49,
    54–55
AO classification of ankle fractures, 325
Apert's syndrome, 244
Apophysis, tibial
  avulsion injury of, 307
  overgrowth of, 310–311
Apprehension sign in knee injuries, 298
Arthritis, 40–55
  of acromioclavicular joint, 200
  degenerative. *See* Osteoarthritis
  differential diagnosis in, 31, 40–48
  of elbow, 251–253
  of glenohumeral joint, 199
  gonorrheal, 43*t*–44*t*
  of hand and wrist, 236, 250, 251–253
  of hip, after posterior dislocation,
    269, 270
  of metatarsophalangeal joint,
    351–352
  psoriatic, 43*t*, 47, 53–54
  rheumatoid. *See* Rheumatoid
    arthritis
  septic. *See* Septic arthritis
  treatment in, 48–55
Arthrodesis
  in calcaneus fractures, 336
  in osteoarthritis, 52
  in rheumatoid arthritis, 51
Arthroplasty, 51, 52
  in femoral neck fracture, 278

Arthroscopy in joint infections, 37
Aspiration of joints, 33, 37, 390–396
   of ankle, 395f, 396t
   of elbow, 391f, 396t
   of fingers, 396t
   of hip, 33, 37, 393f, 394f, 396t
   of knee, 300, 394f, 396t
   in septic arthritis, 52
   of shoulder, 390f, 396t
   of wrist, 392f, 396t
Aspirin, 108t
   in rheumatoid arthritis, 48, 54–55
   in thromboembolism prevention, 110
Atrophy, Sudeck's, 26
Avascular necrosis, 30
   of femur. See Femur, avascular
      necrosis of
   of talus, 338
   in upper extremity, 253f, 253–254
Axonotmesis, 13
Azathioprine in rheumatoid arthritis,
   50

B

Back. See also Spine
   draping of, 382f
   pain in, 178–182
      causes of, 178, 179t
      in disk degeneration, 178–181
      in spondylolisthesis, 181–182
      palpation of, 5
      range of motion measurements,
         362f–365f
Bacterial infections
   antibiotic therapy in. See Antibiotic
      therapy
   osteomyelitis in, 31, 69–72
   septic arthritis in, 31, 40, 45, 46t
      in children, 72–73
   in surgery, prevention of, 131–132,
      133t, 135–137
Bandages, 101
   in athletic injuries, 100
   in plaster casts, application of,
      88–89
   in upper extremity splinting, 78, 80f
Bankart lesion, 192
   reverse, 194
Barlow test in hip dysplasia, 65–66
Barton's fracture of radius, 221f, 223
Baseball fracture of hand, 234
Baumann's angle in humerus fractures, 207
Bennett's fracture, 232
Betamethasone in pseudogout, 53
Biceps brachii
   distal, rupture of, 214, 251

   anatomy in rotator cuff, 192, 197
   rupture of, 195
   tendinitis of, 199
Birth injuries
   of brachial plexus, 244–245
   clavicle fracture in, 245
Bite wounds of hand, 237
Bleeding. See Hemorrhage
Blount's disease, 60
Boähler bow in skeletal traction, 116,
   117f
Body casts and jackets, 90–92, 91f, 92f
   in halo traction, 92, 93f, 121
Bone grafts in fractures, 8, 154–155,
   163
Boutonniere deformity, 234
Bowed legs, 60–61
Bowen wire tightener, 152, 153f
Box sutures, 156, 156f
Braces
   in hip dysplasia, 66
   in kyphosis, 74, 184
   lace-up canvas ankle supports, 81
   in Legg-Calve-Perthes disease, 67
   in osteoarthritis, 52
   in scoliosis, 74, 183
   short leg walkers, 81
   in thoracolumbar spine fractures,
      171, 172
Brachial plexus injuries, 13, 194
   birth-related, 244–245
Breathing, initial assessment and
      management of, 1
Brown-Séquard syndrome, 168
Buck's extension skin traction, 125,
   125f
Bunions, 63–64
Bursitis, 46t
   pes anserinus, 312
   of shoulder, 197–198, 199
      scapulothoracic, 200–201
Burst fracture of thoracolumbar spine,
   169, 171f, 172, 172f, 173
Buttress plates, 145
   in tibia fractures, 314, 316, 316f

C

Calcaneonavicular coalition, flat feet
      in, 62, 63
Calcaneus
   coalition with other tarsal bones, flat
      feet in, 62, 63
   fat pad trauma of, 346
   fractures of, 334–337, 342
      classification of, 334, 335f
      open reduction and internal
         fixation in, 336, 336f
      stress, 351

wire or pin insertion for skeletal
 traction, 119
Calcific bursitis/tendinitis, 46*t*
 of shoulder, 199
Cancellous bone screws, 144
Capsulitis
 of metatarsophalangeal joint, 347
 of shoulder, adhesive, 199–200
Carpal fractures and dislocations, 7,
 227–230, 238
Carpal tunnel syndrome, 19–20, 246*f*,
 246–247
 in Colles' fracture, 222
Carpometacarpal joint
 arthritis in thumb, 251, 252*f*
 dislocation of, 230
Casts, 85–100
 application of, 87–89
 critical setting period in, 85, 89
 equipment in, 86–87
 bivalve or split, 88, 99–100
 body casts and jackets, 90–92, 91*f*,
  92*f*
 in halo traction, 92, 93*f*, 121
 in bone and joint infections, 33
 Dehne and Sarmiento technique,
  97–98, 318–319
 in halo traction, 92, 93*f*, 121
 indications for, 87
 knee cast-brace, 98–99, 317
 knee cylinder casts, 96
 long-leg, 96–97, 317
 materials used in, 85–86
 removal of, 99*f*, 99–100
 equipment used in, 86, 99
 joint mobilization after, 101–102
 short-leg, 92–94, 96
 spica, 92–96
 hip, 94, 95*f*, 288
 shoulder, 94–96, 123–125
 three-point fixation in, 87, 87*f*, 89
 weight-bearing in, 96, 97–98
Catheterization
 urinary, in orthopaedic unit, 110–111
 venous, in shock, 2*t*, 2–3
Cefazolin, 9, 34*t*, 133*t*
Ceftazidime, 35*t*
Ceftriaxone, 35*t*
Cefuroxime, 35*t*
Cellulitis, 31
Central cord syndrome, 168
Cephalosporins, 8–9, 34*t*, 35*t*
 preoperative, 132, 133*t*
Cerclage techniques, 152–153, 153*f*
Cerebral palsy, 75–76, 182, 245–246
Cervical spine
 injuries of, 161–169
  body jacket and casts in, 92, 93*f*,
   121

diagnosis of, 5, 6, 7
 emergency splinting in, 78
 hangman's fracture in, 164*f*,
  164–165
 with head trauma, 5, 165
 hyperextension whiplash, 168–169
 Jefferson fracture in, 161, 162*f*
 in lower cervical region, 165–168,
  166*f*
 odontoid process fracture in, 6,
  161–164
 traction in. *See* Traction, cervical
  spine
 range of motion measurements, 365*f*
Chance fracture of thoracolumbar
 spine, 170, 174*f*
Charnley's traction unit, 125–126, 127,
 128*f*, 129*f*
Children, 16–17, 57–76
 antibiotic therapy in, 32, 34*t*–36*t*
  in osteomyelitis, 71
  in septic arthritis, 72–73
 brachial plexus injuries in, 244–245
 calcaneus fractures in, 337
 cerebral palsy in, 75–76, 245–246
 clavicle fractures in, 185
 femoral fractures in, 16, 287–288
  distal physeal, 307
  intertrochanteric and subtrochanteric, 286
  in neck, 279–280
 foot conditions in, 61–64
 genu varum and valgum in, 60–61
 hip disorders in, 65–69, 272
 humerus fractures in, 207–211
  epiphyseal, 205
 infectious and inflammatory conditions in, 30, 69–73
 intervertebral diskitis in, 31
 intoeing in, 58–60, 59*f*
 knee disorders in, 64–65, 307–308
 kyphosis in, 74, 184
 Legg-Calve-Perthes disease in, 67
 limp in, 57–58, 67
 lordosis in, 74–75
 lower extremity alignment in, 58–61
 metaphyseal fractures in, 8, 17
 Minerva body jacket for, 90–92, 92*f*
 myositis ossificans in, 26
 osteomyelitis in, 31, 69–72
 radial agenesis in, 243–244
 radius and ulna fractures in,
  217–218, 219, 223–224
 rheumatoid arthritis in, 54, 55
 scoliosis in, 73–74, 182–183
 septic arthritis in, 31, 72–73
 spina bifida in, 76
 sternoclavicular joint injuries in,
  187

Children, (*contd.*)
  synovitis in, transient, 73
  tibia fractures in, 17, 307, 319
Chisels, 141, 141*f*
Chloral hydrate, 108
Chlorhexidine gluconate, 136
Chloroquine in rheumatoid arthritis, 50
Chondroitin sulfate in osteoarthritis, 52
Chondrolysis in slipped capital
      femoral epiphysis, 69
Chondromalacia patellae, 64, 311
Chondrometaphyseal dysplasia, 60
Chondrosarcoma of upper extremity,
      255
Christmas disease, 16
Circulation, initial assessment and
      management of, 1–2
Clavicle
  in acromioclavicular joint injuries,
      185, 187–190
  fractures of, 185–186
    birth-related, 245
    splints in, 78, 79*f*, 185–186
  osteolysis of, 200
  in sternoclavicular joint injuries, 187
Claw toe deformities, 347
Clindamycin, 34*t*
Clostridial infections, gas gangrene in,
      37
Clotting factors, in hemophilia, 16
Club foot, 61–62
Club hand, 243
COBB radiography method in scoliosis,
      183
Coccyx, fractures of, 260*t*
Codeine, 109*t*
Colchicine in gout, 52–53
Collagen-vascular disease, 43*t*
Collateral ligament injuries of knee,
      296, 304
  examination in, 305
  instability in, 297, 305
  mechanism of injury in, 305
  in tibia fractures, 318
  treatment of, 306
Colles' fracture, 220–223
  examination in, 220, 221*f*
  reversed, 221*f*, 223
Compartmental syndromes, 20–26
  decompression in, 23–25
  in elbow dislocation, 216
  etiologies of, 21
  locations of, 21, 21*f*, 22*f*
  pain in, 21, 23, 24*t*
  physical examination in, 21–23, 24*t*
  in tibia fracture, 321
  tissue pressure measurements in,
      23, 25*f*, 26*f*
  in traction, 21, 23*f*

Compression fracture of thoracolum-
      bar spine, 169, 170*f*, 172
Congenital disorders
  patella dislocation in, 65
  radial agenesis in, 243–244
  spondylolisthesis in, 181
  syndactyly and polydactyly in, 244
  talipes equinovarus in, 61–62
Connective tissue disease, mixed, 43*t*
Consciousness, level of, 2, 2*t*, 4
Consultations in orthopaedic unit care,
      105
Cortical bone screws, 144
Corticosteroid therapy
  in cervical spine injuries, 167
  in lupus erythematosus, 54
  preoperative and postoperative, 132
  in pseudogout, 53
  in rheumatic fever, 54
  in rheumatoid arthritis, 50–51, 55
  in rotator cuff bursitis/tendinitis,
      197–198
Coxa vara, 60
  in femoral neck fractures, 279
Cricothyroidotomy in initial resuscita-
      tion, 1
Cruciate ligament injuries, 295–296, 304
  in children, 307
  examination in, 305
  instability in, 297, 305
  mechanism of injury in, 305
  in tibia fractures, 318
  treatment of, 306
Cryoprecipitate in hemophilia, 16
Crystal-induced arthritis, 44*t*, 45, 46*t*,
      52–53
Cubital tunnel syndrome, 247–248
Cuboid bone fracture, 338
Cuneiform bone fracture, 338
Cutting instruments
  for bones, 141*f*, 141–142
  for casts, 86, 99

D
Danis-Weber classification of ankle
      fractures, 325, 327*f*
Dantrolene in malignant hyperthermia,
      138
De Quervain's tenosynovitis, 237,
      250–251
Debridement of soft tissue wounds,
      9–10
Degenerative disorders
  of intervertebral disks, 178–181
  osteoarthritis in. *See* Osteoarthritis
  spondylolisthesis in, 181
Dehne and Sarmiento casting tech-
      nique, 97–98, 318–319

Deltoid ligament injuries, 325, 330
Dermatomes, 376f–377f
Dermatomyositis, 43t
Dextran in thromboembolism pre-
    vention, 110
Deyerle technique in femoral fractures,
    277
Diabetes mellitus, 132
Diaphyseal fractures, 8
    of femur, 286–288, 290
    of humerus, 205–207, 212
    of radius and ulna, 219
    of tibia, 318–321
Diphenhydramine, 108
2,3–Diphosphoglycerate levels, 4
Discoid meniscus, 65
Disks, intervertebral. See Interverte-
    bral disks
Dislocation
    of acromioclavicular joint, 188, 189f,
        190
    of carpal bones, 7, 227–230
    of carpometacarpal joint, 230
    of elbow, 211, 214–216, 224
    in foot, 340, 342
        subtalar and talar, 337–338, 342
    of glenohumeral joint, 192–195
    of hip, 266–270, 272
    of knee, 306, 312
        in children, 64, 65
        patellar. See Patella, dislocation of
    of spine, 161–174
    of sternoclavicular joint, 187
Documentation
    on initial assessment and manage-
        ment, 6
    on orthopaedic unit care, 105–106
Donati sutures, 158, 158f
Draping techniques, 132–134, 136,
    382f–386f
Drawer test
    anterior, in ankle injuries, 330
    posterior, in knee injuries, 305
Dressings in soft tissue wounds, 8, 9
Drilling technique for bone screws,
    142–144
Dunlop's traction, 123, 123f, 207
Durkin's compression test in carpal
    tunnel syndrome, 247
Dynamic compression plates, 145, 146f,
    147f, 148f
Dysplasia
    chondrometaphyseal, 60
    of hip, developmental, 65–67
Dystrophy, reflex sympathetic, 26

E
Elbow, 214–219
    arthritis of, 251–253

aspiration and injection of, 391f, 396t
    in biceps brachii rupture, distal, 214
    breadth measurements, 381t
    dislocation of, 211, 214–216, 224
        examination in, 214, 215f
    examination in nonacute conditions,
        242
    in humerus fractures, distal,
        207–211, 212
    in lateral epicondylitis, 248–250, 249f
    Monteggia's fracture-dislocation of,
        218–219
    plaster splint for, 90
    in radius fractures, 217–218, 224
    range of motion measurement, 354f,
        373t
    in ulna fractures, proximal, 216–217,
        224
    ulnar nerve compression at, 20,
        247–248
Elderly
    femoral fractures in, 275, 280, 284
    humerus fractures in, 207, 210
Electromyography, 387, 388f, 389t
Embolism, fat, in fractures, 19
Emergency care, 1–7
    primary survey in, 1–4
    secondary survey in, 4–7
    splinting in, 78–84
Enchondroma of hand, 255, 256f–257f
Epicondyles of humerus
    lateral
        epicondylitis of, 248–250, 249f
        fracture of, 210–211
    medial, fracture of, 211
Epiphyseal injuries, 17
    of femur, 69, 70f, 279, 280
    of humerus, 205, 210
    of radius, 217–218, 223–224
    in sternoclavicular dislocation, 187
Erb's palsy, 244
Etanercept in rheumatoid arthritis, 50
Everting sutures, 156, 157f
Exercise
    in cast removal, 101–102
    in orthopaedic unit, 111
Extension injuries of cervical spine,
    165, 168–169
Extensor pollicis longus rupture in
    Colles' fracture, 223
Extensor tendon injuries
    of hand, 223, 236
    of knee, 298, 307

F
Factors, clotting, in hemophilia, 16
Fasciitis
    necrotizing, 37–38
    plantar, 346

Fat embolism syndrome, 19
Fat pad trauma, calcaneal, 346
Femur
  anteversion of, 58–60
  avascular necrosis of
    in fracture of femoral neck, 278,
      279
    in Legg-Calve-Perthes disease, 67
    in posterior hip dislocation, 269,
      270
    in slipped capital epiphysis, 69
  dislocation of head, in developmen-
    tal dysplasia of hip, 65–67
  fractures of, 7, 275–290
    in children. See Children, femoral
      fractures in
    diaphyseal, 286–288, 290
    distal, 288–289, 290, 307
    fat embolism syndrome in, 19
    of greater trochanter, 284
    in head, 270–271, 273
    intertrochanteric, 280–283, 286,
      289
    knee cast-brace in, 98–99
    of lesser trochanter, 284
    in neck, 7, 275–280, 289
    physeal, 307
    Pipkin types of, 271
    stress, 10, 275–276
    subtrochanteric, 284–286, 290
    Thomas splint in, 81, 83f, 280,
      284, 286
    traction in, 117f, 125, 127–129
    treatment recommendations in,
      289–290
  in genu varum and valgum, 60
  slipped capital epiphysis, 69, 70f
  wire or pin insertion for skeletal
    traction, 118
Fiberglass casts, 85, 88, 89
Fibula
  fractures of, 10, 325, 328
  wire or pin insertion for skeletal
    traction, 119
Figure-of-8 splint in clavicle fracture,
  78, 79f, 185–186
Files, bone, 142
Fingers. See Hand
Finkelstein's test in de Quervain's
  tenosynovitis, 250
Flail chest, 1
Flatfoot, 62–63
  in tibialis posterior rupture,
    347–350
Flexion-distraction injuries of thora-
  columbar spine, 169–170, 173f
Flexor tendons of hand, 236
  tenosynovitis of, 236–237
Fluid management in shock, 21, 2 4

Flurazepam, 108
Foot, 334–343
  calcaneal fat pad trauma of, 346
  claw toe deformity of, 347
  dislocations in, 340, 342
    subtalar and talar, 337–338, 342
  emergency splinting of, 81
  fractures in, 334–343
    of calcaneus, 334–337, 342, 351
    metatarsal, 340–341, 342
    of navicular, cuneiform, and
      cuboid bones, 338
    stress, 347, 350–351
    of talus, 7, 338, 339f, 341, 350
    of toes, 341, 343
    treatment recommendations in,
      341–343
  in hallux rigidus, 351–352
  in hallux valgus, 63–64
  heel pain of, 345–347
  intoeing position in child, 58–60, 59f
  metatarsalgia of, 347
  in metatarsus adductus, 63
  in metatarsus primus varus, 63
  nerve entrapment syndromes in,
    346–347
  overuse conditions of, 345–352
  in pes planus, 62–63
  in tibialis posterior rupture,
    347–350
  plantar fasciitis of, 346
  puncture wound infections of, 32,
    36t
  range of motion measurements,
    370f–372f, 374t
  rheumatoid arthritis of, 51
  in talipes equinovarus, 61–62
  tarsometatarsal joint injuries of, 340,
    342, 351–352
  in tibialis posterior rupture,
    347–350
  turf toe of, 351
  Unna's boot for, 101
Forceps, 139
Forearm
  examination in nonacute conditions,
    242–243
  injuries of, 214–225
    casts in, 89
    compartmental syndrome in, 21,
      21f
    diaphyseal fractures in, 219, 225
    Galeazzi's fracture in, 220, 225
    Monteggia's fracture in, 218–219
    treatment recommendations in,
      224–225
  Madelung's deformity of, 244
  posterior interosseous nerve com-
    pression in, 248

radius in. *See* Radius
range of motion measurements, 354*f*,
    373*t*
ulna in. *See* Ulna
Fractures, 7–10, 16–17
of acetabulum. *See* Acetabulum,
    fractures
of ankle, 325–329, 331–332, 350
bone grafts in, 8, 154–155, 163
of calcaneus, 334–337, 342, 351
casts in. *See* Casts
cerclage techniques in, 152–153
classification of severity, 9, 9*t*
of clavicle, 78, 79*f*, 185–186, 245
delayed primary closure in, 10
diaphyseal. *See* Diaphyseal fractures
external skeletal fixation in, 154
fat embolism syndrome in, 19
of femur. *See* Femur, fractures of
in foot. *See* Foot, fractures in
in gunshot wounds, 14
in hand. *See* Hand, fractures in
healing of, 7–8
in hemophilia, 16
of humerus. *See* Humerus, fractures of
initial diagnosis and management
    of, 4–5, 8
in multiple injuries, 6, 7
in stress fractures, 10
transfusion requirements in, 3
intramedullary nailing in, 153–154
metaphyseal, 8, 17
nerve injuries in, 9, 20
of patella, 296, 299, 300–302
tension band fixation in, 148, 300,
    301*f*
of pelvis, 7, 259–264
plate fixation of, 145–152
of radius. *See* Radius, fractures of
of scapula, 195
of spine, 161–174
stress, 10
of femur, 10, 275–276
of foot, 347, 350–351
of tibia. *See* Tibia, fractures of
traction in. *See* Traction
of ulna. *See* Ulna, fractures of
Frozen shoulder, 199–200
Fungal infections, septic arthritis in,
    45, 46*t*
Furosemide in malignant hyper-
    thermia, 138

G
Gait, 57–60
intoeing in, 58–60, 59*f*
in Legg-Calve-Perthes disease, 67
in tibialis posterior rupture, 348

Galeazzi fracture of radius, 220, 225
Galeazzi test in developmental dys-
    plasia of hip, 66
Gamekeeper's thumb, 235–236
Gangrene, gas, 37–38
Gardner-Wells skull traction tongs,
    119, 120*f*, 163
Gas gangrene, 37–38
Gastrointestinal disorders
in lumbar fractures, 172
in orthopaedic unit, 111
Gentamicin, 35*t*
Genu valgum and varum, 60–61
Gigli's saw, 142
Glasgow Coma Scale, 2, 2*t*, 4
Glenohumeral joint
in adhesive capsulitis, 199–200
anatomy of, 192
arthritis of, 199
dislocation of, 192–195
in humerus fractures, proximal,
    203–205, 211
Glucosamine in osteoarthritis, 52
Glucose
administration in malignant hyper-
    thermia, 138
blood levels in diabetes mellitus, 132
Gold therapy in rheumatoid arthritis,
    49–50, 55
Goldwaithe iron apparatus, 90, 91*f*
Gonorrheal arthritis, 43*t*–44*t*
Gouges, surgical, 141, 142
Gout, 44*t*, 45, 46*t*, 52–53
Grafts, bone, in fractures, 8, 154–155,
    163
Grasping surgical instruments, 139
Gunshot wounds, 14

H
Hallux
rigidus, 351–352
valgus, 63–64
Halo traction, 121–123, 122*f*
body jacket and casts in, 92, 93*f*, 121
in hangman's fracture, 164
in Jefferson fracture, 161
in lower cervical injuries, 167, 168
in odontoid process fracture, 163
Hamate fracture, 230
Hamilton-Russell's traction, 125, 126*f*
Hand, 227–240
arthritis of, 236, 250, 251–253
aspiration and injection of, 392*f*,
    396*t*
bite wounds of, 237
club hand deformity of, 243
examination in nonacute conditions,
    242, 243

Hand (*contd.*)
  fractures in, 231–234, 238, 239
    carpal, 7, 227–230, 238
    metacarpal, 232, 233*f*, 239
    phalangeal, 232–234, 239
  function assessment, 231
  high-velocity injection injuries of, 238
  ligament injuries of, 228, 234–236, 238
  in mallet finger, 234, 240, 251
  nerve injuries in, 238
  plaster splint for, 90
  range of motion measurements, 355*f*–359*f*, 373*t*
  in syndactyly and polydactyly, 244
  tendon injuries of, 12, 223, 236, 250–251
  tenosynovitis of, 236–237, 250–251
  traumatic amputation of, 14, 236, 237*f*, 238
  in trigger finger and thumb, 236, 250–251
  tumors of, 254–255, 256*f*–257*f*
  work-related injuries of, 242, 255
Hangman's fracture, 164*f*, 164–165
Hare splints, 81
Hawkins' classification of talus fracture, 338, 339*f*
Head halter traction, 119
Head trauma, 5, 6, 7
  with cervical spine injuries, 5, 165
Healing of fractures, 7–8
Heel pain, 345–347
Height measurements
  and elbow breadth, 381*t*
  and weight, 380*t*
Hemarthrosis in hemophilia, 16
Hematomas, 13–14
  in hemophilia, 16
Hemolytic disorders, bone and joint infections in, 32, 36*t*
Hemophilia, 16, 132
Hemorrhage
  initial assessment and management of, 1–2, 3
    transfusions in, 2*t*, 3, 4
  in pelvic fractures, 259–260
Hemostats, 139
Hemothorax, 5
Heparin therapy
  in fat embolism syndrome, 19
  in thromboembolism prevention, 110
Herniation of intervertebral disks, 180
Heterotopic ossification, 26–27
  in acetabular fractures, 27, 272
  in elbow dislocation, 216
Hill-Sachs lesion, 192
  reverse, 194
Hip, 266–273

arthritis of, traumatic, 269, 270
aspiration and injection of, 33, 37, 393*f*, 394*f*, 396*t*
childhood disorders of, 65–69, 272
dislocations and fractures of, 266–273
  acetabular fracture, 269–270, 271–272, 273
  anterior dislocation, 266–267
  in children, 272
  classification of, 266
  femoral head fracture, 270–271, 272, 273
  posterior dislocation, 267–270
  sciatic nerve injuries in, 20, 267, 269, 270
  traction in, 125, 272
  treatment recommendations in, 272–273
  draping of, 386*f*
  dysplasia of, developmental, 65–67
  in Legg-Calve-Perthes disease, 67, 68*f*
  range of motion measurements, 366*f*–369*f*, 373*t*–374*t*
  in slipped capital femoral epiphysis, 69
  spica casts, 94, 95*f*, 288
History-taking, 4, 105
HIV infection and AIDS, 32, 47
Hole drilling for bone screws, 142–144
Hospitalization
  operating room equipment and techniques in, 131–158
  orthopaedic unit care in, 104–112
Humerus
  fractures of, 203–212
    diaphyseal, 205–207, 212
    distal, 207–211, 212
    Dunlop's traction in, 123, 123*f*, 207
    epiphyseal, 205
    intercondylar, 210
    of lateral condyle, 210–211
    of medial epicondyle, 211
    olecranon traction in, 123, 210
    proximal, 203–205, 204*f*, 211
    splinting in, 78, 80*f*, 206, 206*f*
    supracondylar, 123, 207–210, 208*f*, 209*f*
  lateral epicondylitis of, 248–250, 249*f*
  Panner's disease of capitellum, 253
Hydrocortisone
  preoperative and postoperative, 132
  in pseudogout, 53
Hydroxychloroquine in rheumatoid arthritis, 50, 55
Hydroxyzine, 108

Hyperextension whiplash injury of
cervical spine, 168–169
Hyperthermia, malignant, 137–139
Hypnotic drugs, 108

I

Ibuprofen, 108t
in rheumatoid arthritis, 49
Ileus, paralytic, in lumbar fractures,
172
Iliotibial band syndrome, 310
Ilium
dislocation of, 266–267
fractures of, 259, 260t, 264
grafts of, 154–155, 163
Immobilization
in bone and joint infections, 33, 38
casts in, 85–100. See also Casts
splints in, 78–84. See also Splints
thromboembolism prevention in,
108–110, 110t
Immunodeficiency virus infection, 32,
47
Immunosuppressive drugs in psoriatic
arthritis, 53–54
Impingement of rotator cuff, 197–198
Indomethacin
in gout, 53
in heterotopic ossification, 27, 272
Infections, 29–38
antibiotic therapy in. See Antibiotic
therapy
in children, 30, 69–73
early diagnosis of, 29
in fractures, 8–9
in hemolytic disorders, 32, 36t
immobilization in, 33, 38
in puncture wounds of foot, 32, 36t
in skeletal traction, 129–130
of soft tissues, 31
in surgery, prevention of, 29, 135–137
antibiotic therapy in, 131–132,
133t
in staff and surgeon exposures, 135
surgical intervention in, 33, 37
Inflammatory bowel disease, spondyloarthropathy in, 48, 48t
Infraspinatus muscle, 192, 197. See
also Rotator cuff muscles
Injection and aspiration of joints,
390–396
Injection injuries of hand, high-
velocity, 238
Inpatient care in orthopaedic unit,
104–112
Insulin
in diabetes mellitus, 132
in malignant hyperthermia, 138

Interosseous nerve of forearm, poste-
rior, compression of, 248
Interphalangeal joint of hand
dislocation of, 235, 239
Wilson's fracture of, 233f, 233–234
Intervertebral disks
degeneration of, 178–181
herniation of, 180
infections of, 31–32
Intoeing in child, 58–60, 59f
Intradermal sutures, 156, 157f
Intramedullary nailing, 153–154

J

Jefferson fracture, 161, 162f
Jones compression splint, 81
Jones metatarsal fracture, 340

K

Kenny Howard sling in acromioclavicular joint injuries, 190
Kidney failure in compartmental
syndrome, 25
Kienböck's disease of lunate, 253, 254
Kirschner traction bow, 115, 116f, 152
Kirschner wires in skeletal traction,
115–116
Klumpke's palsy, 244
Knee, 295–312
acute injuries of, 295–307
anterior pain in, 64
aspiration and injection of, 300, 394f,
396t
cast-brace for, 98–99, 317
childhood disorders of, 64–65,
307–308
cylinder casts for, 96
dislocation of, 306, 312
in children, 64, 65
patellar. See Patella, dislocation of
emergency splinting of, 81
extensor tendon injuries of, 298, 307
in femoral fractures, distal, 288–289,
290, 307
in genu valgum, 60–61
in iliotibial band syndrome, 310
imaging of, 299–300, 309
immobilizers for, 81
instability of, 297f, 297–298, 298f,
305–306
in children, 64–65
ligament injuries of, 304–306
in adolescent, 307
differential diagnosis in, 295–296
examination in, 296, 299, 305–306
instability in, 297, 297f, 305–306
in tibia fractures, 317–318

Knee (contd.)
locked, 296, 311
meniscus of
discoid, 65
injuries of, 296, 303–304
in Osgood-Schlatter's disease,
310–311
in osteochondritis dissecans, 307–308
overuse syndromes of, 295, 308–312
pain referred to, 65
patella in. See Patella
patellar tendon disorders of, 307, 310
patellofemoral pain syndrome of,
311–312
in children, 64
in pes anserinus bursitis, 312
physeal injuries of, 307
range of motion, 296, 374t
strength testing of, 309
in tibia plateau fractures, 7,
314–318, 322
cast-brace in, 98–99, 317
Knock knees, 60–61
Knot strength in cerclage, 152–153
Kyphosis, 74, 183–184

L
Lachman test, 305
Lag screw fixation, 144
Lauge-Hansen classification of ankle
fractures, 325, 326f
Lavage, peritoneal, 5, 6f
Legg-Calve-Perthes disease, 67, 68f
Ligament injuries, 12–13
acromioclavicular, 188–190, 189f
of ankle, 329–331, 332
in fractures and fracture-
dislocations, 325, 328–329
of hand, 228, 234–236, 238
of knee. See Knee, ligament injuries
of
sternoclavicular, 188
Limp in child, 57–58
in Legg-Calve-Perthes disease, 67
Lipoma of hand or wrist, 255
Lisfranc's joint injury, 340, 342
Locked knee, 296, 311
Lordosis, 74–75, 182
Lower extremity
alignment of
in children, 58–61
in overuse syndromes of knee, 308
in patellofemoral pain syndrome,
311
ankle injuries of, 325–332
casts for, 89, 90
Dehne and Sarmiento technique,
97–98, 318–319

hip spica, 94, 95f
knee cast-brace, 98–99, 317
knee cylinder casts, 96
long-leg, 96–97, 317
short-leg, 92–94, 96
total contact, 97, 98f
walking, 96, 97
compartmental syndromes of, 21, 22f,
24t
draping of, 386f
femoral fractures of, 275–290
foot fractures and dislocations of,
334–343
in genu varum and valgum, 60–61
hip dislocations and fractures of,
266–273
knee injuries of, 295–312
neurology of, 180, 181t
overuse syndromes of
of foot and ankle, 345–352
of knee, 295, 308–312
range of motion of, 366f–372f, 374t
splints for
in emergency care, 81–84, 82f–83f
plaster, 90
strapping and taping of, 100
tibia fractures of, 314–322
traction applied to, 125–129
Unna's boot for, 101
Lumbar spine injuries, 169–174
Lunate
avascular necrosis of, 253, 253f, 254
dislocation of, 7, 228
Lunotriquetral ligament injuries, 228
Lupus erythematosus, 43t, 47, 54

M
Madelung's deformity, 244
Maisonneuve fracture, 328–329
Malgaigne fracture of pelvis, 259
Malignant hyperthermia, 137–139
Malleolus of tibia fractures, 325, 328
Mallet finger, 234, 240, 251
Mallets, surgical, 141
Mannitol in malignant hyperthermia,
138
McElvenny's technique in femoral
fractures, 277
McMurray test in meniscus injuries,
304
Median nerve compression in carpal
tunnel, 19–20, 246f, 246–247
Melanoma, 255
Meniscus
discoid, 65
injuries of, 296, 303–304
Mepacrine in lupus erythematosus, 54
Meperidine, 107, 108, 109t

Metacarpal bones
  in carpometacarpal dislocation, 230
  fractures of, 232, 233f, 239
  in metacarpophalangeal joint dis-
    location, 234–235
  wire or pin insertion for skeletal
    traction, 118
Metacarpophalangeal joint
  dislocation of, 234–235
  in gamekeeper's thumb, 235–236
Metaphyseal fractures, 8, 17
Metatarsal fractures, 340–341, 342
  stress, 347, 350, 351
Metatarsalgia, 347
Metatarsophalangeal joint
  capsulitis of, 347
  in hallux rigidus, 351–352
  in turf toe, 351
Metatarsus
  adductus, 63
    intoeing gait in, 58–60, 59f
  primus varus, 63
Methadone, 109t
Methicillin, 34t
Methotrexate
  in psoriatic arthritis, 53–54
  in rheumatoid arthritis, 50, 55
Methylprednisolone
  in cervical spine injuries, 167
  in pseudogout, 53
Meyerding grading of spondylolisthesis,
    181
Mezlocillin, 35t
Milwaukee brace in kyphosis, 184
Minerva body jacket, 90–92, 92f
Mobilization of joints in cast removal,
    101–102
Monteggia's fracture-dislocation of
  elbow, 218–219, 225
Morphine, 107, 109t
Morton's neuroma, 347
Muscle strength testing, 375
  in knee injuries, 309
Musculotendinous junction injuries, 11
Myoglobinuria in compartmental syn-
  drome, 25
Myositis
  ossificans, 26–27, 216
  polymyositis and dermatomyositis, 43t

N
Nafcillin, 34t
Nailing, intramedullary, 153–154
Naprosyn, 108t
Narcotics, 107
Navicular bone
  coalition with calcaneus, flat feet in,
    62, 63
  fractures of, 338, 350–351

Neck halter traction, 119
Necrosis, avascular, 30
  of femur. See Femur, avascular
    necrosis of
  of talus, 338
  in upper extremity, 253f, 253–254
Needle holders, 139
Nerve conduction studies, 387–389
Nerve injuries, 9, 13, 20
  back pain in, 178
  carpal tunnel syndrome in, 19–20,
    222, 246–247
  in cervical spine trauma, 165, 167,
    168
  in Colles' fracture, 222
  in elbow dislocation, 216
  in femoral fractures, 287
  in foot, 346–347
  in hand, 238
  in humerus fractures, 205, 206–207
  in intervertebral disk herniation, 180
  of median nerve, 19–20, 222, 246–247
  in pelvic fractures, 264
  of peroneal nerve, common, 20
  scapular winging in, 201
  of sciatic nerve in hip dislocation,
    20, 267, 269, 270
  in shoulder dislocation, 194
  in thoracolumbar spine fractures,
    171, 173–174
  in tibia fractures, 317
  in traction, 130
  of ulnar nerve, 20, 247–248
Neurapraxia, 13
Neurologic examination, 8
  in primary survey, 2, 2t
  in secondary survey, 4, 5
Neuroma, Morton's, 347
Neuromuscular disorders in children,
    75–76
Neurotmesis, 13
Neutralization plates, 145, 145f
Nurses in orthopaedic unit, role of,
    104–105
Nutrition in orthopaedic unit care, 106

O
Obturator dislocation, 266
Odontoid process fractures, 6, 161–164
Olecranon
  examination of, 242
  fractures of, 216–217
    tension band fixation in, 148, 149f,
      216–217, 217f
  traction through, 123, 124f
    in humerus fractures, 123, 210
    wire or pin insertion in, 118

Operating room equipment and techniques, 131–158
Orbital fractures, 6
Orders in orthopaedic unit, 106
Orthopaedic unit care, 104–112
  activities and physical therapy in, 111
  drug therapy in, 107–108, 108*t*, 109*t*
  initial orders in, 106
  nutrition in, 106
  postoperative, 112
  preoperative, 106–107, 111
  rounds in, 104–105
  skin care in, 106, 111
  thromboembolism prevention in, 108–110, 110*t*
  in urinary retention, 110–111
  workup routines in, 105–106
Ortolani test in developmental dysplasia of hip, 65–66
Osgood-Schlatter's disease, 310–311
Ossification, heterotopic, 26–27
  in acetabular fractures, 27, 272
  in elbow dislocation, 216
Osteoarthritis, 40, 41*t*, 42*t*, 45
  of acromioclavicular joint, 200
  of glenohumeral joint, 199
  of hip, after posterior dislocation, 269, 270
  treatment of, 49*t*, 52
Osteochondritis dissecans, 307–308
Osteolysis of clavicle, 200
Osteomyelitis, 30
  antibiotic therapy in, 30, 31, 32, 36*t*
    in children, 71
  in children, 31, 69–72
  chronic, 37
  in hemolytic disorders, 32
  surgical intervention in, 33, 72
Osteonecrosis, 30
  of femur. *See* Femur, avascular necrosis of
  of talus, 338
  in upper extremity, 253*f*, 253–254
Osteosarcoma of upper extremity, 255
Osteotomes, 141, 141*f*, 142
Overuse injuries
  of foot and ankle, 345–352
  of knee, 295, 308–312
Oxycodone, 109*t*

P
Palsy
  cerebral, 75–76, 182, 245–246
  Erb's, 244
  Klumpke's, 244
  ulnar nerve, 20
Panner's disease of humerus, 253

Patella
  chondromalacia of, 64, 311
  dislocation of, 296, 299, 302–303
    in children, 64, 65
    fractures associated with, 299*f*
    recurrent, 303
  fractures of, 296, 299, 300–302
    tension band fixation in, 148, 300, 301*f*
  imaging of, 299
  instability of, 298
    in children, 64–65
Patellar tendon
  disruption of, 307
  tendinitis of, 310
Patellofemoral joint
  degenerative changes of, 303
  instability in extensor tendon injuries, 298
  pain syndrome of, 64, 311–312
Pavlik harness in developmental dysplasia of hip, 66
Pearson attachment in skeletal traction, 126
Pectoralis major rupture, 195
Pediatric conditions, 16–17, 57–76.
  See also Children
Pelvic bones
  dislocation of, 266–267
  disruption of symphysis pubis, 259, 261*f*
  fractures of, 7, 259–264
    type A, 259, 260*t*, 262–264
    type B, 259, 260*t*, 261*f*, 262*f*, 264
    type C, 259, 260*t*, 263*f*, 264
  iliac grafts, 154–155, 163
D-Penicillamine in rheumatoid arthritis, 50
Penicillin G, 34*t*
Periosteal elevators, 139–141, 140*f*
Peripheral nerves, cutaneous distribution of, 378*f*
Peritoneal lavage, 5, 6*f*
Peroneal nerve, common, compression of, 20
Peroneal tendon
  in ankle sprains, 330
  in talus fracture, 338
Pes anserinus bursitis, 312
Pes planus, 62–63
  in tibialis posterior rupture, 347–350
Phalangeal bones
  of foot, dislocation of, 340
  of hand, fractures of, 232–234, 239
Phalen's sign in carpal tunnel syndrome, 247
Physical examination
  joint motion measurements in, 354–374

in orthopaedic unit, 105
in secondary survey, 4–7
Physical therapy in orthopaedic unit,
    111
Pins
    in external fixation of fractures, 154
    in skeletal traction, 115–119,
        129–130
Pipkin types of femoral head fractures,
    271
Piroxicam, 108*t*
Plantar fasciitis, 346
Plantar nerve entrapment, 346–347
Plaster bandages and splints, 85, 87*f*,
    87–89
Plate fixation, 145–152
    buttress plates in, 145, 314, 316, 316*f*
    contouring of plates in, 148–152,
        150*f*, 151*f*
    dynamic compression plates in, 145,
        146*f*, 147*f*, 148*f*
    neutralization plates in, 145, 145*f*
    tension band techniques in,
        146–148, 149*f*
    in olecranon fractures, 148, 149*f*,
        216–217, 217*f*
    in patella fractures, 148, 300, 301*f*
Pneumatic tourniquets, 134*f*, 134–135
Pneumothorax, 1, 5
Polyarteritis nodosa, 43*t*
Polyarthritis, inflammatory, 43*t*–44*t*,
    45–47, 53–54
Polydactyly, 244
Polymyalgia rheumatica, 44*t*
Polymyositis, 43*t*
Postoperative care in orthopaedic unit,
    112
Prednisone
    in lupus erythematosus, 54
    in pseudogout, 53
    in rheumatic fever, 54
    in rheumatoid arthritis, 51
Preoperative care, 106–107, 131–139
    check sheet on, 111
Presiser's disease of scaphoid, 253
Pressure sores, 111
Primary survey, 1–4
Probenecid in gout, 53
Pseudogout, 44*t*, 45, 46*t*, 53
Psoriatic arthritis, 43*t*, 47, 53–54
Psychogenic back pain, 178
Pubic bones
    dislocation of, 266–267
    disruption of symphysis, 259, 261*f*

Q
Quadriceps tendon injuries, 307

R
Radial nerve injuries, 205, 206–207,
    248
Radiography, 4–5, 7
    in ankle fractures, 326
    in knee injuries, 299, 309
    in limp of child, 58
    in nontraumatic joint conditions, 40,
        41*t*, 72
Radioulnar joint, distal
    in Colles' fracture, 222
    in Galeazzi's fracture, 220
Radius
    agenesis of, 243–244
    fractures of, 224, 225
        Barton's, 221*f*, 223
        Colles', 220–223
        diaphyseal, 219, 225
        distal, 220–224, 225
        epiphyseal, 217–218, 223–224
        Galeazzi's, 220, 225
        of head and neck, 7, 218, 224
        Monteggia's, 218–219, 225
        proximal, 217–219
        Smith's, 221*f*, 223
    Madelung's deformity of, 244
    wire or pin insertion for skeletal
        traction, 118
Range of motion measurements,
    354–374
Record-keeping
    on initial assessment and manage-
        ment, 6
    on orthopaedic unit care, 105–106
Referred pain
    in intervertebral disk degeneration,
        179
    to knee, 65
Reflex sympathetic dystrophy, 26
Reiter's syndrome, 43*t*, 46, 48*t*, 53
Respiratory disorders
    in fat embolism syndrome, 19
    initial assessment and management
        of, 1
Resuscitation measures, 1–4
Rheumatic fever, 43*t*, 47, 54
Rheumatism, palindromic, 46*t*
Rheumatoid arthritis, 40, 41*t*, 43*t*, 44*t*
    of glenohumeral joint, 199
    juvenile, 43*t*, 46*t*, 47, 54–55
    synovial fluid analysis in, 42*t*
    tenosynovitis of hand and wrist in,
        236, 250
    treatment of, 48–51, 49*t*, 54–55
Risser classification of scoliosis, 183
Risser localizer cast, 92
Roller splints, 81
Rotator cuff muscles, 192
    acute tears of, 194, 195

Rotator cuff muscles (*contd.*)
  anatomy of, 192, 197
  bursitis/tendinitis of, 197–198, 199
  impingement syndrome of, 197–198
  nonacute disorders of, 197–199
Rounds in orthopaedic unit, 104–105
Russell's traction, split, 125, 127*f*

S

Sacrum, fractures of, 259, 260*t*, 264
Salter classification of epiphyseal injuries, 17
Saws
  bone, 142
  cast, 86, 99, 99*f*
Scaphoid
  fracture and dislocation of, 7,
    227–228, 238
  Presiser's disease of, 253
Scapholunate dissociation, 228, 229*f*
Scapula
  fracture of, 195
  snapping, 200–201
  winging of, 201, 201*f*
Scapulothoracic disorders, 200–201,
  201*f*
Schatzker classification of tibia
  plateau fractures, 314, 315*f*
Scheuermann's disease, 74, 184
Sciatic nerve injuries in hip dislocation, 20, 267, 269, 270
Sciatica, 178–182
Scissors, surgical, 139
Scleroderma, 43*t*
Scoliosis, 73–74, 182–183
  casts in, 87
  in cerebral palsy, 75, 76, 182
Screws, bone, 142–145
  in plating techniques, 145–152
  types of, 144*f*, 144–145
Secobarbital, 108
Secondary survey, 4–7
Sedative drugs, 107–108
Self-tapping bone screws, 144*f*,
  144–145
Sensory function in compartmental
  syndromes, 21, 23, 24*t*
Septic arthritis, 31, 40, 41*t*, 45
  antibiotic therapy in, 36*t*, 49*t*, 52,
    72–73
  in children, 31, 72–73
  differential diagnosis in, 40, 45, 46*t*
  drainage and irrigation of joint in, 52
  fungal, 45, 46*t*
  radiographic findings in, 40, 41*t*, 72
  surgical intervention in, 33, 49*t*, 52
  synovial fluid analysis in, 42*t*
  viral, 45, 46*t*

Sesamoid fractures, 341, 350, 351
Shock, initial management in, 2*t*, 2–4
Shoulder, 192–201
  acromioclavicular joint in. *See*
    Acromioclavicular joint
  acute injuries of, 192–196
  adhesive capsulitis of, 199–200
  anatomy of, 192
  arthritis of, 199, 200
  aspiration and injection of, 390*f*, 396*t*
  biceps brachii in, 192, 197
    rupture of, 195
    tendinitis of, 199
  bursitis/tendinitis of, 197–198, 199
    scapulothoracic, 200–201
  dislocation of, 192–195, 196
    anterior, 192–194
    emergency splinting in, 78, 80*f*
    inferior, 195
    multidirectional instability in,
      194–195
    posterior, 6, 194
    recurrent, 194
  draping of, 385*f*
  glenohumeral joint in. *See* Glenohumeral joint
  in humerus fractures, proximal,
    203–205, 211
  immobilizers for, 78
  nonacute injuries of, 197–201
  in pectoralis major rupture, 195
  range of motion measurements,
    360*f*–361*f*, 373*t*
  rotator cuff muscles in. *See* Rotator
    cuff muscles
  in scapular fracture, 195
  scapulothoracic disorders of,
    200–201, 201*f*
  spica casts for, 94–96
  traction in, 123–125
Sickle cell disease, 32
Skin
  closure of wounds, 9, 10–11
    delayed, 11, 155
    suture techniques in, 11, 155–158
  preparation in surgery, 136
  pressure sores of, 111
  traction force applied to, 115
    in hip dysplasia, 66
    in upper extremity, 123, 123*f*
Skull
  fractures of, 6
  palpation of, 5
  traction tongs applied to. *See* Tong
    traction
Sling in acromioclavicular joint injuries, 190
Slipped capital femoral epiphysis, 69,
  70*f*

Smith's fracture of radius, 221*f*, 223
Snapping scapula, 200–201
Soft tissues
    infections of, 31
    injuries of, 4, 8–14
        in femoral fractures, 286
    of ligaments. *See* Ligament in-
        juries
    of nerves. *See* Nerve injuries
    of tendons. *See* Tendon injuries
    tetanus prophylaxis in, 14, 15*t*
Spica casts, 92–96
    hip, 94, 95*f*, 288
    shoulder, 94–96, 123–125
Spina bifida, 76
Spinal cord injuries, 168
    in cervical trauma, 165, 167, 168
    myositis ossificans paralytica in,
        26–27
    in thoracolumbar trauma, 173–174
Spine, 161–184
    back pain in disorders of, 178–182
    cervical, 161–169. *See also* Cervical
        spine
    coccygeal fractures of, 260*t*
    diagnosis of injuries, 5, 6, 7
    emergency splinting of, 78, 79*f*
    fractures and dislocations of,
        161–174
    intervertebral disks in. *See* Interver-
        tebral disks
    kyphosis of, 74, 183–184
    lordosis of, 74–75, 182
    range of motion measurements,
        362*f*–365*f*
    sacral fractures of, 259, 260*t*, 264
    scoliosis of, 73–74, 182–183
        in cerebral palsy, 75, 76, 182
        in spina bifida, 76
    spondylolisthesis of, 181–182
    thoracolumbar, 169–174. *See also*
        Thoracolumbar spine
Splints
    in bone and joint infections, 33
    in clavicle fractures, 78, 79*f*,
        185–186
    in Colles' fracture, 221, 222
    in emergency care, 78–84
        of lower extremity, 81–84, 82*f*–83*f*
        of spine, 78, 79*f*
        of upper extremity, 78–81, 79*f*–80*f*
    in humerus fractures, 78, 80*f*, 206,
        206*f*
    in myositis ossificans, 27
    plaster, 85, 89–90, 91*f*
Split Russell's traction, 125, 127*f*
Spondylitis, ankylosing, 40, 48, 48*t*, 54
Spondyloarthropathy, inflammatory,
    48, 48*t*, 54–55

Spondylolisthesis, 181–182
Sprains, 12
    acromioclavicular, 188–190
    of ankle, 329–331, 332
    sternoclavicular, 187
Staff
    occupational exposure to blood-
        borne pathogens, 135
    in orthopaedic unit, 104–105
Steinmann pins in skeletal traction,
    116, 117*f*
Sternoclavicular joint injuries, 187
Straight-leg raising test in knee in-
    juries, 298
Strains, 11
Strapping, adhesive, in athletic in-
    juries, 100–101
Strength testing, 375
    in knee injuries, 309
Stress fractures, 10
    of femur, 10, 275–276
    of foot, 347, 350–351
Subacromial space
    anatomy of, 197
    decompression of, 198, 199
Subscapularis muscle, 192, 197. *See
    also* Rotator cuff muscles
Subtalar joint
    in calcaneus fractures, 334, 336
    dislocation of, 337–338, 342
    in tibialis posterior rupture, 348,
        349, 350
Sudeck's atrophy, 26
Sulfasalazine in rheumatoid arthritis,
    50
Sulfinpyrazone in gout, 53
Supraspinatus muscle, 192, 197. *See
    also* Rotator cuff muscles
Surgery, 131–158
    in amputation, traumatic, 14
    bone cutting instruments in, 141*f*,
        141–142
    bone grafts in, 8, 154–155, 163
    bone saws and files in, 142
    bone screws in, 142–145
    cerclage in, 152–153
    draping techniques in, 132–134, 136,
        382*f*–386*f*
    exposure instruments in, 139–141,
        140*f*
    external skeletal fixation in, 154
    grasping instruments in, 139
    infection prevention in, 29, 135–137
        antibiotic therapy in, 131–132,
            133*t*
        in staff and surgeon exposures, 135
    intramedullary nailing in, 153–154
    in kyphosis, 74, 184
    malignant hyperthermia in, 137–139

Surgery (contd.)
  in open fractures, 9, 10
  orthopaedic unit care in, 104–112
  in osteoarthritis, 52
  in osteomyelitis, 33, 72
  plating techniques in, 145–152
  pneumatic tourniquets in, 134f,
    134–135
  postoperative care in, 112
  preoperative care in, 106–107, 111
  in rheumatoid arthritis, 51, 55
  in scoliosis, 74, 183
  in septic arthritis, 33, 49t, 52
  for skeletal traction, pin and wire in-
    sertion in, 116–119
  in soft-tissue injuries, 10–11
  suture techniques in, 11, 155–158
  thromboembolism prevention in,
    108–110, 110t
Suture techniques, 11, 155–158
  box, 156, 156f
  Donati, 158, 158f
  everting, 156, 157f
  intradermal, 156, 157f
  near-far/far-near, 156–158, 158f
Symphysis pubis disruption, 259, 261f
Syndactyly, 244
Synovectomy in rheumatoid arthritis,
    51, 55
Synovial fluid analysis, 40, 42t
Synovitis, transient, in children, 73

T
Talipes equinovarus, 61–62
Talocalcaneal coalition, flat feet in, 62,
    63
Talofibular ligament injuries, 325, 330
Talus
  avascular necrosis of, 338
  coalition with other tarsal bones, flat
    foot in, 62, 63
  dislocation of, 337–338
  fractures of, 7, 338, 341
    Hawkins' classification of, 338,
      339f
    stress, 350
  instability in ankle sprains, 329–331
Taping of athletic injuries, 100–101
Tarsal bones, 334–337, 338
  calcaneus. See Calcaneus
  coalition of, flat feet in, 62, 63
  cuboid fracture, 338
  cuneiform fracture, 338
  navicular, 62, 63, 338, 350–351
  stress fractures of, 350–351
  subluxation and dislocation of, 340
  talus. See Talus
Tarsal tunnel syndrome, 347

Tarsometatarsal joint injuries, 340,
    342, 351–352
Team approach, 1–7
  in hemophilia, 16
  in orthopaedic unit, 104–105
Tendinitis, 46t
  Achilles, 345
  calcific, 46t, 199
  patellar, 310
  rotator cuff, 197–198, 199
Tendo calcaneus. See Achilles tendon
Tendon injuries, 11–12
  Achilles, 331, 345
  of hand, 12, 223, 236, 250–251
  of knee, 298, 307, 310
  in open fractures, 9
  of tibialis posterior, 347–350
Tenosynovitis of hand and wrist,
    236–237
  de Quervain's, 237, 250–251
Tension band fixation, 146–148, 149f
  in olecranon fractures, 148, 149f,
    216–217, 217f
  in patella fractures, 148, 300, 301f
Teres minor muscle, 192, 197. See also
    Rotator cuff muscles
Tetanus prophylaxis, 8, 14, 15t
Thomas splint, 81, 82f, 83f
  in femoral fractures, 81, 83f, 280,
    284, 286
  in skeletal traction, 126, 127, 128f,
    129f
Thompson's test in Achilles tendon
    rupture, 331
Thoracic spine
  injuries of, 169–174
  range of motion measurements, 364f
Thoracolumbar spine, 169–174
  burst fracture of, 169, 171f, 172,
    172f, 173
  Chance fracture of, 170, 174f
  compression fracture of, 169, 170f,
    172
  flexion-distraction injuries of,
    169–170, 173f
  range of motion measurements, 364f
  translational injuries of, 170, 175f
Thromboembolism prevention,
    108–110, 110t
Thumb
  arthritis of carpometacarpal joint,
    251, 252f
  fracture of metacarpal, 232, 239
  gamekeeper's, 235–236
  range of motion measurements,
    356f–357f
  trigger, 250–251
Tibia
  avulsion injury of, 307

overgrowth of, 310–311
fractures of, 314–322
  ankle ligament injuries in, 325
  apophyseal, 307
  buttress plate fixation of, 314, 316,
    316f
  in children, 17, 307, 319
  complications in, 317, 321
  Dehne and Sarmiento casting
    technique in, 97–98, 318–319
  diaphyseal, 318–321
  external fixation in, 154, 319
  interlocking nails in, 319, 320f, 321
  knee cast-brace in, 98–99, 317
  knee ligament injuries in, 317–318
  in malleolus, 325, 328
  pilon, 329, 331
  in plateau, 7, 98–99, 314–318, 322
  Schatzker classification of, 314,
    315f
  stress, 10
in genu varum and valgum, 60
torsion of, 58–60
vara, 60
wire or pin insertion for skeletal
  traction, 119
Tibial nerve entrapment in tarsal tunnel, 347
Tibialis posterior tendon rupture,
  347–350
Tibiofibular ligament injuries in ankle
  fractures, 325, 328–329
Tinel's sign in carpal tunnel syndrome,
  247
Tobramycin, 35t
Toes. See Foot
Tong traction, 119–121, 120f
  in hangman's fracture, 164–165
  in Jefferson fracture, 161
  in lower cervical fractures and dislo-
    cations, 167, 168
  in odontoid process fracture, 163
Tourniquets, pneumatic, 134f,
  134–135
Toxic shock syndrome, 37
Tracheal intubation in initial resuscitation, 1
Tracheotomy in initial resuscitation, 1
Traction, 115–130
  cervical spine, 92, 93f, 119–123
  halo. See Halo traction
  in hangman's fracture, 164–165
  in Jefferson fracture, 161
  in lower cervical injuries, 167, 168
  in odontoid process fracture, 163,
    164
  tong. See Tong traction
  complications of, 21, 23f, 129–130

in hip dislocation and fracture, 125,
  272
in hip dysplasia, 66
lower extremity, 125–129
  skeletal, 125–129, 128f, 129f
  skin, 125, 125f, 126f, 127f
objectives of, 115
in shoulder dislocation, 193
skeletal, 115–119, 129–130
  for lower extremity, 125–129,
    128f, 129f
  for upper extremity, 123–125, 124f
  skin, 115
  in hip dysplasia, 66
  for lower extremity, 125, 125f,
    126f, 127f
  for upper extremity, 123, 123f
upper extremity, 123–125
  skeletal, 123–125, 124f
  skin, 123, 123f
Transfusions, 2t, 3, 4
Translational injuries of thoracolumbar spine, 170, 175f
Transverse process fractures, lumbar,
  174
Trendelenburg gait, 57
Triamcinolone in pseudogout, 53
Triangular fibrocartilage of wrist injuries, 230
Trigger finger and thumb, 236,
  250–251
Triquetrum fracture, 230
Tuft fracture, 234
Tumors in upper extremity, 254–255,
  256f–257f
Turf toe, 351

U
Ulna
  absence of, 243
  fractures of
    diaphyseal, 219, 225
    distal, 223
    isolated, 220
    Monteggia's, 218–219
    in olecranon, 148, 149f, 216–217
    proximal, 216–217, 218–219, 224
    treatment recommendations in,
      224, 225
  olecranon of. See Olecranon
  wire or pin insertion for skeletal
    traction, 118
Ulnar nerve compression at elbow, 20,
  247–248
Unna's boot, 101
Upper extremity
  acromioclavicular joint injuries of,
    187–191

Upper extremity (*contd.*)
  arthritis of, 251–253
  avascular necrosis of bones in, 253*f*,
    253–254
  casts for, 89, 90
    shoulder spica, 94–96, 123–125
  clavicle fractures of, 185–186
  developmental disorders of, 243–246
  draping of, 383*f*–385*f*
  elbow and forearm injuries of,
    214–225
  examination in nonacute conditions,
    242–243
  hand and wrist injuries of, 227–240
  humerus fractures of, 203–212
  nerve compression in, 246–248
  range of motion measurements,
    354*f*–361*f*, 373*t*
  shoulder problems of, 192–201
  splints for
    in emergency care, 78–81, 79*f*–80*f*
    plaster, 90
  sternoclavicular joint injuries of, 187
  strapping and taping of, 100
  traction applied to, 123–125
    skeletal, 123–125, 124*f*
    skin, 123, 123*f*
  tumors of, 254–255, 256*f*–257*f*
Uric acid levels in gout, 45, 53
Urine output, 7
  in orthopaedic unit care, 110–111
  in shock, 4

V
Vancomycin, 9, 133*t*
Vascular disorders, back pain in, 178
Velpeau's bandages, 78, 80*f*
Vertebral column. *See* Spine

Viral infections, septic arthritis in, 45,
  46*t*
Von Willebrand's disease, 16

W
Walking casts, 96, 97
Warfarin in thromboembolism preven-
  tion, 110
Watson-Jones approach in femoral
  fracture, 277
Weakness in compartmental syndromes, 21, 23, 24*t*
Weight and height measurements, 380*t*
Whiplash injury of cervical spine,
  168–169
Wilson's fracture, 233*f*, 233–234
Winging of scapula, 201, 201*f*
Wires
  in cerclage techniques, 152–153
  in external skeletal fixation, 154
  in skeletal traction, 115–119,
    129–130
  in tension band fixation, 146–148,
    149*f*
Work-related injuries of hand, wrist,
  and elbow, 242, 255
Wrist, 227–240
  aspiration and injection of, 392*f*,
    396*t*
  examination in nonacute conditions,
    242, 243
  ligament injuries of, 228, 238
  median nerve compression at, 19–20,
    246*f*, 246–247
  range of motion measurements,
    355*f*, 373*t*
  tenosynovitis of, noninfective,
    236–237
  tumors of, 255